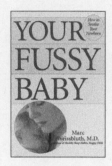
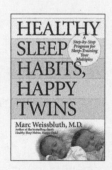

Healthy Sleep Habits, Happy Child

Fourth Edition

Healthy Sleep Habits, Happy Child

A STEP-BY-STEP PROGRAM FOR A GOOD NIGHT'S SLEEP

Fourth Edition

Marc Weissbluth, M.D.

Ballantine Books • New York

This book contains advice and information relating to the care of infants. It is not intended to substitute for medical advice and should be used to supplement rather than replace the regular advice and care of your child's pediatrician. Since every child is different, you should consult your child's pediatrician on questions specific to your child.

2015 Ballantine Books Trade Paperback Edition

Published in the United States by Ballantine Books, an imprint of Random House, a division of Penguin Random House LLC, New York.

BALLANTINE and the HOUSE colophon are registered trademarks of Penguin Random House LLC.

Earlier editions of this work were published in the United States by Ballantine Books, an imprint of Random House, a division of Penguin Random House LLC, in 1987, 1999, and 2003.

Quotes by Carl D. Williams in chapter 4 are from "Case Report: The Elimination of Tantrum Behavior by Extinction Procedures" (*Journal of Abnormal and Social Psychology,* 1959).

LIBRARY OF CONGRESS CATALOGING-IN-PUBLICATION DATA
Weissbluth, Marc.
Healthy sleep habits, happy child : a step-by-step program for a good night's sleep / Marc Weissbluth, M.D.—2015 Ballantine Books Trade Paperback edition, Fourth edition.
pages cm
Includes bibliographical references and index.
ISBN 978-0-553-39480-1 (paperback)—ISBN 978-1-101-96559-7 (ebook)
1. Sleep disorders in children. 2. Children—Sleep. 3. Child rearing.
I. Title.
RJ506.S55W45 2016
618.92'8498—dc23
2015029852

Printed in the United States of America on acid-free paper

randomhousebooks.com

9 8

Book design by Mary A. Wirth

This book is dedicated, with all my love, to Linda

As night falls, the weary creatures of earth,
And the woods and the frothing seas,
Grow calm like the stars as they circle their course,
And sleep with quiet ease.
And so all creatures far and wide,
From the craggy fields to the glassy lakes,
Stretch and live 'neath the silent night,
And sleep takes away their worries and aches.

—VIRGIL, *The Aeneid* (translation by Jed Weissbluth)

Contents

Foreword

A friend recommended this book to me when my first child, Presley, was seven months old. I was still nursing, but getting ready to stop, and definitely ready to stop the 4:00 a.m. feeding. Also, we had let Presley get into the bad habit of only wanting to sleep *on* someone. This was great when I needed an excuse for a nap, but not so convenient on busy days.

I devoured the book back then in a matter of hours and put the principles into practice immediately—with instant results. I especially liked how Dr. Weissbluth taught me to watch out for my child's sleepy signs and then encouraged me to get him to bed before he became overtired. I was also very comforted by Dr. Weissbluth's explanation of sleep as one of your child's basic needs. You offer healthy food to your child when she's hungry. You must also offer sleep when your child is tired—even if she doesn't know it or thinks she doesn't want it (just like my kids didn't usually choose the vegetable on their own!).

As a correspondent for *Good Morning America*, I had the good fortune to interview Dr. Weissbluth as a part of a series called Baby's First Year. He became a trusted resource and adviser, not only on the topic of sleep, but also subsequently on potty training and discipline.

Dr. Weissbluth's philosophy that a well-rested family is the most important thing has stayed with us always. I can't say that my kids never woke up at night or always went to sleep without a power struggle. We had our ups and downs—that's parenthood. But from this book I learned the structure and rhythm of sleep and how to get back into it, an especially helpful skill when I was bleary-eyed at 2:00 a.m. or our schedule got out of balance after traveling or when someone had a cold.

Sixteen years have passed since I became a mother. In fact, my son just got his driver's license. Now, some nights, my husband and I lose sleep for different reasons. But what I have noticed is that even as teenagers both my children are good at reading their own sleepy cues. They seem to remember what it feels like to be well rested, know when they should go to sleep, and don't burn the candle at both ends. This makes for a much happier and harmonious family. I know we are all our best selves when we've given ourselves the gift of sleep. Fortunately, thanks to *Healthy Sleep Habits, Happy Child*, most days (and nights!) we do! Thanks, Dr. Weissbluth!

Cindy Crawford

How to Use This Book

If you are *not yet a parent,* read Chapters 1–3 and 5 first.

Sleep-deprived parents should read only the age-appropriate chapter for your baby at this time. Read Chapter 4, on treating sleep problems, if needed.

Well-rested parents can begin with Chapters 1–3 and the age-appropriate chapter for your baby first. It may also be useful to read the chapters for children younger and older than your child. For example, if your child is 5–6 weeks old (Chapter 6), reading about the first month (Chapter 5) and months 3 and 4 (Chapter 7) may help you understand how your baby's sleep developed and what changes are about to occur. Again, read Chapter 4 if needed.

Skip or skim the studies, numerical data, and parent reports if you wish. They supply added detail and context, but this is not a college textbook! This is a book to aid parents who are looking to establish or restore healthy sleep habits to their growing families.

Author's Note

Throughout the book, I use the terms *fathers, mothers, marriage,* and *marital problems* merely for convenience. I wish to embrace all partner and partner-child relationships.

Introduction

I know from sleep.

I have studied both healthy and disturbed sleep in children as founder of the original Sleep Disorders Center at Children's Memorial Hospital in Chicago (now the Ann and Robert H. Lurie Children's Hospital of Chicago). I have helped thousands of families understand how their children's sleep habits directly impact behavior and school performance. Based on this research, my general pediatric practice spanning more than forty years, and life with my own four sons and eight grandchildren, I have discovered that there is hope for bleary-eyed parents. Both you and your child can benefit from this knowledge. In fact, I personally benefited from my sleep research: when I was younger, I thought that naps were a waste of time. I wanted to spend time with my boys, and I had all those chores to do. The result? I was distracted and irritable from accumulated sleeplessness. But I came to understand that my whole family benefited when I took the naps I needed. I learned not only how to change my own sleep habits for the better but also how to help my children and my patients do the same. Now I am offering those same insights and knowledge to you and your family.

SLEEP DEPRIVATION HARMS CHILDREN
Sleep deprivation can be prevented and treated.

The prevention and treatment of unhealthy sleep habits in infants and young children is important, because if those habits are uncorrected, they will *persist*. There is no automatic correction. Children do not simply outgrow these problems. Adult sleep specialists commonly see incurable adult insomniacs, chronically disabled from sleepiness and dependent on sleeping pills, who correctly describe themselves as never sleeping well as children.

The good news is that the harmful effects of unhealthy sleep are reversible when parents provide treatment. The younger the child, the more successful parents will be in reversing the ill effects of unhealthy sleep. But children of all ages will benefit if parents make an effort to address sleep problems.

Preventing the development of unhealthy sleep patterns is something all parents can do. But it requires that they start early, paying attention to their baby's evolving natural sleep rhythms and synchronizing their soothing-to-sleep behavior with the time when the sleep process first begins. Perfect timing produces no crying. This book is designed to educate parents as to how they can accomplish perfect timing and prevent sleep problems in their child. But to achieve perfect timing requires practice, so it is possible, especially if this is your first child, that there may be a little crying when your baby becomes overtired.

Treatment of sleep problems is more difficult than prevention for the simple reason that both the child and the parents are already stressed from being overtired. Overtired children are fatigued, and the body's natural response to fatigue is to fight it by producing a stimulating chemical. This "second wind" of stimulating energy causes a hyperalert or hypervigilant state that prevents easy entry into sleep or sleeping for long periods. Once upon a time, this response was an important survival mechanism, as primitive humans had to flee, fight, or continue hunting even when overtired. Our bodies are hardwired to respond in certain ways, to certain stimuli, even though the circumstances of our daily lives have changed greatly from the days in which those biological responses first evolved. The same response that once gave a weary hunter the strength to press on after his wounded prey now powers the tired businesswoman laboring to meet a deadline. But it's also the reason why overtired children appear "wired," unable to fall asleep easily or stay asleep.

In the same way that we know how much calcium your baby needs for his bones to grow stronger, we know how important healthy sleep is for the growing brain. Calcium deficiency in childhood harms bone development, but the problems of osteoporosis may not show up until much later in adult life. If your child eats a calcium-deficient diet, a future problem is "hidden" because there are no immediately apparent ill effects. Likewise, sleep deficiency in childhood may harm neurological development; the problems remain "hidden," not showing up until later. I think it is quite possible that unhealthy childhood sleep habits contribute to school-related problems such as attention deficit hyperactivity disorder (ADHD) and learning disabilities. I also suspect chronically tired children become chronically tired adults who suffer in ways we can't measure, including less resiliency, less ability to cope with life's stresses, less curiosity, less empathy, and less playfulness. The message is simple: sleep is a powerful modifier of mood, behavior, performance, and personality. It impacts every area of our lives.

We know that the process of falling asleep and staying asleep is learned behavior, and that the learning will occur naturally, just like learning how to walk, if parents do not interfere. Difficulties in learning how to walk used to occur when walkers were popular, because they interfered with the natural development of a normal gait. Difficulties in learning how to sleep occur when parents do not respect and protect the child's natural, periodic need to sleep. With practice and patience, all parents will clearly see that perfect timing produces no crying!

BE PATIENT

It takes time for your child to develop the strength, coordination, balance, and confidence needed to "learn" to walk. In the same way, it takes time for your baby to develop the night-sleep

consolidation, regular and long naps, and self-soothing skills necessary to "learn" to sleep well.

New parents need to practice before they achieve perfection, and they need to be patient. Because of new parents' inexperience and the baby's shifting sleep rhythms, there will be incidents when the timing will be off and the baby will become painfully overtired. This is not your fault! It is inevitable. This book will coach you to catch the rising wave of sleepiness before your child crashes into an overtired state.

Helping babies and children sleep well is not just mothers' work; fathers also play an important role in helping to establish healthy sleep habits. Traditionally, mothers have suffered the burden of sleep deprivation because they were doing night duty alone. They were on call day and night much more than fathers were, and when there were problems occurring on the night shift, guess who was expected to handle it? When babies do not sleep well, guess who gets the blame? I have tried to correct this situation by discussing how important it is—for the sake of the child, the marriage, and the family—to get the father actively involved.

In this new edition of *Healthy Sleep Habits, Happy Child,* you will learn in detail how to prevent and treat sleep problems in our modern society.

Although children's sleep need is based on biological development, how parents deal with their children's sleep is influenced by society. That is, we are talking about both nature and nurture.

Our society has dramatically changed since 1987, when *Healthy Sleep Habits, Happy Child* was first published. The Internet and social media have enabled mothers and fathers to become much more knowledgeable about parenting. Some of this information is reassuring and factual, based on solid research. But, sad to say, some of it is opinion masquerading as fact. And some of it reflects a trend of labeling many normal behavioral and developmental differences among children as medical problems requiring treatment. Overwhelmed by conflicting advice, many parents are uncertain where to place their trust and are understandably tentative and inconsistent in responding to their children's needs. Additionally, because there is much more easily obtained information online about parenting, parents might feel overloaded with too much information and wind up feeling defeated before they even start.

How are parents able to trust what they read in books, in magazines, or on the Internet? When you compare advice on sleeping and crying from different writers, ask yourself one simple question: on what are they basing their advice? Besides practicing general pediatrics since 1973, conducting and publishing original research, and lecturing on crying and sleep problems in children since 1981, I have helped my wife raise our four sons and have been actively involved in raising eight grandchildren. Believe me, when it comes to sleep problems in infants and children, I have been there!

Modern families are much busier than those of twenty-five years ago because more mothers are working outside the home. Thus, when both parents are at home, it may be hard for them to have a calm focus on their child, even though they quite naturally want to spend quality time with the latest addition to the family. Single-parent families are also far more common today than a quarter century ago. And these days, of course, work often follows parents home in the form of cell phones, email, and Internet connections. Even when parents are physically present with their children, they may be distracted by digital messages and Web surfing. More and more parents work in a global economy that never sleeps. So it is not surprising that one or both parents may suffer from moments of inattentiveness to their child, uncertainty about parenting, inconsistency, and sleep deprivation.

Today's parents are exposed to daily reminders and images that magnify fearfulness about local, international, and environmental dangers impacting their children's safety now and in the future. On top of this feeling of physical insecurity is a heightened sense of academic competitiveness among some parents who view preschool as but the first rung on a ruthless ladder of global competition for good jobs. Early education classes, enrichment programs, and scheduled activities to acquire knowledge and skills are increasingly popular among parents. And school itself has grown more demanding, with children expected to master more knowledge and skills at an earlier age than ever before, to say nothing of the demands placed on students by sports programs and other extracurricular activities. All of this runs the risk of interfering with naps and early bedtimes for children, ironically making it more difficult for them to learn.

Sleep deprivation in parents and children alike, combined with the challenging, technologically complex modern world, has created even more anxiety about parenting. But you are not alone. I know from my practice that countless other parents are experiencing these feelings.

I strongly wish to reassure you now that there will be much less worrying within a well-rested family. With healthy sleep, parents are better able to cope with many of the challenges they face. When families are well rested, they are more able to prevent and correct the inevitable problems that will develop.

Becoming a well-rested family is not really that difficult as long as we don't let our anxiety or exhaustion blind us.

Please don't be scared by the topic of how or when your baby will sleep well. I know that you might be afraid or even desperate; haven't we all heard horror stories of babies who never sleep through the night, are cranky all day, and turn overwhelmed parents into nervous wrecks? But the fact is, you *can* help your newborn to develop good sleep habits, even if your baby turns out to be colicky. In the following pages, I will make this subject simple to understand, and I am confident that you will be successful. *Healthy Sleep Habits, Happy Child* is now easier to read, even if you are crazy busy or short of sleep. There will be no judgment here. Instead, you will find reassurance, support, and guidance, as well as new and trustworthy information about children's sleep.

My goal is to translate facts based on solid scientific research into practical, useful, and concrete advice for parents. You might be desperate to be told exactly the "right" way to get your child to sleep well. But raising a child is not as straightforward and predictable as cooking from a recipe. Let's face it, no parent is perfect, and no baby does exactly what you expect. I will offer guidelines for you to pick and choose from and for you to modify to fit your family. Flexibility is absolutely essential to find what works for you and your child.

Consider the beginning of parenting, around the time when your baby is born. Imagine you are in a hospital nursery viewing newborn babies. Close your eyes and visualize this scene for a moment. You, your family, other parents, and grandparents are on one side of the glass: happy, smiling, and pointing. On the other side of the window, babies are swaddled, on their backs, drowsy or asleep. The babies appear magically calm and content. They seem peaceful, without a care in the world. This is what is meant by "sleeping like a baby." Observing this scene might also make you feel more at peace with the world. Try to remember the sight of the babies in the nursery, as well as how you feel—a little apprehensive, perhaps, but also peaceful.

Now look again at the babies in their cribs in the nursery. Please note that none of them is being held by a nurse or a mother. Yet the babies do not seem to mind. Pause, breathe deeply, reflect on this fact, and remember this observation: for your baby to sleep this well at home, it is not necessary to always hold your baby when he or she is drowsy or sleeping. In fact, moving about with your drowsy baby in your arms or stroller may interfere with peaceful sleep.

This is a small but important lesson. I mention it now because, as you will see, small changes in parenting may have big effects in improving your child's sleep. It's not all that complicated. *Healthy Sleep Habits, Happy Child* will help you create this scene of serenity for your sleeping baby in your home after you are discharged from the hospital. In the pages that follow, I will gently and patiently teach you many such lessons and give you many tips so that when you come home, your newborn will sleep like a baby. Not just for the first days and weeks, but for months to come, setting a pattern in place that will extend throughout childhood . . . and beyond.

When your child sleeps well, you, too, will sleep well, and as a result will be better able to nurture and teach your child, who, in turn, will be better able to learn. Thus, healthy sleep has a mutually reinforcing effect that goes back and forth between parent and child, bringing out the best in everyone. Sleeping well makes your child's brain healthy. Sleeping well allows your child to learn more about people and the world. Sleeping well permits your child to behave and perform at his or her personal best. Sleeping well makes life better. Being well rested provides a necessary foundation for a healthy, happy family.

Now let's take a closer look at sleep in our children.

PART I

Sleep Strategies and Solutions— Understanding Healthy Sleep Habits

CHAPTER 1

What Constitutes Healthy Sleep?

Healthy Sleep

Are your child's sleep patterns healthy? There are five elements of healthy sleep for children:

1. Sleep duration: night and day
2. Naps
3. Sleep consolidation
4. Sleep schedule, timing of sleep
5. Sleep regularity

When these five items are in proper balance, children get the rest they need. Let's first take a look at each one separately. Later, we will see how each element is not really independent of the others but simply part of a package called "healthy sleep."

There are five turning points in the sleep maturation process:

1. At 6 weeks, night sleep lengthens.
2. At 12 to 16 weeks, daytime sleep regularizes, with two major naps and a variable third nap.
3. At 9 months, night waking for feeding disappears, as does the third nap.

4. At 12 to 21 months, the midmorning nap disappears.

5. At 3 to 4 years, the midday nap becomes less common.

As your baby's brain matures, the patterns and rhythm of sleep change. If you adapt your parenting practices to these changes, your child will sleep well. Those parents who do not notice these changes or fail to make the proper adjustments have babies who become overtired. The biological development causing these changes is under the control of two regulatory mechanisms. (Things such as feeding routines, which vary from family to family, do not influence how the brain develops.) Understanding these biological controlling mechanisms will help you organize your thoughts and plan your actions to ensure healthy sleep for your child.

The first regulatory system controls the body's need for sleep and has been called the "homeostatic control mechanism." This system keeps track of how much sleep you need. In a nutshell, it means that the longer you go without sleep, the longer you will subsequently sleep. If you lose sleep, the body tries to restore it. This automatic process reflects an internal biological mechanism that we do not control. It is similar to the body's regulation of temperature; when we get hot, we automatically sweat, and when we're cold, we shiver. It is no different with sleep needs. But since babies cannot use language to inform us of their needs, parents must be on their toes in order not to miss the signs of shifts in sleeping requirements.

The second regulatory system has been called the "circadian timing system." It is also called the "human body's inner clockwork" or "internal timing system" and can be thought of as a dedicated regulatory program that switches specific genes on and off in response to the light-dark cycle. This regulatory apparatus is a molecular clock set to the proper time by sunlight. It automatically tries to ensure that the body is sleeping at the right time, and that when you are asleep, the timing and amounts of different stages and types of sleep are correct. Signals come from a specific area within the brain to make us feel sleepy or wakeful. These signals are present in babies as well as adults, but in babies the patterns change over the weeks, months, and years of growth and maturation. The pace of these changes is especially quick during the first several months, so it is easy for a parent to get a little off tempo. Just when you think you have figured out when your baby needs to nap or be put to bed at night, the circadian timing system sends your baby new instructions!

The internal timing system is under genetic control, so there is individual variation. It takes time for the internal timing system to express itself.

Sleep Duration: Night and Day

If you don't sleep long enough, you feel tired. This sounds very simple and obvious, but how much sleep is enough? And how can you tell if *your* child is getting enough sleep?

The sleep patterns of infants under 3 or 4 months of age seem mostly to reflect the development of the child's brain. During these first few weeks, in fact, sleep durations equal sleep needs, since infant behavior and sleep durations are mostly influenced by biological factors. But after about 3 or 4 months, and perhaps even at about 6 weeks (or 6 weeks after the due date, for babies born early), parenting practices can start to influence sleep duration and, consequently, behavior. As I will discuss later in more detail, I believe parents can promote more charming, calm, alert behaviors by becoming more sensitive to their growing child's need to sleep and by helping to establish and maintain healthy sleep habits. The goal is to recognize and respect your child's need to sleep and not do things that interfere with the natural sleep process.

NEWBORNS AND YOUNG INFANTS

During their first few days, newborns sleep about sixteen to seventeen hours total each day, although their longest single sleep period is only four to five hours. It makes no difference whether your baby is breast-fed or bottle-fed, or whether it's a boy or a girl.

> Nursing mothers often worry unnecessarily that long sleep periods deprive their baby of adequate breast milk. Weight checks with the doctor will reassure you that all is well.

Between 1 week and 4 months, the total daily sleep duration drifts down from sixteen and a half to fifteen hours, while the longest single sleep period—usually the night—increases from four to nine hours. We know from several studies that this development reflects neurological maturation and is *not* related to the start of feeding solid foods.

Some newborns and infants under the age of 4 months sleep much more and others much less. During the first few months, you can usually assume that your baby is getting sufficient sleep. But if your baby cries too much or has extreme fussiness/colic, you might assist Mother Nature by trying the helpful hints for "crybabies" described in Chapter 5.

> When they are 1 or 2 weeks old, many infants begin to have periods of increasingly alert, wakeful, gassy, and fussy behavior. This continues until about 6 weeks of age, after which they start to calm down. This increasingly irritable and wakeful state is often misinterpreted as resulting from maternal anxiety or from insufficient or "bad" breast milk. Nonsense! The culprit is a temporarily uninhibited nervous system that causes excessive arousal. Relax; this developmental phase will pass as the baby's brain matures. It's not your fault.

Young infants are very portable. You can take them anywhere you want, and when they need to sleep, they will. I remember when, as a medical student at Stanford University, I was playing tennis with my wife one day and my first child was sleeping in an infant seat near the fence. A huge dump truck came crashing down the narrow street, making an awful racket. We ran over to our son, certain that he had been jolted from his peaceful sleep, only to be surprised that he slept on blissfully. After 6 weeks of age, he became more socially aware of people around him; after about 4 months of age, he, like all children, became interested in barking dogs, wind in the trees, clouds, and many other curious things, all of which could and did disturb his sleep, either by waking him up or by making him fight to stay awake.

For some infants, the time when the baby first makes a socially responsive smile (usually at 6 weeks of age, or 6 weeks after the due date for babies born early) is when social curiosity or social learning begins. However, under about 3 or 4 months of age, most infants, like my son, are not much disturbed by their environment when it comes to sleeping. When their body says it's time to sleep, they sleep. When their body tells them to wake up, they wake up—even when it's not convenient for their parents! This is true whether they are fed on demand or according to a regular schedule. It is also true even when they are continuously fed intravenously because of birth defects of the stomach or intestines. Hunger, in fact, seems to have little to do with how babies sleep. A much more likely candidate for influencing a baby's sleeping patterns is the hormone melatonin, which is produced by the baby's brain beginning at about 3 to 4 months of age. This hormone surges at night and has the capability to both induce drowsiness and relax the smooth muscles encircling the gut. So around 3 or 4 months of age, so-called day/night confusion and apparent abdominal cramps (colic) begin to disappear.

Furthermore, infants raised in an environment where the lights are constantly on evolve normal sleep patterns, just like babies brought up in homes where the lights are turned on and off routinely. Another bit of evidence to suggest that environment has little effect on sleep patterns in children under 3 or 4 months of age comes from infants born prematurely. A child born four weeks before his due date, for example, reaches the same level of sleep development as a full-term baby four weeks *later* than the child born on time.

Biological sleep/wake development does not speed up in those pree-mies who are exposed to more social stimulation.

What we can conclude, therefore, is that for infants under 3 or 4 months of age you should try to flow with the child's need for sleep. Don't expect predictable sleep schedules, and don't try to en-force them rigidly. Still, some babies do develop regular sleep/wake rhythms quite early, at about 6 to 8 weeks. These babies tend to be very mild, cry very little, and sleep for long periods of time. Con-sider yourself blessed if you are the lucky parents of such an infant!

OLDER INFANTS AND CHILDREN

As children age, the amount of time they sleep tends to decrease. Figures 1 through 3 describe how much daytime sleep, night sleep, and total sleep occur at different ages for older children. The bot-tom curve in each graph means that 10 percent of children sleep less than the amount shown, while the top curve means that 90 percent of children sleep less than the amount shown for each age. These curves were generated by my own research using data collected from 2,019 children, mostly white, middle-class residents of northern Il-linois and northern Indiana, in 1980. These graphs can help you tell whether your child's sleep is above the 90th percentile or below the 10th percentile. (Other studies have used only the 50th percentile, or average values, and do not tell you whether your child's sleep dura-tion is slightly below average or extremely below average.) Interest-ingly, the results of studies of similar social classes in 1911 in California and in 1927 in Minnesota, also involving thousands of children, were the same as those in my study. In addition, studies in England in 1910 and Japan in 1925 showed identical sleep curves.

Thus, it seems that despite cultural and ethnic differences, social changes, and the impact of such modern inventions as television, computers, and cell phones on our contemporary lifestyles, the age-specific durations of sleep are firmly and universally rooted in our children's developing biology.

An exception to this generalization is that adolescents everywhere are now getting less sleep. During the second half of the twentieth century, a trend toward earlier start times for high school developed. This forced children to get up earlier during the school week and reduced the total number of hours available for sleeping. At the same time, it became more popular for teenagers to hold part-time jobs after school, and participation in extracurricular sports became more prevalent and demanding, so teenagers were going to bed later. Further, the amount of homework has increased.

But how long you sleep is not the whole story. In 9- to 16-year-olds, the timing of sleep, not just sleep duration, makes a big difference. Even when the sleep duration is the same, those children who went to bed later did less vigorous exercise each day and had more periods of physical inactivity than children with an earlier bedtime.

My study on sleep duration was in 1980. In 1990, less than 10 percent of children had a TV in their bedroom. However, beginning around 1990, the trend of having a TV in a child's bedroom developed, so that by 2007 about 20 percent of children under 2 years of age and 40 percent of children from 3 to 6 years old had a TV in their bedroom. Having a TV in the bedroom is associated with sleep problems and less sleeping. More recently, cell phone and computer use at night has pushed bedtimes even later. As noted previously, after about 4 months I think parents can influence sleep durations, and as you will see, sleep durations for these older infants, toddlers, and teens are especially important. One easy thing you can do is keep all screen-based media devices out of the bedroom at bedtime.

I studied sixty healthy children in my pediatric practice at 5 months of age and then again at 36 months. At 5 months of age, the infants who were cooing, smiling, adaptable, and regular (their sleep times and hungry times were around the same time every day) and who curiously approached unfamiliar things or people slept longer than infants with opposite characteristics. These easy and calm infants slept about three and a half hours during the day and twelve hours at night, for a total of fifteen and a half hours. Infants who were fussy, crying, irritable, hard to handle, irregular, and more withdrawn slept almost three hours less overall, almost a 20 percent difference (three hours during the day and nine and a half hours at night, or twelve and a half hours total).

In addition, for all the 5-month-olds studied, persistence or attention span was the trait most strongly associated with daytime sleep or nap duration. In other words, *children who slept longer during the day had longer attention spans.*

Figure 1

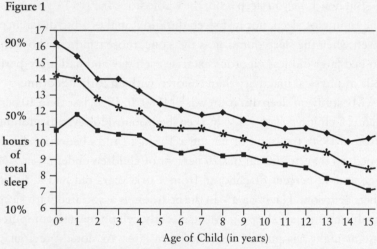

Age of Child (in years)

*Note: 0 represents children between 4 and 11 months of age.

As I will discuss in a later chapter, infants who sleep more during the day are better able to learn from their environment; this is because they have a better-developed ability to maintain focused or sustained attention. They soak up information about their surroundings like a sponge soaking up water. They learn simply from looking at the clouds and trees, from touching, feeling, smelling, and hearing, and from watching their mother's and father's faces. Infants who sleep less in the daytime appear more fitful and socially demanding, and they are less able to entertain or amuse themselves. Toys and objects are less interesting to these more tired children.

By 3 years of age, the easier-to-manage children in my study—

Figure 2

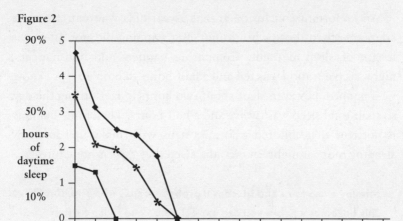

Age of Child (in years)

*Note: 0 represents children between 4 and 11 months of age.

Figure 3

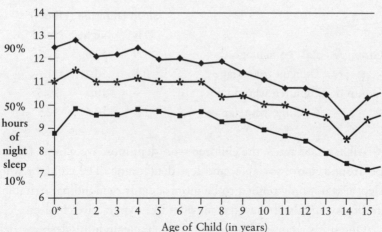

Age of Child (in years)

*Note: 0 represents children between 4 and 11 months of age.

mild, positive in mood, adaptable, and more likely to approach unfamiliar people—slept twelve and a half hours total. The difficult-to-manage children—those who were intense, more negative, less adaptable, and withdrawing—slept about one and a half hours less, almost the equivalent of a daytime nap.

An important conclusion is that 3-year-olds who nap are more adaptable than those who do not. But napping did not affect the length of sleep at night. Comparing nappers and non-nappers, night sleep duration was ten and a half hours in both groups. Those who napped, however, slept about two hours longer during the day, so their total sleep was twelve and a half hours. Therefore, it simply is not true that children who miss naps will "make up" for it by sleeping more at night. In fact, the sleep they miss is gone forever.

Missing a nap here and there will probably cause no harm. But if this becomes a habit, you can expect your child to lag further and further behind in his sleep and to become increasingly difficult to handle in this overfatigued state.

SLEEP DURATION OF 3-YEAR-OLDS

		Sleep Duration (Hours)		
		Day	Night	Total
Group A	Easy to manage	1.9	10.6	12.5
	Difficult to manage	0.9	10.4	11.3
Group B	Children who do not nap	—	10.5	10.5
	Children who nap	2.0	10.5	12.5

All in all, at age 3, the children who slept more were more fun to be around, more sociable, and less demanding. The children who slept less not only tended to be more socially demanding, irritable, and fussy but also behaved somewhat like hyperactive children.

One study examined the effects of a single night of sleep restriction in a group of children between 10 and 14 years old. The researchers noted that there were impairments in verbal creativity, abstract thinking and concept formation, and complex problem solving. These higher cognitive abilities appear to be essential for academic performance and success. In contrast, there were no deficits on rote performance or less complex memory and learning tasks. The ability to maintain routine performance despite being sleepy is familiar to every adult who sometimes gets very tired but nevertheless is able to perform the routine aspects of his or her job fairly well. My interpretation of this study is that chronic sleepiness in infants and young children impairs cognitive development, but this does not become apparent until the child is much older and challenged by more complex tasks. Of course, cognitive development starts in babies, not at 10 to 14 years of age, but the deficits from sleep deprivation remain hidden in young children. When children are younger, the challenges they face are at a much lower level, and these chronically sleep-deprived children may still do well with spelling, writing, reading, and simple arithmetic. Later, when they are older, more demanding academic challenges unmask the cognitive deficits lurking there all along.

Looking at our sleep curves again, we see that throughout early and middle childhood, the duration of sleep declines until adolescence, when the curve shown in Figure 1 levels off and then slightly increases. This increase has been noted in some other studies and suggests that teenagers need more sleep than preteens. Yet, as noted previously, academic demands, social events, and school sports combine during adolescence to pressure teenagers to stay up later and later. Also, there are biological shifts in adolescents that seem to encourage more wakefulness in the evening. This is the time when chronic and cumulative sleep losses begin to take their toll and can make a normally rough period in life unbearably rocky for children and parents alike.

In general, do not pay too much attention to these graphs: they are only rough descriptions of age-specific groups of children. They are not prescriptions for *your* child. The fact is, for any specific age, there are short sleepers and long sleepers. You might wish that your child slept longer, but he might be a perfectly healthy short sleeper. It is much more important to watch your child than it is to watch the clock.

Daytime Wakefulness and Sleepiness

Watching your child carefully allows you to become aware of subtle changes in his wakefulness or sleepiness. We tend to think superficially of being either awake or asleep, as if these two black-and-white states were the only possibilities. But there are gradations of sleep, and of wakefulness, too. Task performance, attentiveness, vigilance, and mood are influenced not only by the quality of our sleep at night but also by the quality of our wakefulness during the day. When we do not feel very awake during the day, we say that we feel "sleepy." Or, to be more precise, studies of adults show that most adults avoid the word "sleepy" and instead use the word "tired," which implies previous effortful behavior or hard work—something to be proud of. It seems that the word "tired" is more acceptable in our culture, and an admission of feeling "sleepy" is something to deny, as if it were a weakness of character. I encourage parents to get into the habit of using the word "sleepy" for their child because it directly implies what is needed: more sleep. Think of excessive daytime sleepiness or impaired daytime alertness as a result of disturbed sleep.

The Stanford Sleepiness Scale is a self-rating instrument developed at Stanford University to describe the different states or levels of daytime sleepiness. Obviously, children who are depressed or irritable due to sleep deprivation will have high numerical ratings.

Level Description
1. Feeling active and vital; alert; wide awake
2. Functioning at a high level, but not at peak; still able to concentrate
3. Relaxed; awake; not at full alertness; responsive
4. A little foggy; not at peak; let down
5. Fogginess; beginning to lose interest in remaining awake; slowed down
6. Sleepiness; preferring to be lying down; fighting sleep; woozy
7. Almost in reverie; sleep onset soon; lost struggle to remain awake

The descriptions in this scale are self-assessments. Because young children cannot articulate what they are feeling, parents have to watch for signs of daytime sleepiness in their children. Okay . . . but what should you be watching for?

Daytime sleepiness resulting from disturbed sleep typically causes adults to feel a mild itching or burning in the eyes. Our eyelids feel heavy. Our limbs feel heavy, too, and we tend to be lethargic. We are less motivated, lose interest easily, and have difficulty concentrating. Our speech slows; we yawn and rub our eyes. As we get sleepier, our eyes begin to close, and we may even find our head nodding. Are these the signs we should look for in our babies and young children?

No. This familiar picture of adult sleep is not usually seen in infants and young children who suffer from disturbed sleep. While it is true that infants who are usually well rested yawn on occasions when they are overtired, it seems that chronically sleepy infants do not yawn much or nod off. Instead, when most young kids get too sleepy, they get grumpy and excitable. At age 3 my first son coined the perfect word to describe this turned-on state: "upcited," a combination of "upset" and "excited," as in "Don't make me upcited!" when we admonished him for behaving like a little monster.

Two very interesting Australian studies on adults have helped to shed light on childhood "upcited" behavior. One study showed that the level of activation of the nervous system was associated with certain personality traits, sleep habits, and activity of the adrenal gland. Poor sleepers were more anxious and had higher levels of the hormone cortisol, which typically rises during stressful situations.

The second study was complex, but I think its results will better help you to understand your child's behaviors. In this study, adult volunteers reported their moods on four scales:

1. Tired to rested
2. Sluggish to alert
3. Irritable to calm
4. Tense to relaxed

The first two scales reflected degrees of *arousal*, while the third and fourth scales reflected degrees of *stress*.

The researchers measured four different hormones (cortisol, noradrenaline, adrenaline, and dopamine) that our bodies make naturally. These powerful chemicals affect our brain and how we feel, and they are related to the four scales in different ways.

For example, fatigue produces an increase in adrenaline concentrations. That is, when we are tired, our body chemically responds with a burst of adrenaline to give us more drive or energy. We become more aroused, alert, and excitable. Concentrations of cortisol also increase with increasing alertness. In children, cortisol concentrations remain high when they do not nap. Perhaps the nap allows the brain to be alert without needing the added boost cortisol provides. Increasing irritability and tenseness—stress factors—are also associated with increasing concentrations of adrenaline, noradrenaline, and dopamine.

These studies support the notion that when an overly sleepy child appears wired, wild, edgy, excitable, or unable to fall asleep easily or stay asleep, he is this way precisely because of his body's response to being short of sleep. Think of how you feel when you work hard and lose sleep in order to finish a major project. You are highly motivated and fight the daytime sleepiness. The impairments of performance and discomfort of sleepiness increase. After a while, you feel keyed up. Thankfully, modern adults are able to get out of this state by taking vacations. But have you noticed how, at the start of a vacation, it takes a few days to unwind? This is the time required for our accumulated nervous energy to dissipate.

REMEMBER
When your infant or young child appears wired, he may actually be tired.

This tells me that our lifestyle and sleep habits can affect our internal chemical machinery, which in turn causes us to feel certain ways. In a study at Dartmouth College, coronary-prone type A students had more night wakings than type B students. A vicious circle could develop whereby fragmented sleep causes increased arousal, the student feels more energized, and, sensing this greater level of energy, the student works even harder late into the night to achieve more, but at the same time loses more sleep.

IMPORTANT POINT
Loss of sleep produces central nervous system hyperarousal.

Infants over 4 months of age as well as older children can push themselves hard fighting sleep in order to enjoy the pleasure of their parents' company and play. The resulting sleep disturbances might produce fatigue, and the body would naturally respond by turning up production of those chemicals, such as cortisol, responsible for maintaining alertness and arousal. Perhaps researchers may someday find that different patterns of sleep deprivation (total sleep loss, abnormal schedules, nap deprivation, or sleep fragmentation) produce different patterns of chemical imbalances. Here are some terms used by professionals to describe the behavior of hyperalert children with disturbed sleep:

Physiological activation
Neurological arousal
Excessive wakefulness
Emotional reactivity
Heightened sensitivity

Parents simply call this behavior "wired."

IMPORTANT POINT
Some chronically sleepy children are always keyed up and never unwind.

So often I have heard comments like "She's so tired, she's running around in circles" or "She wants to fall asleep but can't." This is not a new observation; a classic paper published in 1922 described the "increased reflex-irritability of a sleepy child." In dramatic contrast, over and over again I have seen well-rested children in my practice who spend enormous amounts of time in a state of quiet alertness. They take in everything with wide-open eyes, never missing a thing. They find simple little toys amusing or curious. They never appear bored, even though the toy they pick up may be one they have played with many times.

The good news is that you can help guide your child to healthy sleep and make a big difference. Parents of children 4 to 12 months of age can *dramatically* and *quickly* change their children's mood and behavior depending on how much sleep they allow their kids to get.

For example, in a study published in 2002 of 4- and 5-year-olds, author Dr. John E. Bates stated, "In clinical treatment of young, oppositional children, we have seen some spectacular improvements in manageability associated with the parents instituting a more adequate schedule of sleep for their children. Our clinical impression in these cases was that the changes were too rapid to be accounted for by other changes, such as parental discipline tactics."

REMEMBER AGAIN

A calm and alert state is a sign of sleeping well. Upon awakening, well-rested children are in good cheer and are able to play by themselves.

I believe that in infants and young children, a cause-and-effect relationship exists between disturbed sleep and fitful, fussy behaviors. In addition, as described later, the harmful effects of excessive daytime sleepiness do not stay the same, but rather tend to accumulate. This means that there is a progressive worsening in a child's mood and performance even when the amount of lost sleep each day or night is constant. So a baby becomes increasingly crabby even if her nightly sleep is constantly just a little too brief.

A constant small deficit in sleep produces a cumulative reduction in daytime alertness.

Distinct differences exist between adult insomniacs whose insomnia started in childhood and those whose insomnia started in adulthood. The childhood-onset insomniacs take longer to fall asleep and sleep less than adult-onset insomniacs. I think these data support the hypothesis that the failure to establish good sleeping habits in infancy or early childhood has long-term harmful effects, such as adult insomnia. But the effects go well beyond insomnia. Among psychologically unhealthy adults, the more severe the sleep difficulty, the more severe the degree of mental illness.

Here are some signs that your child is not getting quality sleep: he often falls asleep in the stroller or car when you are out doing errands; he often wakes up crying, grumpy, or painfully confused; and there is usually a "witching hour" in the late afternoon or early evening.

Witching Hour
After 3–4 months of age, if your baby is often fussy during the day, he is most likely short on sleep. But many children suffering from insufficient sleep appear fine during most of the day, only to exhibit the symptoms listed below as the sleep tank begins to go dry near the end of the day (4:00–5:00 p.m. for children under the age of 3 years, and 5:00–7:00 p.m. for children 3 years and older). This is known as the "witching hour." A child experiencing the witching hour may be irritable, easily upset, clinging, whining, fussy, peevish, or, in the words of one mother, "clawing at my breast." He might have a short fuse, be rough around the edges, seem easily frustrated, or be less able than usual to entertain himself. He might be oppositional, defiant, uncooperative, or angry; he might throw tantrums,

be aggressive, display a negative mood, be inattentive or distractible, exhibit learning difficulties, show decreased sociability and physical activity, and be generally depressed or anxious. This is quite a laundry list, but don't despair: very few children demonstrate more than a handful of these symptoms at one time. But any of them, coming during the witching hour, can be a signal of sleep problems that parents should address.

Second Wind

The "witching hour" may be thought of as a second wind or pre-sleep arousal state. Dr. Alice Gregory studied pre-sleep arousals in 8- to 10-year-olds and showed that the arousal was both physical (rapidly beating heart) and cognitive (inability to think). Dr. Julio Fernandez-Mendoza studied 327 children ages 5 to 12 years and showed that children with short sleep durations exhibited hyper-arousal before sleep.

When you are short on sleep, your body reacts in a predictable way. As previously described, you get keyed up because your body produces stimulating chemicals such as cortisol, adrenaline, and noradrenaline. This results in a burst of energy commonly known as a second wind. When you catch your second wind, you are in a state of higher neurological arousal. You might feel more wired, turned on, or full of nervous energy. You also become more prickly or hypersensitive, just as a bad sunburn will make even a light touch painful. This state of hyperarousal is most obvious in a young child in the late afternoon or early evening when his sleep tank is almost empty and he is running on fumes because of missed naps, bedtimes that are too late, or both. Think of how your child might have a total meltdown late in the afternoon at a family holiday involving many hours of travel and many hours without sleep. But while the witching hour occurs near the end of the day, the second wind can occur whenever a period of wakefulness before a nap is too long. The result is difficulty falling asleep for a nap, or the nap is too short, or the nap is missed entirely. If this occurs only occasionally, it is probably not a problem for your child even though your nerves are frayed! But imagine what happens when your child usually goes to bed a little too late or too often misses naps.

When the bedtime is usually or often a little too late, the child wakes up too tired, and this higher neurological arousal then causes him to have difficulty napping well. Not napping well causes his sleep tank to go toward empty by the end of the day and results in an even higher state of arousal, so it now becomes even more difficult for him to easily fall asleep and stay asleep at night. Parents might not appreciate that bedtime battles, long latency to sleep (taking a long time to fall asleep), or night waking result from a bedtime that is too late. Of course, the child eventually crashes. But before he does so, he is in an unhealthy state that gives rise to stressful parent-child interactions, stressful interactions between parents, and stress for each parent as an individual. Additionally, because the bedtime was too late, your child does not receive the benefits of healthy sleep.

Understanding how sleep deprivation causes a second wind that makes it more difficult to easily fall asleep and stay asleep also leads to a deeper appreciation of the opposite situation: being well-rested allows your child to more easily fall asleep and stay asleep.

It's a virtuous circle: sleep begets sleep. It's also a vicious circle: sleeplessness begets sleeplessness.

Naps

Having grown up in a highly achievement-oriented society, most American adults are likely to view naps as a waste of time. We tend to think that adults who nap are lazy, undermotivated, ill, or elderly. In turn, we do not attach much positive benefit to daytime sleep in our infants and young children beyond giving us, the parents and caregivers, a much-needed break. Let me explain why naps are indeed very important for learning, or cognitive development, in children. A study published in 2015 showed that naps enhance the consolidation of memory among infants at 6 and 12 months. Further, infants who have longer naps are better able to remember novel actions than infants who take naps for 30 minutes or less.

Naps are not little bits of night sleep randomly intruding upon children's waking hours. Night sleep, daytime sleep, and daytime wakefulness have rhythms that are partially independent of one another. During the first 3 to 4 months of life, these rhythms develop at different rates, so they may not be in sync. Only later do these sleep/wake rhythms become linked with fluctuations in body temperature and activity levels.

For example, most of us have experienced drowsiness in the afternoon. This sensation is partially related—but only partially—to how long you have been up and how long you slept the night before. Our mental state fluctuates during the day between alert and drowsy, just as fluctuations occur during the night between light and deep sleep stages. As adults, we find a midday nap most refreshing when we take it at the time when we are biologically most drowsy.

If you live in the siesta belt, afternoon drowsiness might prompt you to take a nap, but in the United States, it's time for a coffee break. In England, it's afternoon tea. Both rituals arose to help fight naturally occurring daytime drowsiness through the use of stimulating chemicals such as caffeine.

SLEEP INERTIA

Beyond cultural conditioning, however, there is an important reason some adults do not nap: *sleep inertia*. Sleep inertia is a feeling of disorientation, confusion, pain, discomfort, impaired mood, and the inability to concentrate or think well that occurs upon awakening, especially from naps. Have you ever awakened from a nap with a headache, mental fuzziness, or other unpleasant sensations? With sleep inertia, it appears that sleep is intruding into wakefulness, and this overlap state is painfully uncomfortable.

In children, sleep inertia appears to be more severe and more prolonged for those who are more overtired. One mother described it as a "fugue" state (neither fully awake nor fully asleep), another as a "demonic" state. The children are out of control, panicky, crying, or screaming hysterically. Parents would often call me after three-day holiday weekends, during which their children became severely overtired, and tell me that they were sure their child had a painful ear infection because their child awoke crying. They often added that they were sure their child was not overtired because the child had just completed an extra-long nap! The ears were perfect; the children had simply missed some naps or had been allowed to stay up too late during the holiday, and as a result, sleep inertia was rearing its ugly head.

Sometimes a child shows sleep inertia after a single midday nap, suggesting that the bedtime is too late, but around the end of the day the child seems fine, suggesting that the bedtime is not too late. How to resolve this apparent contradiction? The culprit might be not the bedtime but an interval of wakefulness before the nap that was too long. Trial and error might be needed in adjusting either the bedtime or the nap time or both.

Here is a parent's report:

I was noticing occasional sleep inertia after naps. I assumed it was because the bedtime was too late. However, my sleep logs repeatedly showed that we only got sleep inertia when the wake-up time that day was too early. For example, for the last twelve days we have used super-early bedtimes (6:00–6:15 p.m.) to repay some sleep debt. It has started backfiring, though—this morning the wake-up was 4:45 a.m. And after the nap today—boom! Sleep inertia.

I have seen this again and again. Although sleep inertia might result from cumulative sleepiness from a too-late bedtime, my observation is that it can also result from a too-long interval of wakefulness before the nap.

Understanding that the rhythms of night sleep, daytime sleep, and daytime wakefulness are somewhat independent from one another leads to two important ideas. First, in a child under 3 or 4 months of age, these rhythms are not in synchrony with each other, and the baby may be getting opposing messages from different parts of the brain. The sleep rhythm says "deep sleep," while the wake rhythm says "alert" instead of "drowsy." Wakeful but tired, the confused child cries fitfully; we might call this behavior colic or fussiness. Opposing or overlapping messages from different parts of the brain may cause ambiguous stages such as sleep inertia. In research with adults and animals, this has been called "dissociated states of wakefulness and sleep," or "status dissociatus." Thus, for example, narcolepsy can be seen as the intrusion of REM (rapid eye movement) sleep into wakefulness, while sleepwalking, night terrors, and crying out at night occur during the overlap between wakefulness and non-REM sleep.

We know that adults may have overlapping sleep and wake states, experience incomplete sleep states, or switch rapidly between states. So it is entirely possible that during the first 4 months of a newborn's life, when sleep states are developing, partial states express themselves out of phase and in conjunction with other states, creating overlap problems that we refer to as fussiness, colic, or sleep inertia. For example, it is known that babies can suck, smile, and cry with their eyes open during REM sleep, so while they appear to be awake, they are actually asleep. We can call this "indeterminate sleep" or "ambiguous sleep," which reflects the immaturity of the young brain. After about 4 months of age, these ambiguous states are less common.

Second, if these sleep/wake rhythms are somewhat independent, they may have different functions: learning for the wake cycle, physical and emotional restoration for the sleep cycle. Daytime sleep and nighttime sleep may be different in this regard. I believe that *healthy naps* lead to optimal daytime alertness for learning—that is, naps adjust the alert/drowsy control to just the right setting for optimal daytime arousal. Without naps, the child is too drowsy to learn well.

Also, when chronically sleep deprived, the fatigued child becomes fitfully fussy or hyperalert in order to fight sleep, and therefore cannot learn from his environment.

What happens when a nap is skipped? In toddlers of 30–36 months, Dr. Rebecca Berger experimentally eliminated a single nap. She noted that when only one nap is eliminated, "acute sleep restriction causes dampened positive emotion displays when positive responses are expected (solvable puzzle), as well as increased negative emotion . . . under challenging conditions (unsolvable puzzle)."

In other words, experimental acute nap deprivation revealed that "toddlers [were] neither able to take full advantage of positive experiences nor . . . as adaptive in challenging contexts. If insufficient sleep consistently 'taxes' young children's emotion responses, they may not manage emotion regulation challenges effectively, potentially placing them at risk for future emotional/behavioral problems. . . . Specifically, when children were given the opportunity to complete an age-appropriate puzzle, they showed *less joy and pride* when sleep restricted than when optimally rested. . . . [W]hen children were faced with a puzzle with no solution, they showed significantly *more worry/anxiety* when sleep restricted than when well rested. . . . In sum," Dr. Berger continued, "sleepy children may view and respond to the world differently than children who are well-rested: they may not be able to take full advantage of positive experiences and may not be as able to manage challenges. . . . A lack of sleep in contexts that rely on young children's mastery of new information (e.g., preschool) may have significant and potentially dire long-term consequences."

The takeaway message is that if your child misses a nap now and then, it is not necessarily a big deal, but it will affect your child. Imagine, though, what happens when naps are routinely skipped!

Another study, by Dr. Janice Bell, showed that "insufficient nighttime sleep among infants and preschool-aged children may be a lasting risk factor for subsequent obesity. *Napping does not appear to be a substitute for nighttime sleep*" (emphasis added). One way to think about this is to consider the components of the food we eat. Food contains carbohydrates, proteins, fats, minerals, and vitamins. At different ages, our children need different amounts of these components for healthy growth. But it is not simply a matter of counting calories, and you cannot substitute one component for another even though they may be equivalent in calories. Similarly, at different ages our children need different amounts of naps and night sleep, and it is not simply a matter of adding up the total number of hours asleep. You cannot substitute minutes of night sleep for minutes of naps even though the total sleep duration is equivalent. Whether it be food or sleep, different elements are required for health.

Another feature that distinguishes night sleep from day sleep is that cross-cultural studies show large differences for age-specific bedtimes and evening sleep but not for daytime sleep.

Not only are naps different from night sleep, but not every nap is created equal. There is more REM sleep in the midmorning nap compared to the midday nap. During a nap, the duration of REM sleep within a nap, not simply the total duration of the nap, is related to creative problem solving. Research also suggests that high amounts of REM sleep, under the influence of low melatonin levels, help direct the course of brain maturation in early life. Further, adult studies have suggested that REM sleep is especially important for restoring us emotionally or psychologically, while deep, non-REM sleep appears to be more important for physical restoration. Let's protect opportunities for naps in our children so they can get all the REM sleep they need!

Because naps have their own function and do their job best when they occur at the right time, I suggest that if a nap has been missed, try to keep your child up until the next sleep period in order to maintain the timeliness of the sleep rhythm. This suggestion has to be balanced with the general theme of avoiding the overtired state, so the next sleep period (nap or night) might begin a little earlier.

My studies show that at 4 months of age, most children take either two or three naps. The third nap, if taken, tends to be brief and in the late afternoon or early evening. But by 6 months of age, the vast majority of children (84 percent) are taking only two naps; by 9 months of age, virtually all children are taking just one or two naps. About 17 percent of children have started taking only a single nap by their first birthday, and this percentage increases to 56 percent by the age of 15 months. By 21 months, most children are down to just a single nap.

The midmorning nap develops before the midday nap, but it also disappears before the midday nap. The single nap that is present by 21 months and resurfaces in adolescence or adulthood is always the midday or later-afternoon nap. Infants and young children have much more REM sleep at night than older children, and the midmorning nap has more REM sleep than the midday nap; this suggests that in some infants, the midmorning nap may be viewed as a sort of continuation of night sleep. Later I will discuss how we can help babies sleep better by keeping the interval of wakefulness between the wake-up time and the start of the first nap very short. This strategy may work because we are really allowing night sleep to continue longer.

WARNING
Not all sleep periods are created equal! Long naps do not compensate for late bedtimes. Sleep quality, not just sleep duration, is an essential component of healthy sleep.

Different studies show that longer naps may be associated with later bedtimes even if the wake-up time occurs later. Depending on the bedtime, the wake-up time, and the nap duration, total sleep duration may be the same, less, or more than comparison groups without later bedtimes. But despite longer naps, among children with later bedtimes, problems such as poor diet quality, obesity, and externalizing behavioral problems occur—even if total sleep is unchanged or greater! Why? Late bedtimes rob your child of deep, restorative sleep occurring before midnight, and this lost high-quality sleep is not made up for by lighter early morning sleep or additional daytime sleep. Long naps are not a substitute for less night sleep.

Another thing I've discovered is that up until about 21 months of age, some babies are born to be short nappers and some are inherently long nappers. Some children with normal night sleep tend to have long naps naturally, but parents can interfere with a child's long naps by messing up the child's schedule. However, they cannot make short nappers into long nappers. Here are some important facts about short nappers: at 6 months of age, 80 percent of babies nap between two and a half and four hours total each day. Napping more than four total hours each day occurs in 15 percent of babies. However, in 5 percent of babies, the total daytime sleep each day is less than two and a half hours. If you look at brief naps slightly differently and include babies who sleep a total of two and a half hours or less each day, then 18 percent of babies fall into this category. These short nappers tend to keep this pattern for the next twelve to eighteen months! This truth is especially frustrating to parents and caregivers whose first child was a long napper, accustoming them to long breaks during the day. If their second child is a short napper, they may incorrectly think they are doing something wrong or that there is something wrong with the child.

If parents can cause problems that interfere with good naps, why can't parents make their babies sleep longer? This question provides a good example of the asymmetry between sleep and wakefulness. Sleep is not the absence of wakefulness; rather, the brain automatically and actively turns on the sleep process and simultaneously turns off wakefulness. You and your child can force wakefulness upon sleep, but you cannot force sleep upon wakefulness. You and your child can motivate or force yourself and him into a more wakeful or alert state, but you cannot will anyone into a deeper sleep state. So sleep and wake states are different but not opposite. Parents provide the *opportunity to permit* the maximum amount of sleep to occur; this amount reflects their child's actual need for sleep. As stated before, a baby's nap pattern is largely an individual trait that stays stable until about 21 months. Evidence of the individuality of this trait comes from studies on twins and argues for a strong genetic component to the control of sleep in babies.

At 21 months, the average nap duration is a little less than two and a half hours, but the range is wide: between one and four hours. At this age, some of the children who initially took brief naps are now taking longer naps, and some who had been long nappers are now taking briefer naps. My interpretation is that by 21 months, biology is no longer the primary influence on napping; social factors begin to play a role. For example, events such as the birth of a sibling, an older sibling starting preschool, or the child herself now participating in organized and scheduled activities can cause children who have a biological need for longer naps to take shorter naps. Often, no problems occur if catch-up days are provided, coupled with an extra-early bedtime.

The time of day when the nap occurs is also important. Some studies have suggested that an early nap, occurring in the midmorning hours, is different in quality from a later nap, which occurs in the midday. As mentioned before, there is more active REM sleep than quiet sleep in the first nap, and this pattern is reversed in the second nap. So naps occurring at different times are different! Even for adults, a nap earlier in the day is lighter and less restorative than an midday nap, which consists of deeper sleep.

Long naps occurring at the right time make the child feel rested. Levels of cortisol dramatically fall during a nap, indicating a reduction of stress in the body. Not taking a needed nap means that the body remains stressed. Brief naps or naps that are out of sync with other biological rhythms are less restful, less restorative. But a short nap is better than no nap. It still has a positive effect on alertness.

Children can be taught how to take naps. A nap does not begin and end the way an electric light can be turned off and on. In fact, a nap or night sleep involves three periods of time: the time required for the process called falling asleep, the sleep period itself, and the time required to wake up. One father complained to me, "I can't see the pre-Z's coming out of his head," meaning he had difficulty seeing the lull in activity or quieting that precedes sleep. In later chapters I will show you how to recognize the "pre-Z' s" and teach your children to fall asleep at the optimal time.

> **Do not expect your baby to nap well outside his crib after 4 months of age. If you don't protect your baby's nap schedules, you can produce nap deprivation.**

When children do not nap well, they pay a price. Infants between 4 and 8 months who do not nap well have shorter attention spans or appear less persistent when engaged in activities. By 3 years of age, children who do not nap or who nap very little are often described as nonadaptable or even hyperactive. Adaptability is thought to be a very important trait for school success.

One mother of a nonadaptable child said with a laugh that every morning she prayed to the "nap god" to give her a break. In contrast, another mother described her son as a very easy child as long as she had a bed around. He was such a "rack monster" that she decided he just liked his own company best. Another mother described her son, who napped well, as the "snooze king."

Sometimes it appears that the older toddler needs exactly one and a half naps—while one nap is insufficient, two are impossible to achieve. These children are rough around the edges in the late afternoon or early evening, but parents can temporarily and partially compensate by putting the child to bed earlier on some nights.

An earlier bedtime may become a necessity when your child develops a single-nap pattern, between 15 and 21 months. Earlier bedtimes help prevent bedtime battles, deter night waking, discourage extremely early morning awakenings, and regularize and prolong naps. Why, then, do many parents resist the notion of putting their children to sleep when they first appear tired at night, even though it is clear that the brain is sleep-sensitive?

First, parents naturally want to be with their children and play with them. Second, there is a powerful inhibitory fear that if their child is put to bed very early when tired, she will get up extra early the next day. Third, because I recommend that, along with an earlier bedtime, the parents not go to the child at night except for feeding, parents are frightened about the possibility of prolonged crying when they put the child to bed or in the middle of the night. This fear of possible crying discourages parents from trying for an earlier bedtime. It is a natural fear . . . but in most cases a groundless one. These parents mistakenly think that a later bedtime will make the child more tired and resist sleep less.

Here is an example of how a family started early, at 8 weeks of age, to focus on an earlier bedtime. The baby was not overtired and did not have extreme fussiness/colic, so the transition went smoothly. But 20 percent of babies have extreme fussiness/colic, and for them, this change to an earlier bedtime at 8 weeks of age is not easy, as we shall see later.

When our daughter Jaden was born, we were anxious to start off on the right foot with her sleep habits. We immediately focused on no more than two hours of wakefulness with a bedtime around 10:00 or 11:00 p.m., which was very easy to accomplish. After a few weeks, though, we still weren't really seeing very long nighttime stretches. When Jaden was 8 weeks old, we visited Dr. Weissbluth to discuss her sleeping pattern. Dr. Weissbluth told us that at 6 weeks, we should have incorporated an early bedtime in addition to keeping shorter periods of wakefulness. We left wondering whether an early bedtime would really work for someone so young. We really expected that Jaden would be up within an hour or two after we put her down. We started off with a 7:00 p.m. bedtime. She still woke up in the late evening to eat, but we put her promptly back to bed. There were a few bumps in the road for the first couple of nights—sometimes she would wake up a few times and cry—but we kept at it.

After a few days, Jaden went from sleeping a four-to-five-hour stretch in the evening, to seven, then eight, then nine or ten hours a night. In fact, she seemed happy to be sleeping so much! If she woke up to nurse, she would eat and immediately fall back asleep as soon as we put her back in her crib. We couldn't believe how easy it was. The earlier we got her to bed, the better she slept. Her daytime naps even seemed longer and more restful. She is now 7 months old. We now try to get her down between 6:00 and 6:30 each night, and she is extremely happy about it. (So are we!)

Over and over again I have seen children who are put to bed too late. It becomes a vicious circle: the child's nap schedule is messed up, and the child is fussy in the late afternoon or early evening. This fatigue-driven fussiness ends in a wired state at bedtime, which interferes with the ability to go to sleep easily. As a result, in an attempt to avoid a bedtime battle, the parent keeps the child up until he crashes. The next day the child is still tired, the naps are messed up, and so on. The circle never ends.

The solution is obvious in Meg's story.

We had never been very consistent with Meg's bedtime. We would put her to bed when she appeared tired (rubbing eyes, yawning), anywhere from 7:00 to 7:45 p.m., but occasionally even later. It usually took her between fifteen and thirty minutes of crying to fall asleep. I thought this was normal. She had always gone to bed rather late, and she had always taken a while to fall asleep.

At Meg's 9-month appointment we asked Dr. Weissbluth about her night waking. He made a very simple suggestion. He told us that we should put Meg to bed twenty minutes earlier at night. He said that her night waking would disappear and she would still wake up at a normal hour in the morning. I told him that we had been putting her to sleep when she appeared tired, at around 7:30 p.m., give or take thirty minutes. He said that once she appears tired it is too late and she should already be in bed.

The first night we put her to bed at 6:45. We were very skeptical. We were sad to put her down so early when she seemed so wide awake and happy. She cried for about five minutes and then fell asleep, and with no night waking! The same thing happened the next night—about five minutes of crying and then asleep until morning. Sometimes she would wake up as early as 5:30, but we would give her a bottle and she would fall back to sleep, sometimes until almost 8:00!

It has been almost four weeks since our 9-month appointment. Bedtime is an absolute joy. Meg eats dinner, takes a bath, and is in bed about 6:30 p.m. Sometimes I hesitate to put her down so early when she seems to be in such good spirits, but she cuddles with her blanket and her doll, sucks her thumb, closes her eyes, and sleeps till morning. It's the sweetest thing I have ever seen.

As Meg's parents said about my recommendation for a much earlier bedtime, "He made a very simple suggestion." Sometimes simple approaches work better than complex solutions. And it's normal to be "skeptical" and "sad." Here's another example.

When we met with Dr. Weissbluth, Jared, now 19 months old, was waking up every hour and a half to two hours during the night. He would have to fall asleep while we were walking and carrying him on our shoulder. When placed in the crib, Jared would awaken and abruptly "pop up." He would only sleep in the bed "nest" we created for him on the floor of our family room. We endured three months of the night waking before we consulted Dr. Weissbluth.

We were instructed to place Jared in bed in an awake state between 6:00 and 7:00 in the evening and that we should leave him there until 6:00 in the morning. Our initial reaction was that Jared would carry on relentlessly when placed in his crib so early, and that the recommended approach was too strict and would never work. Much to our shock and delight, the first night we tried the new routine, Jared was asleep after five minutes of crying, and remained asleep for eleven hours, not waking until 5:30 the next morning. During the next two nights, Jared went to sleep on his own, with no episodes of crying. On the fourth night, he lay down in the bed with his favorite stuffed animal under his arm, as he has done since. Our baby was clearly overtired from going to bed at 8:30 p.m. and not being allowed to relax and go to sleep without interference. We never expected it to be so simple and provide such an immediate result. Jared wakes up happy, energized, and ready for a day full of adventures. Now, several months later, Jared is most happy when going to bed at 6:30 p.m., and will go to his bed himself if he is tired.

Probably the most common worry is that the earlier bedtime will produce an earlier wake-up time, as expressed by Anna's story.

At 18 months it became apparent that Anna was ready to make the transition from two naps to one, but would need some help because she fought the midmorning nap. We began, as Dr. Weissbluth suggested in his book, by gradually delaying the midmorning nap till 11:00 or so. Over a two-week window we were able to continue to push back the nap to sometime between noon and 1:00 p.m.

In his book, Dr. Weissbluth suggested an earlier bedtime to help prevent night waking or early morning waking. Anna was going to bed at 6:30 p.m. and sleeping until 7:00 a.m., so we really questioned this theory. My husband and I agreed that Dr. Weissbluth's advice has always been right on the money, so we decided to put her down an hour earlier. We feared that she would wake up at 5:30 or 6:00 a.m. after her usual twelve or thirteen hours of sleep. To our surprise, she awoke at 9:00 a.m., and she was in the most cheerful mood to date!

Family, friends, even strangers constantly tell us what a happy, cheerful child we have. The reality is that she is a very well-rested child.

Not napping means lost sleep. Over an extended period of time, children do not sleep longer at night when their naps are brief. Of course, once in a while—when relatives visit or when a painful ear infection keeps the child awake—a child will make up for lost daytime sleep with longer night sleep. But day in and day out, you should not expect to satisfy your child's need to sleep by cutting corners on naps and then trying to compensate by putting your child to sleep for the night at an earlier hour. What you wind up with is a cranky or demanding child in the late afternoon or early evening. Your child pays a price for nap deprivation, and so do you.

Spending hours holding your child in your arms or in a rocking chair while he is in a light, twilight sleep also is lost sleep because you have delayed the time when he will fall into a deep slumber. It is similar to having a bedtime that is too late. It's a waste of your time as well. Brief catnaps during the day, "motion" sleep in cars or baby swings, light sleep in the stroller at the pool, and naps at the wrong time are all poor-quality sleep.

When your child does not nap well and you keep him up in the evening, he suffers.

MOTIONLESS SLEEP

How well do you nap in a car or on a plane compared to in your bed? I think babies have better-quality, more restorative sleep when they are sleeping in a stationary crib, bed, or bassinet. Vibration or motion during sleep appears to force the brain to a lighter sleep state and reduce the restorative power of the nap. I explained to the mother of one child that her baby would not sleep well while she was shopping, walking in the park, or doing something active with her friends. The mother discovered that this was true, that her baby napped best at home, but she also found it very difficult to spend more time at home during the day, as she and most of her friends were outdoorsy people. On the positive side, after starting to nap at home, her child no longer cried before going down for a nap.

You may wish to use a moving swing or a calm ride in the stroller or car for a few minutes as part of the soothing-to-sleep process, but after your baby falls asleep, drive home, turn off the swing, or stop walking with the stroller. Although your baby may appear to be in an awkward position, don't disturb him if you notice that he always wakes as you try to move him to a crib. It doesn't hurt babies to sleep in their swings or car seats. Your baby might also sleep well outdoors in a stationary stroller, especially if it's a quiet neighborhood. In general, however, as the brain matures, the child's increasing curiosity and social awareness make it more difficult to have good naps outside, so be careful.

When you maintain a healthy nap schedule and your child sleeps well during the day, well-meaning but clueless friends may accuse you of being overprotective. They'll say, "It's not real life," or "Bring her along so she'll learn to play with other children," or "You're really spoiling her." Remember: they are on the outside looking in. Only you know what works best for your baby and your family.

Sleep Consolidation and Fragmentation

Consolidated sleep means uninterrupted sleep, sleep that is continuous and not disrupted by awakenings. Slumber broken by awakenings or complete arousals is known as disrupted sleep or sleep fragmentation. Abnormal shifts of sleep rhythms toward lighter sleep, even if we do not awaken completely, may also cause sleep fragmentation. Ten hours of consolidated sleep is not the same as ten hours of fragmented sleep. Doctors, firefighters, and parents of newborns or sick children who have their sleep interrupted frequently know this very well.

The effects of sleep fragmentation are similar to the effects of reduced total sleep: daytime sleepiness increases and performance measurably decreases. Among healthy adults, even one night of sleep fragmentation will produce decreases in mental flexibility and sustained attention, as well as impairment of mood. Adults with fragmented sleep often fight the ill effects of fragmented sleep with extra caffeine.

> **Let sleeping babies lie! Never awaken a sleeping baby, except to maintain a sleep schedule. Destroying sleep continuity is unhealthy.**

However, it is important to understand that our children, like ourselves, *normally* cycle between deep sleep and light sleep throughout the night. Babies often vocalize with quiet sounds during the light sleep period and then return to a deeper sleep by themselves. If a baby is unable to return to deep sleep unassisted, the child may signal her awakening by crying or calling out. This "signaling," as it is known, may disturb the parents and be considered by them to be a night-waking problem. The real problem is not the night waking per se but how the parents respond to it, as we shall see.

MAJOR POINT
Some arousals from sleep are normal.

Protective Arousals

Sometimes our brains awaken us in order to prevent asphyxiation in our sleep. These awakenings, or protective arousals, occur when we have difficulty breathing during sleep, which can be caused by large tonsils or adenoids obstructing the air passage. (See Chapter 11.) Arousals may also prevent crib death, or sudden infant death syndrome (SIDS), which kills young infants. This tragedy might be caused by a failure to maintain breathing during sleep or a failure to awaken when breathing starts to become difficult.

Sleep Fragmentation

But after several months of age—beyond the age when crib death is most common—frequent arousals are usually harmful, because they destroy sleep continuity. Arousals are complete awakening from either a light, deep, or REM sleep.

Arousals can also be thought of as a quick shift from deep sleep to light sleep without a complete awakening.

Figure 4: Arousals During Sleep

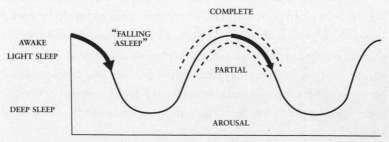

Figure 4 is a simplified illustration of the cycling from deep sleep to light sleep that normally occurs after about 4 months of age. During partial arousals, we stay in a light sleep state and do not awaken. But during complete arousals, or awakenings, we might become aware that we are looking at the clock, rolling over, changing arm positions, or scratching a leg. This awareness is dim and brief, and we return to sleep promptly. The bold arrow in the figure indicates that the process of falling asleep at bedtime and after an arousal is similar and requires self-soothing skills.

As we can see, arousals come in several forms, and depending on which types occur, how many times they happen, and how long they last, we pay a price: increased daytime sleepiness and decreased performance. For example, in a study by Dr. Anat Scher, children of 12–36 months with more fragmented sleep displayed higher cortisol levels upon awakening. The elevated cortisol levels were associated with day care teachers' reports of more negative emotionality and internalizing behaviors such as social withdrawal and appearing or feeling sad, lonely, nervous, or fearful. Some arousals, however, always occur naturally during healthy sleep. The brain, not the stomach, makes arousals. Please don't confuse arousals from sleep with hunger.

It's not just night sleep that can be fragmented. I believe naps can also be fragmented when parents rely on "motion" sleep in a baby swing or car, or when they allow catnaps in the stroller. Holding your dozing child in your arms in a rocking chair during the day also probably prevents good-quality day sleep. These naps are too brief or too light to be restorative. Motionless sleep is best. If you use a swing for soothing, turn it off once your baby falls asleep.

> **After 4 months, naps of much less than one hour cannot count as "real" naps. Sometimes a nap of forty-five minutes may be all your child needs, but naps of less than thirty minutes don't help.**

By 4 to 8 months of age, infants should have at least a midmorning nap and one at midday, and the total nap duration should be about two to four hours. If it is less and your child is well rested, do not worry.

Remember, watching the child, not the clock, is most important.

Night sleep is ten to twelve hours, with one, two, or no interruptions for bottle-feeding. If you are breast-feeding and room sharing, you might feed your baby at night many times. In this situation, both mother and baby may be more asleep than awake during the feeding, and neither suffers from sleep fragmentation. As previously mentioned, some arousals or awakenings at night are normal, and a child returns to sleep unassisted. But in cases of signaling, when the child awakens and cries until the parent arrives for soothing, the real problem is the child's inability to return to sleep unassisted. Until the child learns self-soothing skills, the result will be fragmented night sleep for parent and child.

Some arousals (or awakenings at night) from sleep are normal. Problems occur when children have difficulty returning to sleep by themselves. They "signal" because they have not learned the process of falling asleep.

Sleep Schedule, Timing of Sleep

Figures 5 and 6 show the times when most children awaken or go to sleep. These graphs are based on data from the same 2,019 children referred to in Figures 1 through 3 (see pages 10–11). Looking at the graphs, you can see, for example, that 90 percent of preschool children (those under the age of 6) fall asleep before 9:00 p.m., and 10 percent of children between the ages of 2 and 6 fall asleep before 7:00 p.m.

Figure 5

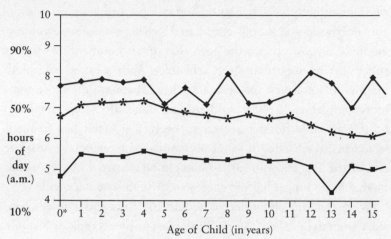

*Note: 0 represents children between 4 and 11 months of age.

Figure 6

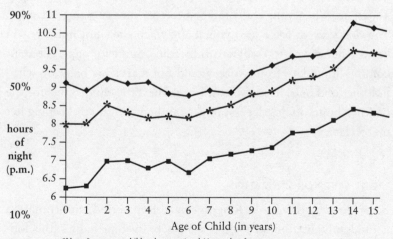

*Note: 0 represents children between 4 and 11 months of age.

MAJOR POINT

When our children are hungry, we feed them without delay. Just as you try not to let your child become overly hungry, so, too, you shouldn't let your child become overly tired.

When sleep/wake schedules are not in sync with other biological rhythms, attentiveness, vigilance, and task performance are measurably decreased and moods are altered. Jet lag syndrome is one example of this. Another is the poor sleep quality some shift workers suffer due to abnormal sleep schedules. Shift workers complain mainly of headaches and stomachaches. These are the most common complaints of older children with unhealthy sleep schedules. So if your child doesn't appear to be very sick but has frequent headaches or episodes of vague abdominal pain, especially near the end of the day, ask yourself if he might be overtired. A clue would be that he no longer has the energy or drive that he once had.

When thinking about sleep schedules in babies and toddlers, consider sleep to be "food" for the brain, just as breast milk or formula is food for the body. You don't breast-feed on the run while doing errands; instead, you find a reasonably quiet space. Same for naps. You don't withhold feeding because it is socially inconvenient; you anticipate when your child might become hungry. Same for naps. You don't try to force-feed your baby when she's not hungry; you know a hungry period will naturally come. Same for naps. A parent coming home late from work would not starve his baby by withholding food until he arrived and could feed the child. Same for the bedtime hour; don't "sleep-starve" your baby's brain by keeping her up too late.

NIGHT-SLEEP ORGANIZATION

Before 6 weeks of age, the longest single sleep period, unfortunately, is randomly distributed around the clock. In some babies, this longest sleep may actually be only two to three hours! But after 6 weeks of age (or 6 weeks after the due date, for babies born early), the longest single sleep period will predictably occur in the evening hours and last four to six hours.

During these early weeks, you may find breast-feeding too demanding or too frequent and think that you might want to quit

so that you can get some rest. On the other hand, you also may want to continue nursing because of its benefits. Hang in there until your baby is past 6 weeks of age. Then you, too, will get more night sleep.

After 6 weeks of age, the peak of wakefulness and fussiness passes, and babies sleep longer at night. So do moms! Also, babies start social smiling at their parents, and they become less fussy or irritable. Life in the family definitely changes after 6 weeks. One exception is the premature baby, whose parents might have to wait until about 6 weeks after the expected date of delivery. Another exception is the extremely fussy/colicky baby, whose parents might have to wait until their child is 3 or 4 months old.

DAY-SLEEP ORGANIZATION

At about 3 to 4 months of age, daytime sleep becomes organized into two or three long naps instead of many brief, irregular ones. Mothers, especially nursing mothers, should learn to nap when their baby naps. You never know what the night will bring; you might be up a lot holding, walking, or nursing.

Abnormal sleep schedules usually evolve in infants and young children when parents keep them up too late at night. Parents do this because they enjoy playing with their baby, they cannot put the child to sleep and instead wait for their child to crash from total exhaustion, or both. Some parents leave work late, have a long commute to the day care site to pick up their child, and then arrive home even later. This lifestyle is extremely difficult for the child if naps are not regular at the day care center and he is put down to sleep too late at night. If it is impossible to have an early bedtime under these circumstances, do the best you can. A bedtime that is only a little late is not as harmful as a bedtime that is way too late. Don't beat yourself up over this, but do your best to protect naps and early bedtimes on weekends. Unfortunately, if both parents are working outside the home, sometimes naps may suffer on weekends because the parents do too many errands with the child or attempt to spend too much time playing with their child to make up for the minimal time together during the week. Sleeping well during the day may also suffer when parents skip naps in favor of organized, scheduled preschool activities. These baby classes are usually fun for both child and parent, but if they take up too much time, the child becomes overtired.

One common mistake is keeping bedtime at *exactly* the same hour every night. Usually this hour is too late and is based more on the parents' wishes than the child's sleep needs. It is important to have a fairly regular routine of soothing events before putting your child to sleep, but it makes biological sense to vary the bedtime a little. The time when your child *needs* to go to sleep at night depends on his age, how long his previous nap lasted, and how long his wakeful period was just before the bedtime hour. The time when he *wants* to go to sleep may be altogether different! If your child is unusually active in the afternoon or if she misses a good midday nap, then she should be put to sleep earlier.

This is true even if a parent returns home late from work. A parent who arrives home late might walk into the house and immediately begin a twenty- to thirty-minute soothing-to-sleep routine without playtime. If the parent returns very late, the child should be put to bed as usual; keeping a tired child up to play with a tired parent does no one any good. At the cost to the parent of having less time with his child, the benefit is no bedtime battles, no nightwaking habits, no early morning arousals, good-quality naps, a well-rested child, a well-rested spouse, and relaxed private time for the parents in the evening. I encourage the parents to also go to bed early so that they are not rushed in the early morning with their baby. Morning time includes bathing, dressing, feeding, and playing, and may substitute for evening time. Because of the family's early bedtime, the weekends are enjoyably relaxed since everyone is well rested.

The completely opposite scenario occurs when one parent, usually the father, demands that the other parent, usually the mother, keep their child up late so that he can play with him or her. Not only does the child suffer, but it is the mother who is the unappreciated victim, because she is trying to maintain marital harmony and trying to keep her child well rested—and she can't do both. Obviously this is not simply a child's sleep problem but a family problem.

To establish healthy sleep schedules at 4 to 8 months of age, become your infant's timekeeper. Set his clock on healthy time.

Allowing brief naps in the early evening or long late afternoon naps in order to keep a child up late at night will eventually ruin healthy sleep schedules. If your child misses his midday nap, it is better—in order for him to be able to fall asleep close to his biological bedtime hour and avoid the overtired state—to have no nap and an early bedtime than a late nap and a late bedtime. Similarly, you may occasionally need to wake your baby in the morning in order to establish an age-appropriate midmorning nap that is needed to set the sleep schedule for the rest of the day.

Sleep Regularity

The best time for your child to fall asleep at night is when she is just starting to become drowsy, before she becomes overtired. For young children in day care, dual-career families with long commutes, and older children with scheduled activities, it may be impossible to catch that magical drowsy state. These children will be better off if the bedtime occurs at approximately the same time every night. In a study conducted by Dr. Yvonne Kelly, children with nonregular bedtimes examined at ages 3, 5, and 7 years had more behavioral difficulties at age 7 than children with regular bedtimes. The effect of nonregular bedtimes was cumulative (the more years of nonregular bedtimes, the worse the behavior). So the effect of nonregular bedtimes builds up throughout early childhood. The good news is that the harm is reversible. That is, when children change from nonregular to regular bedtimes, they show improvements in their behavior. Additionally, behavioral difficulties were more common when the bedtime was after 9:00 p.m.

One study, by Dr. Bates, examined the sleep of 202 children between 4 and 5 years of age. He studied the home environment, behavior at preschool, and sleeping patterns. Here, variability in bedtime was associated with daytime problems described as "less optimal" behavioral adjustments in preschool. For example, these children did not "comply with teacher's urging to join an activity" or "show enthusiasm for learning something." They argued and fought more than other children. Dr. Bates hypothesized that those children with chronically variable sleep schedules might experience states similar to jet lag syndrome, characterized as nagging fatigue and cognitive disorientation. This particular study asked whether behavior problems at school and sleep behavior problems had a common denominator—that is, family stress—and the answer was no. The child's sleep problems seemed to directly cause the school behavior problems. Perhaps in other studies associating family stress with sleep problems, the sleep problems are directly caused by nonregular or too late bedtimes.

For teenagers, this might mean consistent bedtimes throughout the week, with later times on the weekends. In one study, regularity of the bedtime schedule was assessed in 3,119 high school students. The researchers discovered that a more irregular sleep schedule was associated with more daytime sleepiness. These teenagers had lower grades, more injuries associated with alcohol or drugs, and more days missed from school. Going to bed regularly around 11:00 p.m. might produce the same amount of sleep as a schedule in which bedtime is sometimes at 10:00 p.m. and sometimes at midnight, but the more regular schedule is probably better.

Either nonregular bedtimes or bedtimes that are too late can be corrected by parents. One study clearly showed that with parent-set bedtimes, teenagers had earlier bedtimes, obtained more sleep, and experienced improved daytime wakefulness and less fatigue compared to teenagers whose parents did not set bedtimes. Two other experimental studies on college students showed that regularization of sleep/wake schedules is associated with reduced daytime sleepiness (improvements in alertness) and a reduction in negative mood (tension-anxiety, anger-hostility, and fatigue). These studies prove that irregular bedtimes are harmful and correctable.

Yet some flexibility, especially with younger children, is often called for. For example, a bedtime that always puts a preschool child to sleep at exactly 7:00 p.m. does not take into account the biologic variability, from day to day, of activity levels or lengths of naps for that child. So it makes sense to vary the bedtime by thirty to sixty minutes—but no more than that—based on how your child looks and behaves during the late afternoon. On the other hand, for older children who are not napping, having bedtimes that are hours earlier or later from day to day has been shown to be unhealthy.

A regular bedtime may vary by some minutes per night but not hours per night. Even if the bedtime is too late, a regular bedtime is better than an irregular bedtime.

BIOLOGICAL RHYTHMS

To better understand the importance of maintaining sleep schedules, let's look at how four distinctive biological rhythms develop. First, immediately after birth, babies are wakeful; they then fall asleep, awaken, and fall asleep a second time over a ten-hour period. These periods of wakefulness are predictable and not due to hunger, although what causes them is unknown. Thus a partial sleep/wake pattern or rhythm emerges immediately after birth. Second, body temperature rhythms appear and influence sleep/wake cycles. Body temperature typically rises during the day and drops to lower levels at night. At 6 weeks of age, temperature at bedtime is significantly higher than later in the night. After 6 weeks of age, as temperatures fall more with sleep, the sleep periods get longer. By 12 to 16 weeks, all babies show consistent temperature rhythms. It is exactly at 6 weeks of age that evening fussiness or crying begins to decrease from peak levels and night sleep becomes organized, and it is at 12 to 16 weeks that day-sleep patterns become established.

A third pattern is added by 3 to 6 months of age, when production of the hormone cortisol also shows a similar characteristic rhythm, with peak concentrations in the early morning and lowest levels around midnight. Interestingly, a part of the cortisol secretion rhythm is related to the sleep/wake rhythm, and another part is coupled to the body temperature rhythm. I wish Mother Nature were simpler!

Melatonin rhythmicity is a fourth pattern to consider. Initially, a newborn has high levels of circulating melatonin, which is secreted by the mother's pineal gland and crosses the placenta. Within about one week, the melatonin that came from the mother has disappeared. At about 6 weeks of age, melatonin begins to reappear as the baby's pineal gland matures. But the levels are extremely low until 12 to 16 weeks of age. Then melatonin begins to surge at night, and the hormone appears to be associated with evolving sleep/wake rhythms by about 6 months of age. (Note: melatonin supplements should not be given to healthy babies or young children to make them sleep better, as there is no evidence that this is safe.)

Even at only a few months of age, then, interrelated internal rhythms are already well developed: sleep/wake pattern, body temperature, and cortisol and melatonin levels. In adults, it appears that a long night's sleep is most dependent on going to sleep at or just after the peak of the temperature cycle. Bedtimes occurring near the lower portion of the temperature cycle result in shorter sleep durations.

Shift work or jet travel in adults, or parental mismanagement in children, might cause disorganized sleep. What is disorganized sleep? When you are awake but your body clock is in the sleep mode, or when you crash from exhaustion and your body clock is in the awake mode, then wakefulness or sleep is occurring out of phase with other biological rhythms. The result is poor-quality sleep or poor-quality wakefulness. Imagine a choir in which the individual voices, instead of blending harmoniously, blare out in strident dissonance! Many studies have been conducted with shift workers and in sleep labs on the internal desynchronization of circadian rhythms, the uncoupling of rhythms that are normally closely linked, and shifting rhythms that are out of phase with one another. The most common complaints in these adults are headaches and abdominal pain. Such people appear healthy and can function reasonably well except for the fact that they have pain in their head or stomach. Not surprisingly, headaches and stomachaches are the most common symptoms experienced by school-age children whose busy schedules cause them to lose sleep. One parent told of gradually worsening stomachaches in their teen that necessitated repeated visits to the doctor and finally a trip to the emergency room. At no time was a physical cause or illness identified. The stomachaches subsided on their own; only later, when consulting me about sleep issues in a younger sibling, did the parent realize that the stomachaches had coincided with a stretch of difficult schoolwork that had resulted in the teenager staying up later and later, accumulating a substantial sleep debt that manifested itself in these unpleasant physical symptoms.

REMINDER
Never wake a sleeping baby (except to restore a sleep schedule).

I always advise parents to become sensitive to their child's personal sleep signals. This means capturing that magic moment when the child is tired, ready to sleep, and will easily fall asleep. The magic moment is a slight quieting, a lull in being busy, a slight staring off, and a hint of calmness. If you catch this wave of tiredness and put the child to sleep then, there will be no crying. I like the analogy of surfing, because timing is so important there, too—you have to catch the wave after it rises enough to be recognized but before it crashes. But if you allow a child to crash into an overtired state, it will be harder for him to fall asleep, because he is trying to fall asleep out of phase with other biological rhythms. His ride to sleep then will not be easy or pleasant. Timing is most important! Remember, not every sleep wave is the same, and not every child learns quickly how to ride his sleep wave. But as with everything else, after practice it occurs effortlessly.

More Healthy Sleep Issues

CUMULATIVE SLEEPINESS

It's been known for many years that the effect of lost sleep accumulates over time. When you constantly have insufficient sleep, the sensation of sleepiness when you should be awake increases progressively. Let me explain what this means by giving an example. When adult volunteers have their sleep shortened by a constant amount, impairments in their mood and performance can be measured during the day. If the sleep disruption is repeated night after night, the actual measured impairments do not remain constant. Instead, there is an escalating accumulation of sleepiness that produces in adults continuing increases in headaches, gastrointestinal complaints, forgetfulness, reduced concentration, fatigue, emotional ups and downs, difficulty in staying awake during the daytime, irritability, and difficulty awakening. Not only do the adults describe themselves as more sleepy and mentally exhausted, but they also feel more stressed. The stress may be a direct consequence of partial sleep deprivation or it may result from the challenge of coping with increasing amounts of daytime sleepiness. Think how hard it would be to concentrate or be motivated if you were struggling every day to stay awake.

If children have constant sleep deficits, do they show these same escalating problems during the day? Yes! I believe the young child's brain is as sleep-sensitive as an adult's, if not more so. It is also possible that severe or chronic sleep deficits occurring early during the period of rapid brain growth might hardwire neurological circuits to produce permanent effects. This would be difficult to prove, because young children cannot report how they feel and we assume it is "natural" for them to have difficult temperaments, have tantrums, get frustrated, become easily angry, and so forth. In addition, in older children we have learned to accept as "normal" vague neurological differences such as learning difficulties or attention deficit hyperactivity disorder (which, oddly enough, we treat with stimulant medications).

The problem with concluding that constant sleep deficits are associated with these problems is that early nighttime sleep deficits may be mild and masked by long naps. If the brain has been permanently changed due to severe or chronic sleep loss, then, when the naps disappear and school requires more mental vigilance and focused attention, preexisting problems may appear. It is not simply your child's academic performance that might suffer. We do not know the contribution of healthy childhood sleep toward creativity, empathy, a sense of humor, or adult mental health. Part of the problem is, of course, that we don't have yardsticks to measure items such as creativity or empathy, so we do not yet have a way to measure the contribution that healthy sleep during childhood might make.

I do know that many parents keep their child up an extra twenty or thirty minutes at night to have fun, and notice no problems in the beginning. Later they call and ask why their "good sleeper" is now resisting bedtime or is cranky in the morning for "no obvious reason." Because the change in routine was small and in the past, they don't even think about it. But during our conversation they will recall that because of the longer spring and summer days, or because "it didn't seem to cause any problems," they pushed the child's bedtime back. The interval between allowing the too-late bedtime and the emergence of sleep-related problems was months in young children who had always in the past been well rested and were taking good naps, or weeks in children who were always on the edge of being overtired anyway. When these parents were asked if they thought their child appeared able to go to sleep twenty or thirty minutes earlier, the answer was almost always yes.

MAJOR POINT

Small but constant deficits in sleep that accumulate over time tend to have escalating and perhaps long-term effects on brain function.

In older children who have outgrown naps, the interval before the effects of cumulative sleepiness show themselves may be very long because of high motivation in the child and many exciting parent-directed events such as classes, lessons, or excursions, which help mask impaired vigilance or performance. The right bedtime is based on your child's behavior, mood, and performance, especially in the late afternoon.

When parents make the effort to help the child get needed sleep, the child becomes better rested, and it becomes easier for her to accept sleep, to expect to sleep, to take long naps, and to go to sleep by herself. Some parents always have to endure days of disruption following trips, illnesses, or immunizations because any irregularity of schedule upsets sleep rhythms.

Slightly overtired children are more easily thrown off balance and take longer to recover. Well-rested children tend to be more adaptable and take occasional changes of routine in stride.

A well-rested baby with a healthy sleep habit awakens with a cheerful, happy attitude. A tired baby awakens grumpy.

SLEEP POSITIONS AND SIDS

A common myth held by Western parents is that all children sleep better on their stomachs. Yet a Chinese mother whose baby preferred to sleep on her stomach said she knew something was very wrong with her infant, because all Chinese babies sleep on their backs! She truly worried that stomach sleeping was unhealthy.

The truth is that some babies seem to sleep better and fuss or cry less when asleep on their backs. Contrary to many parents' fears, sleeping on the back does not cause a misshapen skull. In the past, tradition and social circumstances dictated which sleeping position most parents selected. Now it appears that *sleeping on the back is healthier because it helps prevent sudden infant death syndrome.* Fortunately, most babies sleep equally well on their backs as on their stomachs.

A variant of the myth that babies sleep better on their stomachs is that when a 5-month-old child rolls over, away from the sleeping position selected by the parents, the parent has to intervene and roll the child back. Actually, leaving the child alone allows the child to learn to sleep in different positions. If you roll your child back and he instantaneously returns to sleep, obviously there is no problem. On the other hand, going to your child to roll him back can become a game for the infant by 5 months of age. Games should occur at playtime, not when it's time to sleep. Remember, not going to your baby allows him to learn to roll back alone, learn to sleep in the new position, and learn to remember the next night not to roll in the first place.

Likewise, when the older child pulls herself to a standing position in her crib, parents do not need to help her get down. A child might fall down in an awkward heap, but she will not hurt herself. Next time she will think twice about standing up and shaking the crib railings, or she'll be more careful when letting go.

Parents who rush in to roll the baby over or to help a child down run the risk of reinforcing this behavior, encouraging it to be repeated night after night. Children are very crafty and learn quickly how to get parents to give them extra attention. Don't deprive your child of the opportunity to learn how to roll over or sit down unassisted at night. These small triumphs of self-sufficiency set the stage for later behavioral accomplishments.

Prevent SIDS

The American Academy of Pediatrics recommendations for preventing sudden infant death syndrome are:

Place your baby to sleep on his back for every sleep up to 1 year of age. If he rolls onto his stomach by himself, he may be left in that position.

Place your baby to sleep on a firm sleep surface.

Keep soft objects, loose bedding, or any objects that could increase the risk of entrapment, suffocation, or strangulation out of the crib.

Place your baby to sleep in the same room where you sleep but not the same bed.

Breast-feed as much and for as long as you can.

Schedule and go to all well-child visits.

Keep your baby away from smokers and places where people smoke.

Do not let your baby get too hot.

Offer a pacifier at nap time and bedtime.

Do not use home cardiorespiratory monitors to help reduce the risk of SIDS.

Do not use products that claim to reduce the risk of SIDS.

Some parents wish to co-sleep with their child but are worried about SIDS. There are bassinet-like stands, called co-sleepers, that abut the parents' bed. They allow the nursing mother to feed her baby at night without having to leave her bed. Please discuss safety concerns with your pediatrician.

The last item on the above list is extremely important because of hazards of strangulation. For example, in 2014, there was a recall of a baby monitor because the wires could be separated from a sensor pad.

MODERN LIFE, SLEEP BLINDNESS, AND THE POWER OF SMALL CHANGES

The single most important fact to remember is that the time when sleep occurs may be more important than the duration of the sleep period. You can't fight circadian rhythms! We all have internal clocks that are genetically controlled and evolved from dark (night)/light (day) cues. These clocks create an internal timing mechanism for sleep. The power of this mechanism should never be underestimated, because it is very primitive and caused by the rotation of the earth on its axis. All living creatures are affected by it. Sleep that occurs in sync with circadian rhythms is more restorative and of better quality than sleep that occurs out of sync with circadian rhythms. Jet lag syndrome is an example of sleep not in sync with circadian rhythms. Additionally, a bout of sleep that is continuous (consolidated) is much more restorative than a bout of sleep that is interrupted (fragmented). *Quality sleep means consolidated sleep occurring in phase with circadian rhythms.*

None of this is new information. In 1927, Dr. Lewis Terman, who co-invented the IQ test that we still use today, wrote the following:

> Sleep is one of the many biological rhythms stamped into the organism by the movement of the planet on which we live. To interfere unduly with such an ancient and physiologically established rhythm would, theoretically, appear sufficient to menace the stability of the or-

ganism. Sleep is an instinct which involves the entire body, and is not simply a function of the brain. . . .

An explanation for the lack of correlation we have found between school success and hours of sleep [is] that large quantitative differences in sleep may be fully offset by qualitative differences. If this is true then sleep cannot be accurately measured in units of time alone. . . . There can be little doubt that qualitative differences do exist.

He knew that sleep duration (quantity) does not tell the whole story about sleep quality. He also wrote:

Many children secure insufficient sleep merely because they are not put to bed early enough. . . . The time lost in this way cannot be fully made up in the morning because of the disturbance caused by the early rising of parents and because of the necessity of getting to school at a given hour. In other words, the hours set apart for the sleep of children are not those best adapted to insure a sufficient amount. Even the families who set a reasonably early hour for the children to retire usually permit so many irregularities that, as one writer puts it, "the law is more observed in the breach than in the performance."

Sleep ranks with food as one of the most imperative needs of the human organism, and like the latter it has its educational and economic aspects as well as its physiological and biological. But while diet has long received a liberal share of attention from economist, hygienist, and biologist, the scientific study of the hygiene of sleep has hardly more than initiated. We seem to have rested content in the supposition that sleep of satisfactory quantity and quality can always be had when needed.

Theoretically, and under natural conditions, this may be true. *Under the conditions of modern life it is not true.* In this respect the problem is analogous to that of ventilation. The ocean of fresh air is always at hand, but the problems of the ventilating engineer are none the less real. (Emphasis added)

As early as 1927, "modern life" was being blamed for causing children's sleep problems. Consider that most of rural America did not have electricity until 1935! Even so, Dr. Terman noted that natural conditions were no longer of paramount influence in setting the sleep habits of children, and that "scientific study . . . of sleep has hardly more than initiated." Why, nearly a hundred years later, are we still struggling with sleep issues in our children? One answer is that when we are often mildly to moderately sleepy, we might not sense that we are short on sleep or appreciate the consequences of not being optimally alert. In other words, we tend to be subjectively blind to our own sleep deficits.

A review article in 2013 described a 2003 study in which adults who were experimentally sleep deprived and showed the expected decreases in performance lacked subjective feelings of sleepiness. The authors, Drs. Hans Van Dongen and David Dinges, wrote "that those who are *chronically* sleep deprived may no longer be capable of reliably appraising their own sleepiness. . . . [This] may explain why sleep restriction is widely practiced: People have the subjective impression they have adapted to it because they don't feel particularly sleepy." If parents lack self-awareness about their own sleep loss, then it should come as no surprise that they fail to appreciate subtle harmful effects of sleep loss in their children.

This is such an important point, I wish to restate it: *It is possible that some parents are so unaware of how impaired they are by their own sleep deprivation that they are unable to appreciate the extent to which sleep deprivation is harming their child.* I suspect that this explains why otherwise observant and loving parents (who are nevertheless short on sleep themselves) allow their child to become sleep deprived, with all of its attendant problems. And if the children are too often mildly short on sleep, they themselves might not develop a strong sense of how different it feels to be completely well rested versus mildly sleepy. This subjective blindness to one's own sleep deficit might continue as these chronically slightly sleepy children become adults, or it might be prevented by ensuring healthy sleep for your child. Reports by parents on their preteens and teens who successfully prevented subjective blindness to sleep deficits appear in Chapter 2.

Another answer to why sleep issues in children have been present for many generations may be that we tend to not appreciate the power of small changes. What we do day by day often has a rhythm, and there is a natural temptation to assume that small changes in our routines are probably not very important. It's human nature for adults to vary our patterns of behavior by twenty or thirty minutes and correctly think, "What's the big deal?" In our young children, however, this may be a fallacy, because biologic processes often operate as if they were a finely tuned machine with many interacting parts. Like the famous "butterfly effect" in meteorology, in which the movement of a butterfly's wings in Asia produces a hurricane in the Midwest, an extremely tiny change may produce dramatic damage.

Here is another helpful analogy. Our healthy body temperature is about 98.6 degrees Fahrenheit. When our temperature is greater than 104 degrees, it usually means that there is a serious or perhaps life-threatening illness. However, when our temperature is only slightly elevated, say 99.6 degrees—an increase of just over 1 percent—we still might have a life-threatening disease! A low fever does not necessarily mean a mild medical problem. The thermometer is a useful tool that measures body temperature, but it does not tell the whole story.

Unfortunately, we do not have a "sleepometer" to measure sleepiness. Nevertheless, consider that the work of healthy sleep is to keep the nerve cells in the brain functioning optimally. What happens if your child needs ten hours of sleep but you keep him up just an extra twenty minutes later every night? Twenty minutes seems like a small amount, but this represents a 3.3 percent loss of sleep every night. In one study, as little as nineteen minutes of lost sleep cumulatively was shown to be harmful (see page 207). You have to ask yourself whether this slight sleep deficit might produce a chronic but mild impairment or blunting of function in your young child's developing brain.

But here's the good news: we know now that the brain primarily makes up for sleep loss by increasing sleep *intensity* (slow-wave EEG activity during non-REM sleep), and not necessarily by increasing sleep *duration*. Again, this suggests sleep quality might be more important than sleep quantity. So if your child gets acutely short on sleep, sometimes a brief nap might be sufficiently restorative.

Dr. Terman blamed "modern life" as contributing to sleep problems in 1927; I just suggested that the real problem may be that we are subjectively blind to our own sleep deficits, and that it is part of human nature to simply not pay close attention to the details of our children's sleep. But there have been real changes in modern life since 1927. If we look closely at many published reports, it appears that children today are getting less sleep than in the past, even though that did not appear to be the case when I first studied this subject in 1981. More children have a television in their bedrooms and use their computers or cell phones at night, causing the bedtime to be later. More mothers with young children are in the labor force, and the use of center-based day care has increased, rendering quality naps and early bedtimes more difficult to obtain. So "modern life" today is really different from what it was in 1927, and it seems likely that many of these differences have had increasingly adverse effects on our children's sleep.

RISK FACTORS

Research on why children do not sleep well focuses on risk factors. When risk factors are present, it means that there is a higher likelihood that there will be sleep problems in some children. The mere presence of a risk factor does not automatically mean that your own child will have a sleep problem. If your child does have a sleep problem and some of these risk factors are present, please mention them when you discuss your child's sleep problem with your child's health care provider.

Family conflict and *marital strife*. Family conflict at ages 7–15 years predicts insomnia at age 18, and marital strife at age 9 months predicts a child's sleep problems at 4½ years.

Emotional unavailability of the mother at bedtime (measured by using multiple video cameras) predicts infant sleep quality for children 1–24 months of age. The emotionally unavailable mothers gave stern directives regarding sleep, while the emotionally available mothers talked directly and gently while gazing at the child's face.

Maternal depression and *maternal separation anxiety* are discussed in Chapter 3.

Feeding or attending to the child whenever the child vocalizes, even though the child has recently been fed, is discussed in Chapter 3.

Parental presence in bedroom until child falls asleep.

Maternal smoking during pregnancy.

Television in the child's bedroom.

Caffeine consumption in older children.

Eczema and *snoring* should be discussed with your child's health care provider.

Bed sharing during the first 6 months is associated with chronic awakenings. The longer the infant shares a bed with a parent, the higher the risk of nightly awakenings one year later. As discussed earlier, bed sharing has also been implicated as a risk factor for SIDS.

Sleep Recommendations

Lisa Matricciani's 2013 review of the literature concluded that published recommendations for children's sleep are not based on empirical evidence (see Chapter 9). She wrote that "sleep timing [the time when sleep occurs] may be even more important than sleep duration."

There are several reasons published recommendations for sleep are not very useful for your child. At every age, individual children vary widely regarding the duration of night and day sleep and bedtimes. Also, for young children, there is a wide range at many ages in how many naps occur per day and how many children are sleeping through the night. And for older children, there is a wide range at many ages in how many children are still napping and, for those who still nap, in how many naps occur per week. Furthermore, results from different studies vary widely depending on the social class of the families and whether they were conducted many years ago or more recently. There is even variation in results from country to country.

The take-home message is that what commonly occurs regarding sleep among your relatives, friends, and neighbors might not be what is right for your child. Ignore what they recommend and what you read about bedtimes, naps, and total sleep needs. Instead, *watch your child*. Remember, late bedtimes usually cause less night sleep. In addition, sleeping out of phase with the body's natural rhythms, as shift workers do or as travelers do when crossing time zones, is as unhealthy as jet lag syndrome.

Don't be surprised if your child needs an earlier bedtime and takes longer naps than other children. Also, don't be surprised if you are criticized by others for being too careful regarding early bedtimes and protecting naps.

Summary and Action Plan for Exhausted Parents

Think of healthy sleep as a collection of several related elements grouped together to form a package. All must be present to ensure good-quality, healthy sleep. The elements of healthy sleep are:

1. *Sleep duration: night and day.* Does your child sleep as long as she needs for night sleep and for naps? How long your child needs to sleep depends on her age and temperament. Restricted sleep impairs mood, performance, development, and cognitive ability.

2. *Naps.* Is your child taking naps, or do you sometimes or often skip naps? If a nap is missed, try to keep your child up until the next sleep period in order to maintain the timeliness of the sleep rhythm. If needed, move the next sleep period a little earlier before your child becomes extremely overtired. If the naps are too long because your child has become overtired, you might have to wake him from a nap in order to maintain the timeliness of the sleep rhythm at night. The midmorning nap develops before the midday nap and disappears before the midday nap. Not all naps are created equal. Babies are born to be short or long nappers. An earlier bedtime may be required when two naps are needed but you can get only one.

3. *Sleep consolidation.* Is the sleep interrupted (fragmented) or uninterrupted (consolidated)? Arousals from sleep are normal. Some arousals are protective. Too many arousals, for example, from unnecessary intervention by parents, fragment sleep, and this causes impairments in mood and performance.

4. *Sleep schedule, timing of sleep.* Do naps start and bedtimes begin just when your child is becoming drowsy? A bedtime

that is too late will produce an abnormal daytime sleep schedule. Variability in activity and length of naps causes some variability in the bedtime. Watch your child more than the clock.

5. *Sleep regularity.* Do naps or bedtimes occur at approximately the same times? Even if the bedtime is a little too late, regular bedtimes are better than irregular bedtimes.

These five elements are not independent of each other; each influences the others. So if sleeping is out of kilter, look at all five elements. If you focus on and correct only one element, you might not achieve permanent success, because another element that needed attention was inadvertently ignored.

6. *Prevent sudden infant death syndrome (see page 54).* Recommendations by the American Academy of Pediatrics include room sharing but not bed sharing, and having the baby sleep on its back, not its stomach or side.

Sleep is a natural process, and there will usually be few difficulties if we are patient and don't interfere. Timing is most important, but there are genetically controlled individual differences among children regarding when their sleep rhythms develop and how long they sleep, so don't compare your child with other children. Naps and night sleep are related, and both need to be in place to avoid sleep problems. Our goal is to have well-rested families. But always remember, the amount of sleep our children need is measured by mood, behavior, and performance, not by hours on a clock. The best advice I can give parents is this: let your child's natural sleep rhythms do their job without unnecessary interference!

CHAPTER 2

Why Healthy Sleep Is So Important

Infants and children who are still of tender age [may be]
attacked by . . . wakefulness at night.

—Aulus Cornelius Celsus, A.D. 130

Sleeplessness in children and worrying about sleeplessness in children have been around for a long time.

Healthy sleep appears to come easily and naturally to newborn babies. Effortlessly, they fall asleep and stay asleep. Their sleep patterns, however, shift and evolve as the brain matures during the first few weeks and months. Such changes may result in "day/night confusion"—long sleep periods during the day and long wakeful periods at night. This is bothersome, but it is only a problem of timing. The young infant still does not have any difficulty falling asleep or staying asleep. After several weeks of age, though, parents can begin to shape natural sleep rhythms and patterns into sleep habits.

It comes as a surprise to many parents that healthy sleep habits do *not* develop automatically. In fact, parents can and do help or hinder the development of healthy sleep habits. Of course, children will spontaneously fall asleep when totally exhausted—"crashing" is a biological necessity! But this is unhealthy, because extreme fatigue (often identified by "wired" behavior immediately preceding the crash) interferes with normal social interactions and even learning. You should not assume that it is "natural" for all children to get peevish, irritable, or cranky at the end of the day. Well-rested children do not behave this way.

Nature or Nurture

What do we mean when we say that a certain item is "natural"? For example, breast milk is natural and infant formula is not. So when thinking about rearing children, it might be useful to separately consider items based on biology—that is, your child's *nature*—and, in contrast, the variety of ways parents *nurture* children based on the customs of their society. Obviously, it would be false to assume that everything that is natural is healthy; think of naturally occurring poisonous plants. It would equally be false to assume that there is only one healthy way to nurture your child. Parenting customs change over time, and at any given time there are differences in parenting practices between societies and even within them.

For some parents, there is the temptation to judge some preindustrial parenting practices as more "natural" and therefore best for babies. But parenting practices performed in traditional cultures are not necessarily more biologically based or more "natural" simply because they have the weight of tradition behind them. For example, breast-feeding frequently day and night and sleeping with your baby, wearing your baby in a sling or soft carrier, always being close to your baby, and always responding to your baby may be common in some traditional societies, but there is no scientific evidence that they are superior to other, more modern parenting practices. In addition, modern science has shown that some traditions are potentially harmful: the increased risk of SIDS associated with bed sharing is a prime example. Further, traditional practices may not be practical for today's families.

Some parents may uncritically accept currently popular beliefs about child rearing. Once, mistakenly, it was widely believed that the early introduction of solid foods helped babies sleep better and, separately, that fatter babies were healthier babies. At that time, the dangers of food allergies and obesity were not recognized. Today, the harm from late bedtimes is not widely appreciated. Before the days of electricity, radio, television, computers, smartphones, or commuting long distances to work, some children went to sleep earlier than children do today. Our current popular late bedtimes are no more "natural" than the outdated and false "natural" belief that fatter babies are healthier babies.

Focusing on what is natural and on the challenges to nurture our children may clarify some of the goals and difficulties of child rearing:

Universal Natural Factors
All babies have spells of fussing and crying.
These spells distress all parents.
All parents want to soothe their baby.
The more the baby fusses or cries, the less she sleeps.
The less she sleeps, the less the parents sleep.
The less the parents sleep, the harder it is for them to soothe
    their baby.
Relatives and friends want to help soothe the baby and are
    expected to assist parents.
Breast-feeding, rocking, and holding your baby closely are
    powerful ways to soothe your baby.

Challenges to Nurture Babies
Urban stimulation (noises, voices, delivery trucks, shopping
    trips, errands) may interfere with the baby's sleeping.
Day care (not being able to put your child to sleep when she
    is just starting to become tired, or too much stimulation)
    may interfere with the baby's sleeping.

Social isolation (forcing only the mother to be wholly responsible for the baby's soothing and sleeping) may cause intense stress for the mother.

Busy modern lifestyles mean that parents have many things
to do and little time to do them; sometimes they have to
take their baby with them even at sleep times.

Fathers or mothers who have a long commute and return
home from work late want to play with their baby, and so
they keep their baby up too late at night.

Digital and social media distraction interferes with healthy
sleep routines.

Dr. Christian Guilleminault, who along with Dr. William C. Dement was the founding editor of the world's leading journal of sleep
research, taught me to consider five fundamental principles of understanding sleep:

1. The sleeping brain is not a resting brain.
2. The sleeping brain functions in a different manner than the
   waking brain.
3. The activity and work of the sleeping brain are purposeful.
4. The process of falling asleep is learned.
5. Providing the growing brain with sufficient sleep is necessary
   for developing the ability to concentrate and fostering an easier temperament.

Function of Sleep

Why do we need to sleep? The most recent research, by Dr. Giulio
Tononi, tells us that the purpose of sleep is to weaken or prune the
unimportant noise coming into our brain so that important signals
remain stronger. Here's an example. You are practicing a musical
instrument and you hit the wrong note. The wrong note does not fit

well with previous, older memories of hitting the right note, and sleep erases the memory of hitting the wrong note, leaving behind a stronger memory of hitting the right notes. During sleep the brain is refreshed by eliminating memories of insignificant events, but memories of more important or salient items will be preserved.

This theory, in Dr. Tononi's words, "predicts that sleep is especially important in childhood and adolescence, times of concentrated learning. . . . In youth, [connections between nerve cells] are formed, strengthened, and pruned at an explosive rate never approached in adulthood. . . . One can only wonder what happens when sleep is disrupted or insufficient during critical periods in development. Might the deficit corrupt the proper refinement of neural circuits? In that case, the effect of sleep loss would not merely be occasional forgetfulness or misjudgment but a *lasting* change in the way the brain is wired" (emphasis added).

LOCAL SLEEP

This targeted removal of irrelevant, redundant, or not useful memories explains a curious observation called "local sleep." The more a portion of the brain is used in a task, the more likely it is that this particular area might need to shut down to take a break and do some pruning. So local groups of nerve cells in a tiny area might go offline—that is, go to sleep for a very short nap! This occurs when you think that you are fully awake. Local sleep is a by-product of a local increase in learning. Local sleep occurs in adults and is more likely when we are short on sleep. Dr. Tononi wrote, "One wonders how many errors of judgment, silly mistakes, irritable responses, and foul moods result from local sleep in the brains of exhausted people who believe they are fully awake and in complete control."

Perhaps local sleep occurs more commonly during childhood and adolescence, when learning is especially intense. Also, as mentioned in Chapter 1, it is common for adults to be subjectively blind to their sleep deficits, so the attribution of errors of judgment, mistakes, irritability, or foul mood due to lack of sleep is unlikely. Finally, the idea of optimal wakefulness might be thought of as a midpoint where you are not drowsy from insufficient sleep and you are not up so long that local sleep takes place.

OPTIMAL WAKEFULNESS

As you will discover in reading this book, when children learn to sleep well, they also learn to maintain *optimal wakefulness*. The notion of optimal wakefulness, also called optimal alertness, is important, because we tend to think about the states of sleep and waking in polarized terms, as if people are either one or the other. But just as our twenty-four-hour cycle consists of more than the two states called day and night—dawn and dusk, for instance—so, too, are there gradations in sleep and wakefulness.

In sleep, the levels vary from deep sleep to partial arousals; in wakefulness, the levels vary from being wide awake to being groggy.

The importance of optimal wakefulness cannot be overemphasized. If your child does not get all the sleep he needs, he may seem either drowsy or hyperalert. If either state lasts for a long time, the results will be the same: a child with a difficult mood and hard-to-control behavior, unable to enjoy himself or get the most out of the myriad of learning experiences placed before him.

Sleep is the power source that keeps your mind alert and calm. Every night and at every nap, sleep recharges the brain's battery. Sleeping well increases brainpower just as lifting weights builds stronger muscles, because sleeping well increases your attention span and allows you to be physically relaxed and mentally alert at the same time. Then you are at your personal best.

Personal Best

An athlete's best time in a particular event is called her "personal best." Child development is not an athletic contest, and parenting is not a competitive sport, but all parents want to raise their children to achieve their own unique "personal best."

At any age, different children will need different amounts of sleep to achieve their personal best. All children are born with different temperaments, skills, and endowments; ask any mother of fraternal twins! These individual differences are part of the joys and challenges of parenting. As previously discussed, there are also individual differences in nap duration, so that at 6 months of age some children take long naps and others take short naps, and these patterns are stable over time until about 2 years of age.

At any age, the effects of being a little short on sleep will affect different children differently. Adult research has shown there are individual differences in how resilient we are to performing on not enough sleep. A study by Dr. John Groeger found that "sleep deprivation–induced performance deterioration is more marked in some individuals than in others. These inter-individual differences in response to sleep deprivation have trait-like characteristics consistent with a genetic basis." We should assume that some children pay a higher price than others when they are short on sleep.

So in families or cultures where babies and children are allowed to sleep out of sync with biologic circadian sleep rhythms (unhealthy sleep), I'm sure that this harms some children more than others. But I cannot imagine that unhealthy sleep, if chronic and severe, is good for *any* child. Sleep deprivation is never good for children. You can't fight circadian rhythms!

Without healthy sleep, all the resources of parents, family, and culture will not be sufficient to allow every baby and every child to be at her own "personal best." Sweet, bright, and caring children who are receiving unhealthy sleep will become even sweeter, brighter, and more caring when they get healthier sleep. My research shows that sleep modulates temperament, so sleeping better makes children more adaptable, cooperative, and calmer.

With our busy lifestyles, how can we keep track of nap schedules and regular bedtime hours? Is it really true that I can harm my baby by giving him love at night when he cries out for me? How can I be sure that sleep is really that important? Am I a bad parent if my child cries? If he cries at night, isn't he feeling insecure? Many frustrated parents ask me these questions. They often mention that articles, books, or Internet posts they have read advocate conflicting ideas, and so they conclude by throwing up their hands and saying that since the whole issue is "controversial," they might as well let matters stay as they are. But if your child is not sleeping well, how long would you be willing to wait for improvement to occur? Three months? Three years? If you are following the opinion of a professional who says you must spend more time with your child at night to make him feel more "secure," and yet the results seem to be rather the opposite, ask that professional, "When will I know we are on the right track?" Don't wait forever! Consider what Dr. Charles E. Sundell, the physician in charge of the Children's Department in the Prince of Wales General Hospital in England, wrote in 1922: "Success in the treatment of sleeplessness in infants is a good standard by which to estimate the patience and skill of the practitioner." He also wrote: "A sleepless baby is a reproach to his guardians, and convicts them of some failure in their guardianship." But isn't this outmoded advice? Absolutely not. Sometimes scientific progress forces us to reevaluate the wisdom of the past. Other times, it reinforces it.

The truth is, modern research regarding sleep/wake states only confirms what careful practitioners such as Dr. Sundell observed more than ninety years ago. He wrote:

> The temptation to postpone the time for a baby's sleep, so that he may be admired by some relative or friend who is late in arriving, or so that his nurse may finish some work on which she may be engaged, must be strongly resisted. A sleepy child who is kept awake exhausts his nervous energy very quickly in *peevish restlessness,* and when preparations are at last made for his sleep *he may be too weary to settle down. . . .*
>
> *Regularity of habits* is one of the sheet-anchors by which the barque of an infant's health is secured. The

reestablishment of a regular routine, after even a short break, frequently calls for *patient perseverance* on the part of the nurse, but though the child may protest vigorously for several nights, *absolute firmness seldom fails to procure the desired result.* . . . Our aim should be merely to re-establish the normal *habit* of sleep in the child. (Emphasis added.)

So we see that healthy sleep habits were recognized all the way back in 1922!

Each baby is unique. They're like little snowflakes. Babies are born with individual traits that affect the amount of physical activity, the duration of sleep, and the length of periods of crying they will sustain. But babies also differ in more subtle ways. Some are easier to "read"; they seem to have predictable schedules for feeding and sleeping. These more "regular" babies also tend to cry less and sleep more. They are more self-soothing; they fall asleep easier, and when they awaken at night they are more able to return to sleep unassisted. But don't blame yourself if you have an "irregular" baby who cries a lot and is less self-soothing. It's only luck, although social customs may affect how you feel about it.

In those societies where the mother holds the baby close all the time and her breasts are always available for nursing and soothing, there are still great differences among babies in terms of fussiness and crying. The mother compensates by increasing the amount of rhythmic, rocking motions or nursing. She may not even expect the baby to sleep alone, away from her body. As she grows up, a child might share the bed with her parents for a long time. So not only do babies sleep differently, but every society's expectations condition parents' feelings in different ways. Remember, there are no universally "right" or "wrong" ways, or "natural" versus "unnatural" styles, of raising children. Less-developed societies are not necessarily more "natural" and thus "healthier" in their child-rearing practices. After all, strychnine and cow's milk are equally "natural," but they have altogether different effects when ingested.

How much we are bothered by infant crying or poor sleep habits might partially reflect our own expectations about how to be "good" parents. Do we want to carry the baby all the time, twenty-four hours a day, or do we want to put the baby down sometimes to sleep while we carry on with our own responsibilities?

Here's a true story. A Saudi Arabian princess came to my office for a consultation, accompanied by her English-trained Saudi pediatrician, her English-trained Saudi nanny, and two other women, to discuss sleeping habits for the royal family's children. I listened in amazement as the pediatrician described the family's child care arrangements: they were identical to those popular among British aristocrats of the nineteenth century! Like trained baby nurses serving aristocratic families in Victorian England, the Saudi Arabian nanny was expected to hold the princess's baby while the child was asleep, in effect becoming a kind of living cradle. The reason the nanny could do it was that she had servants of her own! These subordinate nannies, not as well trained, were assigned the menial domestic chores associated with child rearing.

But the majority of parents do not have child care staffs. They have to rely on their own skills. So if we are greatly bothered by our baby's crying or our guilt about not being "good" parents, this may interfere with our developing a sense of competence. We may feel that we cannot influence sleep patterns in our child. Unfortunately, this way of thinking can set the stage for future sleep disorders.

Sleep problems not only disrupt a child's nights, they disrupt his *days*, too, by making him less mentally alert, more inattentive, unable to concentrate, and easily distracted. They also make him more physically impulsive, hyperactive, or logy. But when children sleep well, they are optimally awake and alert, able to learn and grow up with charm and humor. When parents are too irregular, inconsistent, or oversolicitous, or when there are unresolved problems between the parents, the resulting sleep problems converge, producing excessive nighttime wakefulness and crying.

A common misconception among parents is that since children pass through different "stages" at different ages, each of these stages must inevitably create its own sleep problems. In fact, after 3 or 4 months of age, all children can begin to learn to sleep well. The learning process will occur as naturally as learning how to walk.

The bad news is that some *parents* create sleep problems. The good news is that parents can prevent sleep problems as well as correct any that develop.

Sleep Is Brain Food: Healthy Sleep Is Like Healthy Food

Food and sleep are similar. You would not starve your child by withholding food; try to not let your child get short on sleep.

Think about food and food quality. Food is a biological need. Food is energy for the body. Poor-quality food or junk food damages the body by causing medical issues such as malnutrition, anemia, diabetes, heart disease, and obesity. A little junk food is okay. A lot is not. Fortunately, we can read the labels on our food in order to satisfy ourselves that we are eating healthily.

Now think about sleep and sleep quality. Sleep is also a biological need. Sleep is energy for the brain; poor-quality sleep harms the brain. Poor-quality sleep is junk sleep. Junk sleep is just as bad for our children as junk food. A little junk sleep is okay. A lot is not. However, unlike food, there are no labels to read with sleep. You have to watch your child, especially at the end of the day or in the early evening, for telltale signs of junk sleep. Junk sleep causes many problems.

Sleep deficiency is a serious medical problem. We should not be surprised that sleep deficiency is dangerous, because we know that iron deficiency in babies can cause permanent harm. Specifically, iron-deficient babies become adolescents with poorer cognitive functioning and then become adults with poorer emotional health, more negative emotions, and feelings of isolation. Sleep, like iron, is a biological necessity. Both are important for brain development.

Please do not worry if now and then your child gets a little short on sleep but is well-rested most of the time. But I would worry if sleep problems are persistent and severe. In the extreme, long-term sleep deprivation in laboratory animals has been shown to permanently damage the brain and even cause death. Short-term sleep deprivation for airplane pilots, doctors in training, and truck drivers is so dangerous that sleep requirements for these occupations are highly regulated. It's not just how much they sleep: it's also *when* they must sleep. For example, truck drivers opposed new sleep restrictions that were based on the body's natural tendency to sleep at night. In 2013, they sued the government. But the United States Court of Appeals upheld the federal sleep requirements that were based on solid scientific research. However, in 2014, for *commercial* reasons, the trucking industry successfully blocked some of the key regulations. This illustrates the practical difficulties that often accompany attempts to modify cultural or commercial behaviors based on scientific data. But that does not invalidate the data. And the data are clear that long-term and short-term sleep deprivation is at least as harmful to children as it is to truck drivers!

Here is a summary of some benefits of healthy sleep and problems associated with unhealthy sleep that cross over all ages. Please note that all of these items are based on peer-reviewed published research and are not merely my opinion.

SOCIAL AND EMOTIONAL DEVELOPMENT

From 12 to 36 months, children with more fragmented sleep displayed higher levels of cortisol (indicating more stress), and this was associated with teachers' ratings of more negative emotionality and internalizing behaviors such as social withdrawal and appearing or feeling sad, lonely, nervous, or fearful. At 18 months, total sleep duration of ten or fewer hours or awakening three or more times a night predicts emotional and behavioral problems at age 5 years. Children age 2 to 3 years who had problems getting to sleep and staying asleep had higher levels of both internalizing and externalizing behaviors (externalizing behaviors are directed against others or things and might manifest in such ways as overactivity, anger, aggression, impulsivity, tantrums, and annoying behavior). And the day after a single laboratory sleepover, 14-month-olds demonstrated poorer emotional regulation and showed special difficulty in recovering from negative emotions.

In a study by Dr. Salome Kurth, connections between the right and left sides of the brain increased as much as 20 percent over a single night's sleep in a group of children 2 to 5 years old. Connections strengthened as the children aged. "Sleep is a key environmental contributor to brain optimization processes . . . [and] plays a crucial role in brain maturation," Dr. Kurth concluded. "In critical phases of development [walking, talking, problem solving], the maturation of skills not only require cortical activity during waking but also a subsequent period of sleep. . . . There are strong indications that sleep and brain maturation are closely related. . . . I believe inadequate sleep in childhood may affect the maturation of the brain related to the emergence of development or mood disorders."

A study of almost nine thousand 4-year-olds showed that about 16 percent were short on sleep. These children were more likely to show externalizing behaviors. Another study showed that children exhibited externalizing behaviors when night sleep was short even though these children had longer naps, so their total sleep over a period of twenty-four hours was the same as for children without these problems. In other words, total sleep duration does not tell the whole story. Night sleep is especially important, and napping more is not a substitute for short night sleep!

Disrupted sleep in 4- and 5-year-old children directly causes difficulties in adjusting to preschool. Less sleep is associated with aggression, defiance, noncompliance, oppositional behavior, acting out, and hyperactivity. Dr. John E. Bates wrote, "In clinical treatment of young, oppositional children, we have seen some spectacular improvements in manageability associated with the parents instituting a more adequate schedule of sleep with their children.

Our clinical impression in these cases was that the changes were too rapid to be accounted for by other changes, such as parental discipline tactics." Sleeping better directly causes better behavior in preschool.

Short sleep duration in 7- and 8-year-olds predicts *hyperactivity/ impulsivity* in adolescence. And in children 7–11 years, a study by Dr. Reut Gruber experimentally adding or eliminating one hour of sleep over five nights showed that fifty-four minutes of sleep restriction resulted in "a low threshold for expression of negative affect (irritability and frustration) and is associated with difficulty in the modulation of impulse and emotion . . . [and] a cumulative extension of sleep duration of **27 minutes** was associated with a detectable improvement of emotional lability and restless-impulsive behavior . . . and a significant reduction of reported daytime sleepiness . . . [C]umulative *small* additions to sleep duration potentially improve functioning in school" (emphasis added). I know it goes against the grain of human nature to believe that such small changes could have such a profound impact, but the data bear it out (see Chapter 1).

Sleep problems at age 8 years predict depressive symptoms at age 10 years. Among teenagers with nightly sleep problems, females were two to six times more likely to develop depression or attempt suicide, and males were more likely to use alcohol, cannabis, or other drugs at follow-up at age 21 years.

Experimentally changing the bedtime over four nights to be only *one* hour earlier or *one* hour later for children 8–12 years showed that the later bedtime caused impaired functioning on measures of positive affective response, emotion regulation, memory, and attention. Also, adolescents age 14–17 experimentally slept six and a half hours a night for three nights and demonstrated worsening of mood and decreased ability to regulate negative emotions. In young adults 18–25 years, experimental sleep deprivation in an affective face-recognition task clearly showed that sleep deprivation impairs the accurate judgment of human facial emotions.

Late bedtimes in seventh grade predict emotional distress (feeling sad, depressed, cried more than once a week) six to eight years later. Although late bedtimes (at or after 11:45 p.m.) were linked to shorter amount of total sleep time, total sleep time was not linked to emotional distress. So sleep before midnight is associated with better emotional health independent of total sleep time!

In adults, one night of sleep loss results in increased impulsivity to negative stimuli, increased failure to inhibit a response, and faster incorrect responses. Experimental sleep deprivation studies in adults show that sleep deprivation temporarily changes brain function. These changes can manifest as impairments in interpersonal functioning, such as reduced empathy toward others.

MEDICAL HEALTH

Short sleep duration in adolescents is associated with higher blood pressure, higher cholesterol, and higher insulin resistance (a risk factor for developing diabetes). Increased susceptibility to infection, increased stress hormone, and systemic inflammation also result from not sleeping well. Separately from short sleep duration, habitual loud snoring is associated with hyperactivity, depression, and inattention. Additionally, habitual snoring has been shown to be a factor in fragmented sleep.

OBESITY/OVERWEIGHT

Most, but not all, research papers describe short sleep duration as a risk factor for obesity/overweight (see Chapter 10). If true, this is a major public health problem, because the percentage of children between 12 and 19 years old who were obese increased from 5 percent in 1980 to almost 21 percent in 2012. There is an epidemic of obesity and a famine for sleep, and it would appear that the two are not entirely unrelated! Obesity may increase the risk for developing diabetes, heart disease, and stroke. Short nighttime sleep under age

5 years predicts obesity by ages 5–9 years. Naps have no effect on the development of obesity and are not a substitute for insufficient nighttime sleep. Naps reduce cortisol levels in infants. Naps in preschool children boost memory. In adults, naps enhance creative problem solving.

TEMPERAMENT

Temperament means behavioral style and is discussed in detail in Chapter 7. Your child's temperament may be modulated by sleep in the same manner that adjusting the volume, bass, or treble controls makes a piece of music sound different—the basic musical composition has not changed, but the listening experience has. One study of infants at 3, 6, and 11 months of age showed that increased night sleep is associated with increased likelihood of approaching new and strange people and things. But fragmented sleep between 6 and 36 months of age is associated with a more difficult temperament.

Another study of infants at 4 to 10 weeks old observed that longer naps, but not night-sleep duration, is associated with a more positive temperament (less active, more approaching, milder, and less distractible). You can ask yourself, what is the magical power of a nap that turns a raving, manic, out-of-control 2½-year-old into a sweet Prince Charming?

ATHLETIC PERFORMANCE

College basketball players showed enhanced performance with a faster-timed sprint, free throw percentage, and three-point field goal percentage with experimental sleep extension. The opposite, experimental sleep restriction, impairs serving accuracy in tennis players.

COGNITIVE PERFORMANCE

Do sleep patterns really affect learning in children? Yes! Different studies of children at different ages all agree on this central point. As one study put it, "Sleep is universal, strictly regulated, and necessary for cognition. . . . Sleep consolidates memories, whereas sleep deprivation interferes with memory acquisition." Or, as another study put it, more succinctly, "Sleep is important for memory consolidation." Focusing on perfectly normal, healthy children, let's consider the data by age groups: infants, preschoolers, and school-age children.

Infants

A study at the University of Connecticut showed that there was a strong association between the amount of time infants were in REM sleep and the amount of time they spent when awake in the behavioral state called "quiet alertness." In the quiet alert state, babies have open, bright eyes, they appear alert, their eyes are scanning, their faces are relaxed, and they do not smile or frown. Their bodies are relatively quiet and inactive. One mother described her 4-month-old, who was frequently in this quiet alert state, as "a looker and a thinker." She's right! These infants don't miss a thing. Another study showed that naps with REM sleep enhance "the integration of unassociated information for creative problem solving." A separate study of sleep development at Stanford University showed that environmental factors, not simply brain maturation, are responsible for the proportion of time infants spend in REM sleep. Unfortunately, the exact environmental factors were not identified, but presumably parental handling could influence all of these items: sleep patterns, the proportion of REM sleep, and the amount of time the child is in the quiet alert state. Also, as mentioned in Chapter 1, naps longer than thirty minutes enhance the consolidation of memory among infants at 6 and 12 months.

Infants who are notoriously *not* quiet alert are those with colic or a difficult temperament. Their fussy behavior may be due to imbalances of internal chemicals such as progesterone or even cortisol. High cortisol concentrations in infants have been shown to be associated with decreased duration of non-REM sleep. So, even in infants, as in adults, there seem to be connections between internal chemicals, sleep patterns, and behavior when awake. Also, these fussy children tend to have irregular schedules and short attention spans. Among 2- to 3-month-old infants, one study showed that the more irregular and less persistent the child was, the slower the rates of learning and the more difficulty in learning to fall asleep unassisted. Thus they easily could become sleep deprived, fatigued, and hyperactive older children.

I think naps are especially important for infants. In my own studies, I've found that how long the infant sleeps during the day is strongly associated with persistence or attention span. Infants who take long naps have longer attention spans. They spend more time in the quiet alert state and seem to learn faster. Infants who do not nap well are either drowsy or fitfully fussy, and in either case they do not learn well.

Naps promote optimal alertness for children. Children who nap well spend relatively more time in the quiet alert state when awake.

It is a myth that long naps interfere with acquiring socialization skills or infant stimulation. While it's true that "rack monsters" are less available for all the classes or activities that abound today— swim gym, mom-and-tot and pop-and-tot groups, or infant-stimulation groups—is that so bad? Do infants suffer because they don't participate in so many activities? Are they less likely to get into the right preschool, which feeds to the right nursery school, which feeds to the right private school? No.

Please do not confuse the quantity of time spent in these organized activities with the high-quality social awareness that well-rested children exhibit. The truth is that these infant-stimulation groups are often not important for infants but instead serve legitimate parental needs by allowing mothers and fathers to meet other parents and escape from their isolation at home.

Preschool Children

Three-year-old children who nap well are more adaptable. (Adaptability means the ease with which children adjust to new circumstances.) *Adaptability is the single most important temperament trait for school success.* The briefer the naps, the less adaptable the child. In fact, the major temperament feature of 3-year-olds who do not nap at all is nonadaptability. It is exactly these non-napping, nonadaptable children who also have more night wakings!

My research has shown that when infants who are easy at 5 months of age develop into crabbier, more difficult 3-year-olds, it is because they have developed a pattern of brief sleep. In contrast, difficult infants who mellow into easier 3-year-olds have developed a pattern of long sleep. I think that parents' helping or hindering regular sleep patterns caused these shifts to occur.

Children 1–3 years of age with more fragmented sleep had higher cortisol level upon awakening when compared to children with fewer awakenings during sleep.

Four-year-olds who, for at least a month, took more than thirty minutes to fall asleep or had five or more night awakenings (of a duration of at least ten minutes) a week or had difficulty waking up at least three times a week were found to be at an increased risk for psychiatric symptoms at age 6.

Short nighttime sleep under age 5 years predicts obesity by ages 5–9. "Napping had no effects on the development of obesity and is not a substitute for sufficient nighttime sleep," noted the authors of one study.

School-Age Children

One study found that "sleep problems in childhood predict neuro-psychological functioning in adolescents." This was supported by another study that showed "short sleep duration in 7- to 8-year-old children predicts hyperactivity/impulsivity."

A third study indicated that children "with more fragmented sleep displayed higher awakening cortisol levels [which] were correlated with [more] internalizing behavior and negative emotionality." And a single night of restricted sleep in 10- to 14-year-olds impairs verbal creativity and abstract thinking even when routine performance is maintained.

In 1925, the father of the Stanford-Binet Intelligence Test, Dr. Lewis M. Terman, published his landmark book, *Genetic Studies of Genius*. He compared approximately 600 children with IQ scores over 140 to a group of almost 2,700 children with IQ scores below 140. For every age examined, the gifted children slept longer.

Two years later, about 5,500 Japanese schoolchildren were studied, and those with better grades slept longer.

Even ninety years later, Dr. Terman's study stands apart in design, execution, and thoroughness. A 1983 scientific sleep laboratory study from Canada has provided objective evidence confirming Terman's result, that children of superior IQ had greater total sleep time. Both studies agreed that brighter children slept about thirty to forty minutes longer each night than average children of similar ages.

Another study from the University of Louisville School of Medicine examined a group of identical twins that were selected because one twin slept less than the other. At about 10 years of age, the twin with the longer sleep pattern had higher total reading, vocabulary, and comprehension scores than the twin with the shorter sleep pattern.

More recent research supports these studies. One paper showed that 7- to 11-year-olds with short sleep had poor performance on IQ measures, and another paper showed that 7-year-olds with irregular and later bedtimes had impaired cognitive performance. The research papers agree that healthy sleep enhances cognitive development because sleep incorporates learning into permanent memory or causes memory consolidation, and that sleep enhances organizational skills, planning, multitasking, and executive functioning.

> **Please don't think there is no lasting effect when you routinely keep your child up too late—for your own pleasure after work or because you want to avoid bedtime confrontations—or when you cut corners on naps in order to run errands or visit friends. Once in a while, for a special occasion or reason, it's okay. But day-in, day-out sleep deprivation at night or for naps, as a matter of habit, could be very damaging to your child. *Cumulative, chronic sleep losses, even of brief duration, may be harmful for learning.***

Children diagnosed with attention deficit hyperactivity disorder or learning disabilities have been shown to have sleep-related difficulties, though we don't know which came first. Nevertheless, one careful intervention study showed that improvements in sleep dramatically improved peer relations and classroom performance for these children.

Research on creative adults supports the concept that originality of ideas and the quality of experiences suffer when you cut back on sleep. What you lose in waking time is made up in terms of a richer life. Have you ever nodded off at an evening event that you really wanted to attend but were too tired to fully enjoy?

There are many other studies that show an association between sleeping and school performance, but these involve children with allergies or large adenoids. (These problems are discussed in Chapter 11.)

SLEEP PROBLEMS AND BENEFITS PERSIST

Sleep problems such as difficulty falling asleep at 6 months of age may persist to age 3 years and beyond. One study showed that among children 3–6 years of age, sleep problems persist for at least four years, and those children with persisting problems were more likely to have aggressive symptoms, attention and social problems, and anxious or depressed mood.

Healthy Sleep in Young Children Has Carryover Benefits in Adolescence

Benefits from early healthy sleep habits persist in preteens and teenagers who continue, pretty much on their own, to get healthy sleep.

Previously, I have presented many facts and figures from published reports describing how healthy sleep benefits your child. In this section, I will shift gears and give you a look into the future as described by parents of older children. In many ways, the experiences of preteens and teenagers are universal and highly predictable, so it is fair to say that it is inevitable that your family will be similar to the families that have shared their stories with us. So sit back, relax, soften your focus, and soak up what veteran parents have learned about the benefits of early sleep training. But first, let me give you some background on how I collected these stories.

I often tell parents of young children that it is worthwhile to put a lot of effort into healthy sleep training because it will help to steer their child away from the icebergs that lie ahead on the voyage toward adolescence and adulthood. Teenagers who do not get enough sleep are at risk for a whole host of problems (see Chapter 10), and if early healthy sleep helps prevent a *Titanic* scenario for your child, then the inconvenience is worth it! But although I practiced pediatrics for forty years and published my first paper on sleep in 1981, I did not actually study the long-term effects of early sleep training. Nobody else did, either. My belief was based on caring for many children from birth to college age. For the revised edition of this book, I decided to find out whether my impression was true.

I sent a survey to parents of preteens and teenagers whom I had cared for since birth and whom I knew had worked hard to help their young children sleep well. All the parents had two or more children, and the median age of the oldest child in each family was 17 years, while the youngest was 13 years.

I asked them whether or not there had been any carryover effect to the preteen and teenage years from the efforts they had put forth in the early years to ensure healthy sleep in their children.

The parents' responses overwhelmingly supported the following simple conclusions:

1. Because your older child appreciates how she feels better with healthy sleep, she strives for sleep.

> *They feel the benefits and know the difference between being rested and being tired on their own because of the healthy sleep habits when they were young and strive for it even today.*

> *I also believe that the children can sense my conviction, and they know that their healthy sleep is important. Perhaps because they grew up and experienced the feeling of being drained by sleep deficit versus the feeling of being well rested, this was internalized by them over time. Maybe this experience is the underpinning for the young adult to regulate independently his/her sleep habits going forward.*

> *We see a definite carryover from their early years' sleep habits, as they view going to bed early as a reward and not a punishment. On school nights, they both look forward to finishing their work so they don't have to stay up late. They also both recognize that they reach a point where they*

know they are tired and going to sleep is the best option. They associate negative behavior and irritability with being tired; our boys realize without a good night's sleep, it is much harder for them to make it through their busy days.

Julia (age 16) says, "I think about how I am going to feel the next day before I decide what time I am going to bed. When I don't get enough sleep, my anxiety skyrockets, and I have a hard time dealing even with simple things."

2. **Healthy sleep continues in the older child because the parents have established a foundation for it:**

Routines

Our five children now range from 27 to 20. When I first wrote a narrative for your book, they ranged in age from 15 to 8 years. I went back and reread the summary—one of the main ideas was routine. I asked each of our grown children what they remember about bedtime and sleep. I spoke to each child separately, and they all spoke of our "routine." As our children grew and schedules changed, we were cognizant to keep a routine. They learned to budget their time to include their obligations, especially their regular attendance at nightly family dinner. I believe a key to this success is the fact that we, as parents, had never given the kids a choice in regard to this routine. Times and events changed as they aged, but the main idea was still the same: consistency in our healthy choices—food, exercise, and sleep. We did not specifically have to tell our high school or college age children to go to bed; it was a routine that grew with our family.

Exceptions derail sleep, but parents get back on track with sleep routines.

When I struggle with their sleep from time to time, it is often after staying up too late, changing the routine, being on a vacation, or just doing something different. What I do see is that it gets easier and easier to get them back on track again, the older they get and the more times we have done this. It is easier for both because of their age but even more because of the early sleep training we did.

It is inevitable they will have some late practices or games and the bedtime will get pushed out. What we learned very early on was to stick to a schedule a majority of the time, and when the exceptions happen, the healthy habits are still intact.

Of course, children go through different stages—nightmares, illnesses, travel, and jet lag—and each of those situations requires special attention, but over the years, I've always tried to get back to our routine—not letting my children stay up so late to the point where they are overtired. Now they are 12 and 14. They usually go to bed around 10:00 p.m., but there are certainly times where, because they are in tune with their own bodies, they put themselves to sleep early. On the flip side, there are other nights where they are wired from too much homework, school drama, or extracurricular activities. We all try to go with the flow on those nights as well. Kids learn best from following an example, so I try to model healthy sleep routines myself. Go to bed early, read rather than watch TV before bed, and keep the bedroom for sleeping and quieter activities.

Establish Priorities

There is an absolute carryover effect from the efforts we put forth during the early years to ensure healthy sleep. As parents, we were in 100 percent agreement that our children's sleep was the priority. We adjusted our dining and socializing and never regretted these changes for one minute. We didn't lose any friends or miss any social opportunities that were important to us because of their napping or early bedtimes. In fact, we believe it helped us learn how to prioritize how, when, and where we spent our time. As a result, we see our children making similar choices on their own. They will adjust their homework rituals during the week or weekends if they know they have to be up early for a sporting or school commitment. As long as they feel we are respectful of their desire to stay up for a special event or TV, a social commitment or weekends and holidays, they never challenge us during the week. The number one reason, we believe, the bedtime process is relatively easy is 100 percent a result of the commitment and understanding from the early months and years. They love to sleep. They find their beds a safe and restful place. The children know their own sleep needs and do not like the feeling of being tired.

Having three children in three and a half years, we learned three basic principles in those earliest days of parenting that we never forget: your child needs a great deal of sleep, your child will be happy and healthy when they are rested, and your family will benefit from rested children. Through those simple directives, we established some very basic priorities for our family that continue to guide us almost thirteen years later.

Family Values

I do feel that getting the appropriate amount of sleep was instilled in them when they were young and the effects did and do carry through. It is almost as if getting appropriate amounts of sleep became a family value for us. I do not think that the importance of that can be overstated. When our daughters were able to catch up on sleep on the weekends, they always did so and were refreshed and ready to go. They both love their sleep and know how vital it is.

Alice is now a freshman at college. I attribute Alice's knowledge of her sleep need to her early training and the importance we as a family placed on getting a good night's sleep. Alice frequently brings up sleep in conversation with us. Sometimes I think she does this for the affirmation that it is okay for her to go to bed earlier than her peers. She does not need us to tell her to go to bed earlier. She knows what she needs to do.

My sense is that we had created a house so centered on balance (sleep and healthy activities) that we have had an easier time sustaining the conversation on the importance of sleep. I think that it would be very hard to employ rules and expectations around decent bedtimes for our teenagers had we not had such a strong sense of sleep when we were raising the little boys!

3. **Among older children who appreciate feeling better when well-rested and who have a family foundation for sleep, there is less resistance and more self-direction regarding sleep.**

I think that the carryover effect has helped somewhat, although I cannot imagine not getting any resistance from a preteen/teen on bedtime. Most of their peers do not sleep much. I do think that I get a lot less resistance because the healthy sleep habits were established when the children were so young and emphasized and maintained throughout their experience.

I believe that their ability to self-monitor their sleep habits as teenagers was a result of having enforced healthy sleep habits and having been taught about the benefits of proper rest over the course of their childhoods.

We worked hard with Trystan to have a regular nap and nighttime schedule when he was young. He is now 13, and even with his homework load, a five-nights/week swim schedule, and weekly youth group participation, Trystan "owns" the decision to head up to bed by 9:00 p.m. each evening. Trystan recognizes the need for sleep in order to perform at school, be in a good mood, and be as strong as he can be. Trystan said that the reason he focuses so much on sleeping is because "sleeping is awesome! It is what lets me grow and get strong while I sleep. Things that I learned during the day have time to sink in. I learn when I sleep. I am a nicer person when I get sleep, and if I miss some, I can try to make up for the sleep I miss if I have to get up early. But I have to do it the same day or I don't feel as good. I can always DVR a show that is on late. It's more important to get the sleep and watch the show the next day or look at my phone or play a game."

4. Helping older children sleep may be difficult, but it is not impossible. Early sleep training makes it easier to help older children sleep. Expect to experience resistance from friends and family when your child is young and from your child when he or she is older.

In the beginning, it may not be easy to follow guidelines for healthy sleep because family and friends will resist your emphasis on healthy sleep schedules. They do this because your child's need-to-sleep schedule may conflict with their social schedule. They will accuse you of being too rigid, for reasons I will explore in more depth below. Later, with more scheduled activities for your older child, he or she will resist more having to take a nap or going to bed early. So it is inevitable that keeping him better rested becomes more difficult, but it is not impossible. Remember, the key message is that there will be *less* resistance from your older child because he or she will have developed more self-awareness or body awareness regarding how it feels to be well rested versus short on sleep.

Also, with very young children, you have more control over naps and bedtimes. But, sad to say, some older children develop common chronic medical problems, such as severe allergies, eczema, or asthma, during early childhood that may interfere with sleep. In addition to the expected adolescent issues revolving around independence versus dependence, sometimes school/educational/learning issues and emotional health issues surface during the preteen and teenage years. However, all preteens and teenagers have to get up early to start school, end school later, and have more difficult classes with more homework, not to mention jobs, sports, and music, social, and religious activities. Sure, a teenager's life is ruled by a calendar of activities, often with irregular schedules, but this doesn't mean you lose all influence over your child's sleep schedule. Rather, parents shift from an authoritative approach with their younger child to a more nudging, reminding approach for their older child. This shift respects your child's growing independence. After all, how better for the preteen or teenager to learn the consequences of staying up too late than for him to feel the pain of being sleep deprived the next day?

It may also be more difficult helping your preteen and teenager sleep well for many other reasons, such as the need to care for other younger children or for aging parents, or a mother who begins to work full-time outside the house after all the children are in school. But again, I want to emphasize that when family routines and consistency in living according to your family values are practiced *from the beginning*, the preteen and teenage years are *more* manageable.

> *I observed and appreciated the enormous benefits of healthy sleep habits and a well-rested family from the beginning. It was not always easy to follow the guidelines I had established, because I encountered significant resistance from family and most friends. Their routines and schedules were very different from ours. Our children, when very young, went to bed so early that few could relate to our schedule. I think that our healthy sleep habits helped our children in a myriad of ways: to explore school, to foster creativity, to face frustration, and develop adaptability. I know that sounds like a lot, but I really do believe that consistent healthy sleep habits are the foundation for the full engagement of one's resources.*

> *We have five children ranging in age from 8 to 18 years old. My husband and I were the first in our respective families to have children. Our family members gave us a hard time when we insisted on starting a gathering later or ending it earlier so that our children could take naps at the right time. After our siblings became parents themselves, however, they admitted to us that up until then they thought we were going overboard about protecting our children's nap times. Now they realize how important sleep is for children and how they really can become completely different people when they are sleep deprived. They aren't "brats"; they just need to take their nap. Getting enough sleep is a constant struggle for all of our children. As parents, we can see that the importance we placed on sleep when they were younger gave them a solid base to draw from: a calm disposition that*

good sleep habits seemed to foster and a healthy attitude toward going to bed.

We have tried to encourage healthy sleep habits in both girls (ages 19 and 17) since birth. I think there is definitely a carryover effect. When they were babies, my husband and I made the mental shift from "sleep is good" to "sleep is critical and essential to our child's health." It became something we both made a priority and have worked to maintain. It helps to have a well-rested 2-year-old to avoid turmoil and tantrums, and I believe it's the same with teenagers. They need rest to be happy and to do their best. They need to be focused to navigate all the difficult challenges and pressures they face at this difficult age. We had to modify the sleep schedule as our girls got older and their schedules have been demanding, but we were constantly trying to encourage more sleep. An early bedtime has been what we have always done, so it was easier to enforce. At times, it has been a struggle because they'd compare us longingly with more permissive parents. Sometimes they would protest with things like "unfair, everybody else or nobody else does that." We had to reinforce the benefits of sleep, things like not having shadows under their eyes, keeping the diary of how much better they felt when well rested, and performing better in sports. In high school, we made exceptions for special things like dances or an occasional concert that ended at midnight. But we all noticed that the high school sleep habits continued into college.

Having four kids—8, 11, 12, and 14 (yikes!)—the sleeping habits that were started from birth have had a huge impact on them today, and all in a good way! Friends would give me a hard time that I was putting my kids to bed at like 6:30 p.m. I would kindly tell them they are not going to miss anything if we stay up later other than a good night's sleep. Bottom line: when my kids do not get the sleep they need, they are not fun to be around. They are cranky, whiny, and pouty— who wants to be around that? Not me. ☺ You tweak as you go, but it is so much easier when the foundation has been laid down. The 8- and 11-year-olds love and cherish their sleep time, and the effort put forth early is still obtainable with little or no resistance. It has been part of their world since they were born that sleep is imperative to be a happy and productive person in our home and in life. The 12- and 14-year-olds need a lot more time to shut down these days, but it has been ingrained in my children from an early age that sleep is important for the obvious reasons! They know how amazing they feel when they get the sleep they need. They have figured out rather quickly that when they are well rested, they are happy. What parent wouldn't want that?

I know that as a new parent, you are probably struggling to keep your eyes open to read. But honestly, no other parenting advice book conveys the real-life messages contained in these parents' comments! So I think it is worthwhile to take a break and then go back and reread the parents' reports supporting these four conclusions. If you find these parents' reports worthwhile, please look ahead to Chapter 10, where these same parents write about their teenagers and reflect on the experiences of the early years.

Healthy Sleep in Children Helps Prevent Maternal Depression

Three separate studies by Dr. Harriet Hiscock showed that healthy sleep in the child helps prevent depression in the mother. One study of 156 mothers of infants aged 6 to 12 months with severe sleep problems used controlled crying (graduated extinction) to help solve the problems. This intervention improved sleep problems in the children and reduced symptoms of depression in the mothers. Unfortunately, the benefits for the child and the mother lasted only about two months.

Another study looked at 738 mothers of infants age 6 to 12 months, 46 percent of whom reported their infant's sleep as a problem. The researchers described a strong association between the maternal report of infant sleep problems and depression symptoms in the mother. After looking at all the variables that might have contributed to maternal depression and the observation that the better the child slept, the less likely the mother was to be depressed, they concluded that teaching mothers how infants sleep should decrease or help prevent maternal depression.

A third study consisted of 114 mothers enrolled when their infants were 8 to 10 months old; the mothers were again studied when their children were 3 to 4 years old. The researchers concluded that infant sleep problems tend to persist or recur in the preschool years and are associated with more child behavior problems and maternal depression. Analysis of their data led to the conclusion that the maternal depressive symptoms were a result, rather than the cause, of the children's sleep problems.

It is uncommon for so many studies to be in agreement!

WARNING
Sleep problems in children may cause depression in mothers.

However, maternal depression may also cause sleep problems in children (see Chapters 1 and 5).

Healthy Sleep and Public Awareness

Now that you understand why healthy sleep is so important for your child, I want to explain why many other parents and your relatives may not appreciate these benefits and why they may make it challenging for you to obtain healthy sleep for your child.

IT TAKES A LONG TIME TO APPRECIATE HEALTHY SLEEP BENEFITS

When there is a scientific observation regarding a health benefit from sleep, it may take a long time for the public to become aware of the benefit and even longer for the information to be acted upon. Here are three examples.

In 1914, a major medical textbook warned of the dangerous symptoms associated with snoring (see Chapter 11), and in 1976, *Pediatrics,* the official journal of the American Academy of Pediatrics (AAP), published a careful clinical study documenting the seriousness of the problem (hyperactivity, depression, and inattention). But it took until 2002, twenty-six years later, for the AAP to publish clinical practice guidelines regarding screening for snoring and sleep-related breathing problems. These guidelines were revised in 2012, almost a hundred years after the 1914 report!

In 1985, it was first observed that sudden infant death syndrome was less frequent in children who slept on their backs. The AAP waited until more evidence was available and finally recommended back or side sleeping in 1992; their recommendation for back sleeping alone did not come until 1996, twenty-one years after the original report. Over a fourteen-year period, from 1992 to 2006, the percentage of children put to sleep on their backs increased from 13 percent to 76 percent. Initial opposition that may have slowed widespread acceptance to this recommendation included an unwarranted fear that the baby might vomit and aspirate the vomit, or develop a flattened skull.

In 1998, it was first observed that a later start time for school for teenagers produced benefits for the children (see Chapter 10). But it wasn't until 2014, sixteen years after the original report, that the AAP finally recommended that all schools for teenagers start later (after 8:30 a.m.). Initial opposition to this recommendation includes the unwarranted fear that teenagers will simply stay up later, that sports practices will be significantly disrupted, and that school bus schedules will be impossible to manage.

Separately, there are two well-documented sleep issues in children for which there are no AAP recommendations or acknowledgment by some other professional organization and, hence, these issues are not widely recognized or acted upon:

1. In 2003, it was first observed that among children 5 years old and younger, there was a trend toward later bedtimes and less sleep that began between 1974 and 1978. The list of problems associated with chronic sleep loss in adolescents (see Chapter 10) led the AAP to recommend a later start time for schools. But there is no AAP recommendation regarding bedtimes in preschool children. Hence, many parents do not appreciate the harm from chronic sleep loss caused by bedtimes that are too late.

   A little history might help explain why we are blind to this obvious problem. After the 1880s, when electric lights began to become commercially available, nighttime activities took off. Nighttime entertainment, sports, and socializing are so common today that we don't even think about it. But it wasn't always so. I suspect that most adults used to have an earlier bedtime, and I suspect that very young children who were too young to do chores or work by candlelight also went to bed earlier than today. Modern pressures on school-age children and adults are real, and later bedtimes may be unavoidable, but how about our preschool children?

   It took twenty-one years to get the message out that back

sleeping was good and sixteen years to recommend that school start times for teens should be later. Although eleven years have passed since the first report regarding the development of later bedtimes in preschoolers, maybe in the future there will develop a more general awareness that late bedtimes and less sleep are harmful.

2. In 1988, it was reported that 10 percent of 3- to 10-year-old children had a TV in the bedroom. In 1999, it was reported that more television viewing was correlated with less sleep and more sleep problems; also, 26 percent of 4- to 10-year-old children had a TV in the bedroom. By 2005, 40 percent of 3- to 6-year-old and 18 percent of children under 2 years of age had a TV in the bedroom. Studies published in 2013 confirmed that more television viewing was associated with less sleep and later bedtimes. This trend of more school-age and preschool children having television in the bedroom began twenty-six years ago, and the fact that this is harmful was known fifteen years ago, but this has not led to a general public awareness campaign that parents should not allow a television in their child's bedroom. Hopefully in the future it will become common knowledge that television does not belong in your child's bedroom. In fact, *all* screen-based electronic media used by children at night may cause the bedtime to become later.

CHALLENGES FROM FRIENDS AND RELATIVES

These examples show how long it can take for scientific findings to make their way into general circulation and result in widespread, commonly accepted behavioral changes. So do not be surprised if your friends or relatives do not agree with your practice of early bedtimes or limiting television and all other electronic screen-based media. Similarly, friends and relatives who are unaware of the health benefits from sleep might complain that you care too much about early bedtimes or naps.

Striving toward a balance between attending social events and keeping your child well rested may create tension between parents themselves or between both parents and their relatives and friends. Social events are important, family harmony is important, but a well-rested child is also desirable. So the goal is to include your child's sleep needs in the equation. Many parents in my practice who utilize early bedtimes feel like pioneers in their circle of friends and relatives because their desire to protect an early bedtime and naps may run counter to how other families live. Occasionally they feel a little like outcasts because they refuse to frequently socialize late at night with other parents or relatives with their child. Sometimes not attending late night events or leaving early may have social costs. Similarly, parents may choose not to participate in playdates as frequently or go to family barbeques on weekends if they interfere with naps. These comments are not intended to suggest that you never allow your child to stay up late or skip naps; rather, look at the big picture of how well rested your child is most of the time and how disruptive a particular social event might be to your child's sleep schedule.

When in doubt about whether to attend a social event with your child that will cause a late bedtime or a missed nap, I always encourage a family to attend the event. After the event, I recommend they consider a super-early bedtime for one night only, to repay a sleep debt. Then I suggest that the parent observe how well rested the child is after the event or how long it takes to recover from the sleep loss from the event. Finally, I ask the parents to decide, "Was it worth it?"

Summary and Action Plan for Exhausted Parents

1. Good sleep quality permits optimal wakefulness, which allows you to be at your personal best.
2. Healthy sleep is good for the brain; junk sleep is bad for the brain.
3. Healthy sleep in children helps prevent maternal depression.

Sleeping is not a completely automatically regulated process, like the control of body temperature. Sleeping is more like feeding. We do not expect children to grow well if all they eat is junk food. Children need a well-balanced diet.

The same is true for sleep. Healthy sleep benefits the child socially, emotionally, medically, physically, athletically, and cognitively. Moreover, the benefits of sleeping well in early childhood carry over into adolescence and even beyond.

CHAPTER 3

Preventing Sleep Problems

There never was a
Child so lovely but his
Mother was glad to see him asleep.

—Ralph Waldo Emerson

In 1957, a famous pediatrician, A. H. Parmelee Jr., wrote, "Parents are never truly prepared for the degree to which the babies' sleep/wake patterns will dominate and completely disrupt their daily activities." That was then. Today, I believe that parents *can* prepare and take charge to ensure a well-rested family. The good news is that most sleep problems in children can be prevented or treated. That does not mean that the road will be easy for all families, but be confident that we have learned a lot since 1957!

Let's start with a basic question: why do some children have difficulty falling asleep or staying asleep? Temperament is part of the answer. In 1981, I discovered that 4-month-old infants with an easy temperament had long durations of sleep. Infants with the opposite temperament had short durations of sleep, and many of these infants had colic during their first few months. About 20 percent of all infants have colic, and they appear to be at a higher risk for the later development of sleep problems that persist well beyond early childhood. So colic, in addition to temperament, is part of the answer.

The fundamental problem is that colicky infants have difficulty falling asleep easily after several minutes of parental soothing with rocking or lullabies (see Chapter 5). This lack of self-soothing ability directly causes them to have difficulty returning to sleep unassisted when nighttime arousals naturally occur and parents are not present. Heroic parental efforts are required to soothe colicky babies to sleep and keep them asleep; the lucky parents of those 80 percent of babies that do not have colic have no clue how utterly exhausting this is. Parents vary in their ability to soothe their babies and cope with the stress of their own sleep deprivation. So when colic subsides at 3 to 4 months, some post-colic babies and their parents are well rested, while others are horribly sleep deprived.

Around this time, in order to prevent subsequent sleep problems, parents need to allow their colicky babies to learn some self-soothing skills by reducing their efforts to soothe their babies to sleep and not responding to signaling behaviors. This reduction might be very gradual or abrupt and may or may not be associated with crying. Because parents are already familiar with the phrase "toilet training," I call my suggestions to help babies learn self-soothing "sleep training."

This phrase first appeared in 1987 in the first edition of *Healthy Sleep Habits, Happy Child*. Now, many years later, it has become popularly misunderstood to mean *only* a "cry it out" approach. Nothing could be further from the truth. But because controversy regarding this subject has overshadowed my original sleep training suggestions, I think it's important to reintroduce these simple steps that parents can take—steps that have proven successful in preventing sleep problems in the 80 percent of infants without colic. *Our general goal for non-colicky babies is to prevent sleep problems by teaching self-soothing early.* The adage "start as you mean to go on" applies to these non-colicky babies, who are more able to learn self-soothing early; however, for babies with colic, teaching self-soothing when your child is older may be more appropriate and is discussed in Chapters 5–7. However, because colicky behavior develops only after the first week and becomes more apparent after a few additional weeks, it makes sense to attempt to teach self-soothing early to *all* babies and, if needed, temporarily abandon these attempts if your child develops full-blown colic. Another reason it makes sense to try to teach self-soothing early in all babies is that there is no sharp distinction between babies without and with colic; rather, children lie along a spectrum of behaviors. Thus, early sleep training might prevent or ameliorate the development of colicky behavior in some babies.

Teach Self-Soothing

Self-soothing is the ability of your child to fall deeply asleep with or without a pacifier or swaddling after becoming drowsy from a parent's soothing efforts. The drowsy child is placed in a crib before she is in a deep sleep and allowed to fall asleep on her own, without parental intervention. A child who is not colicky will learn naturally how to self-soothe. All parents have to do is set up the proper conditions and get out of the way. Self-soothing is absent when your child *always* falls asleep at your breast, on your chest, in a parent's arms, or in a moving swing or car. By giving your baby the opportunity to learn self-soothing, you help prevent sleep problems. Parents who always soothe their baby into a deep sleep before putting her down to sleep deprive her of the opportunity to learn self-soothing skills. Not allowing your baby the opportunity to practice self-soothing will usually result in a baby or child who is entirely dependent on being parent-soothed. Subsequently, she may have difficulty falling asleep alone at sleep onset (bedtime battles) or during naturally occurring arousals at night (night awakenings).

It is common for most parents to spend ten to twenty minutes soothing before they put their baby down drowsy but still awake.

However, the motion of rocking or pushing your baby for hours in a stroller for "soothing" might rob your baby of more restorative deep sleep even though he is in light slumber.

My impression is that self-soothing skills are a prerequisite for long-term healthy sleep habits, and the earlier they are developed, the easier it is for the entire family. But remember: about 20 percent of babies—those who are colicky—will likely have difficulty learning self-soothing until about 3–4 months of age. That is not your fault. That is not the babies' fault. It is just nature's roll of the dice.

START EARLY

The ability to fall asleep and stay asleep unassisted is learned behavior. The earlier you start to help your baby acquire these skills, the easier it is for your baby to learn them. Yes, initiating lactation or feeding your baby or perinatal issues such as prematurity are more important than thinking about sleep, but do not ignore sleep completely. Try the suggestions below as soon as you can—even, if possible, on the first day home from the hospital.

Waiting weeks or months to begin helping your baby learn self-soothing might result in your baby becoming accustomed to falling asleep only after feeding, or in your arms, a swing, or a stroller, or on your chest. When older, he will have to unlearn these expectations or associations. I cannot emphasize enough how important it is for parents to start early to help their child learn to sleep well.

In the late 1970s and early 1980s, to help direct my research career, I read all the papers published in English about children's sleep. This review led to this recommendation in my first book on colic, *Crybabies,* published in 1984: "The *three- or four-month birthday* appears to be an important milestone for sleep development. At this point, infants' sleep patterns tend to resemble those of adults," and parents can actively help their child learn to sleep well. For premature babies, it is three to four months after the expected due date. Subsequently, in 1987, in the first edition of *Healthy Sleep Habits,*

Happy Child, the section "How to Teach Your Baby to Sleep or to Protect His Sleep Schedule" started at 4 months of age. This early approach was based on the fact that at that age the sleep machinery in the brain was developed to the point where parents needed to pay closer attention to circadian rhythms for night and day sleep or else the child would be more likely to develop a sleep deficit. When I did my research for *Healthy Sleep Habits, Happy Twins,* which was published in 2009, I used the 4-month mark to divide early and late parental efforts to help the twins sleep better. What I discovered was that parents who started helping their child sleep better at or before 4 months described better sleeping in their children than those parents who started after 4 months. This validates the notion that starting early is better than starting later.

Now we have research from 2010 by Dr. Jacqueline Henderson that more fully supports this concept. She discovered that "the longest self-regulated sleep period"—that is, the maximum length of night sleep plus quiet wakefulness plus reinitiation of sleep without parental intervention (self-soothing)—rapidly increases during the first 3 months. Dr. Henderson found that falling asleep before midnight and sleeping until 6:00 a.m. from "4 months of age also has implications for interventions intended to prevent infant sleep difficulties." She concluded: "Prevention should occur in synchrony with developmental tasks, which in this case is the task of self-regulating sleep throughout the night. . . . To achieve this, prevention interventions should target the management of infant sleep in the first 3 months of life . . . [because t]he most rapid consolidation in infants' nocturnal sleep occurs within the first 4 months of life. . . . *Prevention efforts should focus in the first 3 months, beginning as early as 1 month* for intervention to be synchronous with the onset of sleeping through the night" (emphasis added).

While it is never too late to help your child sleep well, research and experience demonstrate that it is also never too early. If your child is older and has more ingrained habits, it may take longer to unlearn the old habits and the process may be more stressful for the parents—but it can be done!

If you start early with teaching self-soothing, you will be well along the path to preventing sleep problems.

MANY HANDS

If your baby always falls asleep in his mother's arms after feeding, then he is less able to develop self-soothing skills because he learns to fall asleep only in association with his mother's body odor, skin contact, heartbeat and breathing rhythm, and rocking motions. After breast-feeding, the mother should sometimes pass her child to someone else for soothing to sleep. Or, if the child is bottle-fed, allow others to feed him before soothing to sleep. Try to get both parents as well as grandparents, aunts, uncles, friends, or nannies involved in soothing before sleep.

Father Care: Our Secret Weapon for Soothing

How important is the father? One scientific paper, by Dr. Liat Tikotzky, emphasized the role of the father and concluded, "Paternal involvement in infant care may contribute significantly to the development of infant sleep . . . because fathers in general may endorse to a higher degree of limit-setting approach that encourages the infant to self-soothe. . . . A higher involvement of fathers in infant care predicted and was associated with fewer infant night-wakings and shorter total sleep time," perhaps because the children spent more time asleep at night with better-quality consolidated night sleep. In one study, by Dr. Klaus Minde, of children 1 to 3 years of age, sleep problems were solved when fathers took over the management of the bedtime routine and night awakenings: "The reason for this suggestion [that fathers manage the bedtime routine and night wakings] came from clinical experience which indicated that fathers, partly because of their overall designated caretaking role in the family, and partly because of their more limited contact with their children during the day, were able to relate to them in a more forthright and authoritative fashion. In contrast, mothers often felt tired and spent in the evening and perceived their toddlers as particularly difficult at that time. It was of interest that most fathers were willing and even enthusiastic about this new role. Mothers were initially sometimes doubtful either of their husband's coping or of their own ability to tolerate these new arrangements." Research suggests that mothers play the role of "gatekeeping," either encouraging or inhibiting the father's involvement.

But many mothers may say, "I want to do it all by myself because I can do it better than anyone else." It is completely normal for mothers to feel uncomfortable with fathers playing a major role at bedtime. As one mother stated, "I struggled to trust other people to put my baby to sleep." But remember, falling asleep under different conditions promotes the learning of self-soothing skills. Dads might be available only on weekends and only for naps. No matter. Some attempts are better than none. So get dads, or others, on board!

Before the baby is born, fathers should make the decision to become involved in child care right from the start. Some fathers hold back initially, afraid they might "do the wrong thing" when holding, burping, bathing, changing, or feeding the baby. After mothers get their strength back, they should deliberately leave the house on a weekend, when Dad pulls nap duty, for a few hours to visit a friend, hang out with the older kids, get their hair done, go to a movie, or go shopping at a time when they expect the baby to go through a cycle of feeding, changing, bathing, and putting to sleep. Guess who has to do the work then? Often a father will feel more comfortable doing these things when the "expert" is not looking over his shoulder. Moms deserve to take breaks to get their batteries recharged. This strategy is smart, not selfish, because moms do the heavy lifting when it comes to baby care and a sleep-deprived mom is not at her personal best. Remember the safety advice on the airplane: you put on your oxygen mask first so you can take care of your child second. So the first point is for fathers to start early in practicing baby care.

Second, fathers should plan ahead for the six-week peak of fussing/crying that occurs in all babies. They should come home early or take a few days off from work if they are able. Make adjustments if your baby is born before or after the expected date of delivery, because the six-week peak is counted from the due date. At 6 weeks of age, babies fuss/cry more and sleep less. Less sleep for the baby means less sleep for the mother. All mothers need help in caring for their six-week-old and themselves. Fathers should give mothers a well-deserved break at this time by taking the baby out for long walks or car rides in the evening or night. The baby might not sleep well during these outings, but at least the mother gets a break.

The third point is that fathers can practice and learn how to help their baby fall asleep. For example, after nursing her baby, the mother could pass her son to the father, who then rocks his baby gently for a while and puts him down to sleep or lies down with him in their bed and they both snooze. (This may only occur on weekends, when the father is around at nap times and bedtime.) The participation of fathers in putting their babies to sleep will help them gain confidence in becoming a parent. If the mother is giving expressed breast milk in a bottle, fathers and babies may have an easier time accomplishing the feeding if the mother actually leaves the house. This is because the baby can smell the mother's presence and might resist taking the bottle if he knows his mother is home. So, maybe on weekends, when it's time for the baby's nap, Mom leaves the house and has fun while Dad gives the bottle and puts his baby down to sleep.

Fourth, fathers can learn how to soothe baby fussiness and crying and spend lots of time doing the soothing. For example, fathers can learn infant massage. Classes are offered everywhere; call your local maternity hospital or go online. Fathers can learn lullabies (your baby will not care how well you sing). A baby bath might be especially soothing, and fathers can spend time letting the warm water calm the baby. A father can learn to do everything a mother does to soothe the baby except breast-feed. For babies 6 months of age or older, fathers can attempt to help lengthen naps by responding immediately as a mini-nap nears its end (baby just begins to whimper or cry) by attempting to soothe the baby back to sleep for a nap extension. If mothers do this, it might be more stimulating than soothing and lead to an unnecessary feeding that is more likely to awaken the child.

Lastly, a father can request to help feed or soothe the baby in the middle of the night when the mother needs extra sleep. This is a little bit tricky because many mothers have the attitude that nobody can do the soothing as well as they can, and also that dads need their rest so they can go out to work well rested in the morning. With this attitude, the mother rejects or resists the idea that baby care in the middle of the night should be a shared experience. For some families, this might be the right course of action. But if the mother is distressed, exhausted, sleep deprived, or going through baby blues, then extra help at night from the father is absolutely needed to give the mother a little more sleep. After all, no matter how stressful his job might be, the father at work always gets some breaks. A mother with a baby might not get any breaks during the day.

Fathers need to understand that when children are overtired and not sleeping well, it is sometimes useful to go to a *temporarily* ultra-early bedtime to repay the sleep debt. The child awakens better rested, then learns to nap better, and later is able to have a later bedtime. If fathers refuse to help prevent and solve sleep problems, then they have to accept responsibility for their overtired child's behavior—and not blame the mother!

The contribution of the father is especially important if your baby develops extreme fussiness/colic (see Chapter 5). Here is one parent's explanation of why fathers are helpful:

> I think part of the reason that dads can be so good at soothing is that they, especially with newborns, often have greater internal resources for it. If a mother is nursing, she is up often, and is "on call" 100 percent of the time for months on end. Dad is not worried about being on call with baby all the

time. He's not worried that baby might cry all night and keep him up for hours and hours when he's already been up for the last month! Dad isn't worried that he's going to have to nurse, and nurse, and nurse (sometimes painfully, in the beginning!) if there is no other way to soothe the baby. Dad is often pretty logical and unemotional—babies cry, babies are soothed, babies sleep. If babies are not ever soothed, maybe they are sick. This is not true for all dads and all moms, of course! But it is my observation that the combination of male tendencies toward logic/unemotionalness + not being awake since the birth + not nursing + not being on call for baby 100 percent of the time = greater ability to calmly, successfully soothe a baby.

DROWSY BUT AWAKE

As your baby begins to show signs of becoming drowsy, you should begin a soothing-to-sleep routine in any way that calms him. These signs usually appear after one or two hours of wakefulness. The 20 percent of babies that have colic may not show these drowsy signs, so you have to watch the clock more carefully with them. If your child often shows signs of fatigue, note how long he has been awake and the next time begin the soothing-to-sleep routine about twenty minutes earlier. It is not necessary for your child to always be drowsy and awake when you put him down. Sometimes your baby goes from drowsy to asleep very quickly, and there is no reason why some books suggest that you should then wake up your baby and put him down in a more wakeful state. Your baby may become drowsy after being awake only forty-five minutes; if so, begin your soothing-to-sleep routine then.

If he makes quiet sounds such as whimpering or low-level fussing, wait and watch as long as you feel comfortable. He might fall deep asleep. Or, instead of just waiting, send in Dad for brief and minimal soothing such as gently patting or rubbing the baby, jiggling the crib, or shushing, but not picking up. There is nothing wrong if your newborn sometimes or usually falls asleep at your breast, in your arms, on Dad's chest, or in the swing, car, or stroller. If he falls asleep during feeding, do not awaken him.

But here is the problem: if he is *always* in a deep sleep state when you put him down, then he has no opportunity to learn self-soothing skills. So I suggest that you sometimes put him down after soothing, drowsy but awake. You might be comfortable just trying it maybe only once a day. That's okay. Maybe you will have to shorten the duration of soothing to accomplish this. There is no rule regarding the time of day when you should attempt this or how many attempts you should make in a day.

However, you might be more successful if you try this *within one hour of the baby waking in the morning,* because your baby will be best rested from night sleep. That is, do the changing, feeding, a little playing, and soothing *all within one hour.* Look at the clock when you think your baby awakens to start the day; this time may vary from day to day. On a weekend, have Dad, if available, put him down in a dark and quiet room, drowsy but awake. For these attempts, maybe Mom should leave the house. This often produces more sleep and less crying.

Think of "drowsy but awake" as somewhere between the extremes of fully awake and completely asleep. Please don't overthink or obsess about the exactitude of what "drowsy but awake" means. Just watch your baby for drowsy cues.

Here is a report by a parent who usually had good timing, so most drowsy cues were absent:

Drowsy in this context doesn't mean about to fall asleep (half closed eyes, barely able to keep open). When my son was a baby he would become very still about 10 minutes before he fell asleep—he is a wiggle worm, so it was noticeable. He would also gaze for long periods of time at something. This was the window when he needed to be put down for his nap. If I waited until it passed and he was really tired, he would fight sleep. So when "the stare" appeared, I would check his diaper, swaddle him, and put him down. He would gaze at his mobile for a while and then fall asleep.

The baby should be awake when you put her down for her nap. You aren't trying to ease her down and then sneak out—you want her to be able to fall asleep on her own, without rocking, patting, and so on. Try to catch her in that drowsy pre-sleep period—for many babies it is right around one to two hours after waking for the day. Start watching for signs at around thirty to ninety minutes, and I bet you will soon be able to tell when she is ready to go down. Good luck!

DROWSY SIGNS

Drowsy Cues or Sleepy Signs as He Becomes Drowsy:

Moving into the Sleep Zone

Decreased activity, less animated, becomes quieter
Eyes less focused on surroundings, appears glazed over
Eyelids drooping
Pulling ears
Slower motions, less social, less vocal
Less interested in toys or people
Sucking is weaker or slower
Yawning

Past Drowsy: Short on Sleep (SOS) Distress Signs Begin to Appear

Fatigue Signs: Entering Overtired Zone. Becoming Overtired

Mild fussiness, irritability, cranky

Crying upon awakening

Rubbing eyes

Think of these symptoms of overtiredness as signaling the distress of being *short on sleep* (SOS): "Help me, I need sleep!"

Remember, to avoid junk food, you read the nutritional label. Junk sleep has no label to read, so instead you must learn to "read" your child. Even when there is not a full-blown "witching hour," a child might often have mild fussiness or irritability in the late afternoon. Why is this deterioration in behavior and mood at the end of the day often not recognized by some parents as being directly caused by junk sleep or lack of sleep?

Some parents deny their child is suffering from SOS distress because they are not present when it is full-blown in the late afternoon and he is in day care or nanny care. When parents return home from work, naturally there is intense excitement as they reconnect with their children, play, and have dinner, so some of these distress items are masked. Other parents do not see these SOS signs because their child is pacified and distracted by being parked in front of television or a video game. Or the parents are digitally distracted. Other parents have been sleep deprived themselves for much of their life and do not appreciate the power of healthy sleep because they have not experienced it. Or they think it is normal for children to have a "witching hour." A study of children at 3, 6, and 11 months of age showed that increased night sleep is associated with an increased likelihood of approaching new and strange people and things. But fragmented sleep between 6 and 36 months of age is associated with a more difficult temperament.

What if your baby cries when you put him down drowsy but awake? When you first try to put him down drowsy but awake, he might be almost completely asleep, but with practice you will be able to put him down in a more wakeful state. When you put him down drowsy but awake and he cries hard, immediately pick him up for more soothing and try again some other time that day or the next day. If he makes very quiet sounds, wait and see. He might drift off to sleep or begin to cry hard. If he now begins to cry hard, quickly pick him up. Don't be disappointed if he does not fall asleep when you first start to practice putting him down drowsy but awake; it just takes practice. Expect to become frustrated, because initially you may be successful only about 10 percent of the time during the first week. But by the end of the second week, you may be successful 20 percent of the time. This percentage may double each week, so after a few more weeks it becomes much easier. Be optimistic! After a few months of practice and the maturation of sleep rhythms, you will develop an anticipatory sense of when he will need to sleep. Later, when he is completely well rested, don't be surprised if drowsy signs disappear altogether because you have successfully synchronized the timing of your soothing to sleep with the beginning of his emerging sleep wave. It's like being good at surfing; you catch the wave for a long ride. Patience, practice, timing, and trial and error will guarantee success.

You might be more successful with putting your child down drowsy but awake in the early morning, when he is best rested from the previous night's sleep, especially if the interval of wakefulness between the wake-up time and the first nap is very brief (thirty to ninety minutes). Nursing mothers might have more success if they leave the home and let the father put the baby down drowsy but awake with a bottle of expressed breast milk. The baby senses that Mom is gone, and he knows that Dad cannot breast-feed. He is tired anyway, so he might as well go to sleep. Why not?

Drowsy signs might be absent when a child has colic or is extremely overtired and instead crashes directly from a wakeful state to showing fatigue signs. Also, drowsy signs might be absent in the well-rested child with good self-soothing skills who is put down to sleep just as she is becoming sleepy. This suggests that drowsy signs really are mild expressions of becoming overtired (sleep deprived), not simply tired.

As previously mentioned, drowsy signs might not be noticed by parents because of their own digital distractions (TV, smartphone, or computer). Maybe take a weekend break from all such distractions and simply watch your child for drowsy signs.

Also, signs of drowsiness and fatigue may be masked by parents' intensive play or the child being distracted with video games, TV, or a DVD. Please observe how your child appears and plays independent of digital distractions, especially near the end of the day.

Why does a child become parent-soothed and not learn self-soothing?

Parental sleep deprivation, excitement, or medical conditions push the topic of sleep for the child off the parent's radar.

Thinking that feeding directly causes sleeping causes parents to focus only on feeding.

Distraction interferes with appreciating signs of drowsiness.

Colic interferes with learning self-soothing.

Soothing

What exactly is soothing to a drowsy state? Soothing is restoring a peaceful state. To soothe your newborn is to render her calm or quiet, to bring her to a composed condition by reducing the force or intensity of fussiness or crying. Soothing brings comfort to your baby, a cessation of agitation. Snuggled close to your body, she feels your warmth and senses your affection and protection. Cuddling is the close embrace you do with someone you love. Sometimes you just want to nestle with her as you take a cozy position and press her close to you or lie down close to her. At best, when a child is tired, we hope to lull her into a relaxed, sleepy state.

Bodily contact, sucking, and gentle rhythmic motions over long periods of time seem to work best for soothing. Sometimes loud mechanical sounds like the garbage disposal or hair dryer seem to help. Be careful, however, not to bombard your baby with stimuli. Initially, try to appeal to one sense at a time: tactile (massaging, rubbing, kissing, rocking, patting, changing from hip to shoulder), auditory (singing, humming, playing music, running the vacuum cleaner), sight (bright lights, mobiles, or television; or dim light or darkness when drowsy), or rhythmic motion (swings, cradles, car rides, going for a walk). Sometimes doing too many of these things simultaneously or with too much force has a stimulating effect rather than a relaxing one. However, if your baby remains fussy, try combinations of these different modalities.

Try to synchronize your actions with your baby's rhythms. If he is tense and taut, with deep exhausted heaving sobs and little physical movement, try rubbing his back ever so gently or moving your cheek over his in a slow rhythm that coincides with his breathing pattern. If he is boxing with his fists, jerking his legs, and arching his back, maybe a ride on your shoulders will grab his attention and arrest the spell. You will find that after a while you become attuned to the nuances of your baby's rhythms and respond accordingly.

Each parent should experiment to see what soothing method works best and then try to be somewhat consistent so that your child learns to associate certain behaviors with falling asleep. But it is not necessary that Mom and Dad have the same soothing style.

Rhythmic Rocking

Rhythmic motions are one of the most effective methods of soothing your infant. Use a cradle, rocking chair, baby swing, or Snugli; take the baby for automobile rides, dance with her, or simply walk with her. Rocking motions may be gentle movements or vigorous swinging, depending on what your child responds to. Gently jiggling or bouncing may calm your baby. Some parents claim that raising and lowering the baby like an elevator is effective. Perhaps these rhythmic movements are comforting because they are similar to what the baby experienced in the womb.

Swing, Stroller, Car, and Carrying

Rhythmic rocking motions might occur in an old-fashioned cradle, a swing, a stroller, your car, or when your baby is carried in your arms or an infant carrier. These activities are fine for soothing, but not for sleeping. Sure, your baby can fall asleep in the moving cradle or swing. But it will probably be a light sleep, and your child will miss the full restorative benefit of deeper sleep. Remember, think of sleep *quality*, not just sleep *quantity*.

In your home, perhaps sleeping in a gently moving swing in a dark and quiet room is very similar to motionless sleep in a crib. If this is how your child sleeps best, then sometimes turn off the swing after your child falls asleep and leave him there until he awakens. Later, try to make a transition to placing him in his crib without the swing. For a colicky child, this might only work around 3 to 4 months of age, when the colic is winding down.

Outside your home, the rhythmic rocking motion of a stroller might lull your child to a drowsy state, and you might find a quiet park to stop to let him enjoy motionless sleep while you enjoy the fresh air. But in a bright and noisy shopping environment or public place, I suspect that the naps might be less restorative and maybe shorter.

As a generalization, I think that planning for naps at home helps parents organize schedules and think about consolidated sleep, naps in sync with biologic rhythms, and reasonably early bedtimes. In contrast, I think that frequent napping in shopping malls and other busy places is associated with children who tend to be chronically mildly short on sleep, so they crash despite all the stimulation around them. So when I encourage motionless sleep in the crib or bed over sleep in motion, I am thinking more about discouraging sleeping outside than swings at home.

Sucking

Anything you can do to encourage your baby to suck will help soothe her. Offering the breast, bottle, pacifier, finger, or wrist usually helps calm your baby. If you are breast-feeding, one way to help distinguish between sucking for soothing and sucking for hunger is that the sucking for soothing is often rapid, repeated sucks with very little swallowing. If your baby is hungry, the pattern is usually a rhythmic suck-swallow, suck-swallow, and so forth. But the fussy baby does not suck-swallow in a rhythmic steady fashion; she sucks more than swallows; she starts and stops, twists and turns. If you are bottle-feeding, do not always assume that when your baby eagerly takes several ounces, this means she is hungry. Many babies with extreme fussiness/colic suck more than they need and spit up a lot.

Because sucking is such a powerful way to calm a baby, and babies often fall asleep with sucking, I think it is unnatural and unhealthy for parents to deliberately do things that interfere with sucking. One popular book that promotes "no-cry sleep solutions" tells parents to remove the breast while the baby is sucking, before she falls asleep, and if she continues to want to suck after the removal, the book tells parents to hold her mouth closed to prevent it! Another popular book describes sucking as one of the major ways that babies can calm themselves, but then goes on to recommend that you wake your baby up during sucking if he falls asleep at the breast. Furthermore, the author instructs you to begin this practice at 1 month of age! Both books make the assumption that if the baby falls asleep while sucking, you will be creating a sleep problem. There is no good evidence to support this assumption. Mothers in my practice do not deliberately interfere with sucking at the time of soothing to sleep, and their babies sleep well. Both books also incorrectly assume that feeding and sleeping are tightly linked. So both encourage you to force-feed your baby in order to help him sleep longer. Phrases like "cluster feed," "top off the tank," or "awake when hungry and asleep when full" reveal a profound ignorance about how the developing brain, not the stomach, controls sleep/ wake rhythms. I believe it is much healthier and more effective to follow your baby's needs. If your baby is hungry, feed him. If your baby is fussy, soothe him. If your baby is tired, put him to sleep. If you're not sure what he needs, encourage sucking at the breast or bottle until he seems satisfied because he is full or calm or asleep.

Non-nutritive sucking

Sometimes, try to give your baby a chance or chances to self-soothe to sleep without feeding during the day or night: this means that you do some soothing and then your baby is put down drowsy but awake before falling asleep. Some mothers feel more comfortable trying this than others, and some babies accept this more than others, so try to do what feels right for you and your baby without making comparisons to others. Try to remember that breast-feeding is first of all feeding.

But as long as some chances to self-soothe are offered, I do not think there is a problem using the breast to soothe to sleep when necessary, especially when other soothing methods are not effective. This might occur when your child develops a second wind and becomes overtired, your baby is about 6 weeks old and at the peak of fussiness/crying, or your baby has colic—or anytime mom is desperate for sleep herself. So what if sometimes you might be soothing to sleep using breast-feeding and sometimes you might use other methods to soothe to a drowsy but awake state? This is parenting, not the military!

Pacifiers may help babies sleep and reduce the risk of SIDS. If you have to replace the pacifier once or twice during a night to get great sleep, do it. But if replacing pacifiers occurs many times throughout the night, then one or both parents will be short on sleep. Maybe it is time to teach more self-soothing skills. When your child is older and throws the pacifier out of the crib, instead of going back in to pick it up and return it, just buy a dozen pacifiers, or use one with a ribbon substantially shorter than the circumference of your child's neck (to prevent strangulation) that has an alligator clip allowing you to attach it to your child's pajamas. That way the child will learn self-soothing with the aid of a pacifier.

Swaddling

Gentle pressure, such as that experienced when embraced or hugged, makes us feel good. Swaddling or gentle wrapping, sleeping in a car seat, or being held in a soft baby carrier or sling are other ways to exert gentle pressure. Here, too, perhaps the sensation of gentle pressure resembles a state of comfort that the baby feels before he is born. Both rhythmic motions and gentle pressure may be effective because human babies are born too early. Wait a minute: of course premature babies are born early! No, not just premature babies—*all* babies. The theory is that human babies are born earlier compared to other primate babies because as human pelvic bones evolved to support an upright posture, they became narrower. Thus human babies had to be smaller at the time of birth in order to pass through the pelvic opening. If this theory is correct, then it is likely that rhythmic motions and gentle pressure exert their soothing effects because they partially re-create the sensations experienced by the baby in the womb.

Swaddling should be attempted if it appears to help your child sleep better. Just as with pacifiers in the preceding section, if you have to reswaddle a baby once or twice a night in order to get great sleep, it is worth it. But if swaddling occurs many times throughout the night, then one or both parents will be short on sleep, and this is not good. It is time to allow your child to learn some self-soothing. When your child appears to want to kick free and not be swaddled, then stop.

Massage

Massaging babies has been practiced in many different cultures and has a long history. It is not just a new fad. One particular advantage to massaging your newborn is that the mother or father also directly benefits from this activity. While lovingly stroking your baby, you smile at your baby, talk softly, or sing or hum. These efforts, while focused on your baby, also relax you, too! As your child bonds with you through the close contact, you bond with your child. Since fathers cannot breast-feed their babies, I encourage them to develop an intimate bond with their newborn by practicing baby massage right away—even before any fussiness begins. Using a natural cold-pressed fruit or vegetable oil, gently stroke the skin and gently knead your baby's muscles. All the movements are performed gently— books with pictures and online videos are available to assist you. Baby massage is not a gimmick. Nor is it a cure for extreme fussiness. But it does soothe babies. Equally important, it provides you with a singular opportunity to be completely focused on your baby—turn off the phones. Both you and your baby might even enjoy listening to relaxation music at this time. You are doing something quite different from feeding, changing, and bathing. Comforting your baby this way will give you an inner calmness that will help you get through possible rough times when your baby is extremely fussy and not very soothable. Think of it as making deposits to an interest-bearing account that you will need to draw upon in more difficult times. Only instead of money, it is love that you are putting in the bank.

Sounds

What is the power of a lullaby? Babies calm down and slip into slumber; parents relax and feel more at peace with themselves and their baby. Lullabies, such as those found on my CD *Sweet Baby Lullabies to Soothe Your Newborn,* are the universal language of parents loving babies. Lullabies, music, songs, humming, reading, talking, or nature sounds may have a soothing effect on your baby. One study suggested that music that has a wide dynamic range with lots of loud and quiet elements was not as soothing as music that varied little in intensity, such as harpsichord or guitar pieces. Noise machines may be useful for soothing and for masking street noises. For safety, noise machines should be on their lowest setting and as far away from the child as possible. Maybe gently stroke or massage your baby when listening.

Other Soothing Methods

Be skeptical about the supposed miracles accomplished with crib vibrators, hot-water bottles, herbal teas, or recordings of heartbeat or womb sounds. There has been a great deal of nonsense written about burping techniques, nipple sizes and shapes, baby bottle straws, feeding and sleeping positions, lambswool pads, diets for nursing mothers, special formulas, pacifiers, and solid food. There is no good evidence that chiropractic spinal manipulation helps babies. These items have nothing to do with extreme fussiness, crying, temperament, or sleeping habits.

Many useless remedies can be purchased without a prescription. Anti-gas drops, such as simethicone, have not been shown to be more effective than a placebo in well-conducted studies. One popular pellet contains chamomile, calcium phosphate, caffeine, and a very small amount of active belladonna chemicals (0.0000095 percent). Another remedy contains natural blackberry flavor, Jamaica ginger, oil of anise, oil of nutmeg, and 2 percent alcohol. Maybe enough alcohol will sedate some infants! Please read labels carefully—any natural substance, flavoring agent, or herb can have pharmacological effects. Call a school of pharmacy or a medical school to locate experts in pharmagnosy, the study of natural herbs and plants, to find out if a particular plant or herb is dangerous. Don't assume that if it is safe for adults, it must be safe for infants.

Beware of gimmicks. Newborns have been drowned in rocking waterbeds, strangled in trampoline-like crib platforms, and suffocated by pillows. Beware of prescribed drugs. A London *Times* headline of May 22, 1998, screamed, "Baby Died After Drop of Medicine for Wind." A midwife had "diagnosed trapped wind" and prescribed what was thought to be peppermint water.

Also be cautious in using home remedies. One mother almost killed her baby by giving a mixture of Morton Salt Substitute with *Lactobacillus acidophilus* culture, as prescribed in a popular book. A good rule of thumb here is: when in doubt, don't!

Everything Works . . . for a While

When you believe that something is going to calm your baby—herbal tea, womb recordings, lambswool blankets, you name it—often it appears to work . . . for a while. You are emotionally expecting relief because you trust the advice of an authority. Your fatigue may breed inflated hopes for a cure, and the day-by-day variability in infant crying creates the illusion that a particular remedy works. What is really happening is a placebo effect, the emotional equivalent of an optical illusion.

Mothers may initially fool themselves into believing their babies are better because of a new formula or special tea. Of course, reality sets in after a few days and shatters the illusion. Some doctors believe the mothers' reports and agree that the babies really did improve for a day or two because the babies received novel stimulation.

Novelty is unlikely to be important, because parents report that upon reintroduction, weeks after the special tea or gimmick was discarded, they see no improvement. In other words, there was no placebo effect the second time around. Naturally, if the baby coincidentally outgrows extreme fussiness/colic when a useless remedy is introduced, the mother, the family, and even the doctor might become convinced that the useless remedy actually cured the extreme fussiness/colic!

SOOTHING

There are many ways to soothe babies but only a few major themes.

1. Rhythmic rocking: swings, cars, arms, rocking chairs, stroller rides, crib, swaying to and fro
2. Sucking: breast, bottle, pacifier, wrist, fingers
3. Gentle pressure: swaddling, massage, soft cloth carriers
4. Sounds: lullabies (for example, my CD, *Sweet Baby: Lullabies to Soothe Your Newborn*), nature sounds, music, quiet talking, shushing

Soothing and Crying

I asked a group of new parents in my practice how they soothed their babies when fussy or soothed them to a drowsy state before sleep. The group seemed to agree that slow, rhythmic stroking and rocking was usually more effective than rapid bouncing or patting. But one mother described how the intensity and rapidity of her movements increased when her baby became fussier. This seemed to help calm her baby, and the mother felt this was because she had become more attuned to her baby. However, other new parents in the group did not find this helpful. One mother felt that she increased the intensity and rapidity of her movements when her baby became fussier because she was becoming more stressed herself, not because it was helping her baby calm down. Another mother said that she felt her style of soothing was organically part of who she was, and although she had tried different methods suggested by books and friends, she ultimately did what felt comfortable to her. Perhaps there is no "best" way, but every mother and baby discovers what works for them.

The group also agreed that dads sometimes seemed more effective in soothing because they had a more matter-of-fact approach and talked to the babies as if they were adults. "Here's the deal: I'm going to rock you for a while and then you're going to be put down to sleep because it's time to sleep. Got it? So don't give me any problems."

Some mothers in the group started teaching self-soothing when their babies were only a week old, after hearing from other moms how they had also started early. One mother described how, after feeling comfortable with some successes, she decided that she would let her baby cry at night to learn some self-soothing for night sleep. Her baby cried quietly one night only for twenty minutes and then slept well at night and has slept well since. She did this at age 4 *weeks,* and her baby was now 5–6 months. There were no gasps or astonished looks but simply smiles and nods from the more experienced mothers. I think that more mothers and fathers might experiment with a few minutes of quiet crying to allow self-soothing at night in the newborn period if they feel comfortable. I pointed to a couple present with 38-week newborn twins and described how when attending to one twin, the other might cry and then stop crying and fall asleep before you could get to the crying twin. My impression is that ten to twenty minutes of low-level or quiet crying cannot be harmful.

But here is a curious observation: in the office, after soothing a two-week-old following an exam, I put the baby down on the examination table, and the baby began whimpering and quietly crying. I said to the mother, "Let's watch the minute hand and leave your baby for one to two minutes, as long as the crying does not become loud or strong, to see if your baby might fall asleep." Her immediate response was, "Isn't she crying hard?" I pointed out that hard crying occurs after an immunizations shot, and this was quiet crying. So it appears possible that some mothers, in the beginning, are less able to make the distinction between very quiet crying or whimpering and hard, loud crying and are therefore loath to allow any crying to occur in the context of allowing a child to learn self-soothing. I asked the parents in the group about this and their experiences with teaching self-soothing, and here are some representative responses:

I wanted to respond to your comment about the mother who felt her baby was crying hard. I can relate to this and found with my baby at the start that his crying would actually "hurt" me. My partner, in contrast, didn't know what my problem was and didn't feel he was crying particularly hard (other people also commented that he didn't sound very loud or upset). For me, I feel that the combination of sleep deprivation, hormones, and the overwhelming responsibility of being a first-time mum meant that I overreacted to every single cry, and this has gradually reduced with time and experience.

I am a frequenter of the new parent group at Dr. Weissbluth's office and have had tremendous success with letting my now 11-week-old daughter cry it out. I let her do it the first time for twenty minutes at 4 weeks of age and had success pretty immediately. After about four nights the crying was either extremely limited or nonexistent. Some people might think it's crazy or terrible, but I feel as though I was able to help my daughter sleep and feel better. I limit her to short periods of wakefulness (thirty to forty-five minutes usually), put her to bed early (5:30–6:30 p.m.), and let her cry it out when she needs to. She is now 11 weeks, sleeps twelve to fourteen hours each night, naps really well, and is just the happiest little girl. In addition, I am well rested, happy, and am able to give her my best self. I think you need to be comfortable and do what you believe is the right thing. But no, I don't think it's too early to let her cry it out. My opinion is to put her to bed in a dark, quiet room well fed with a clean diaper and close the door. Turn the baby monitor off and the TV up for twenty to thirty minutes and see what happens.

Resources for Soothing

Some families have vast resources to invest in soothing their babies, but other families are not so fortunate. Twenty percent of babies have colic and require much more soothing, and families with a col-

icky baby and limited resources to soothe might easily become overwhelmed and frustrated. The other 80 percent of babies are more
easily soothed and usually do not overly stress their parents. So you
want to pay attention to whether your child has colic or not, and
take some time to reflect on how able you will be to enlist help to
soothe your baby. It is often more than a one-parent job! If you have
a baby who fusses and cries a lot and is difficult to console, and your
available resources for soothing are limited, you might modify some
of the plans you made before your child was born regarding a family
bed or crib.

Consider a balance between the baby's disposition to express distress and the parents' capability to soothe their baby. Not only do
babies vary in their expression, but parents also vary in their capability to soothe. The resources for parents' ability to soothe fussiness and crying and promote sleep in their baby include the
following.

RESOURCES FOR PARENTS' ABILITY TO SOOTHE

- Father involvement versus absent father
- Agreements or disagreements between parents regarding child
  rearing, such as breast- versus bottle-feeding or crib versus
  family bed
- Absence or presence of marital discord
- Absence or presence of intimacy between wife and husband
- Absence or presence of baby blues or postpartum depression
- Absence or presence of other children requiring attention
- Ease or difficulty in breast-feeding
- Absence or presence of medical problems in child, mother,
  father, or other children
- Number of bedrooms in the home
- Absence or presence of relatives, friends, or neighbors to help
  out
- Help or interference with sleep routines from grandparents
- Ability or inability to afford housekeeping help

- Ability or inability to afford child care help
- Absence or presence of financial pressures such as mother having to return to work soon

MANY NAPS

Immediately after the baby is born, you will see what people mean when they say "sleeping like a baby." For a few days, babies sleep almost all the time. They barely suck and normally lose weight during this time. (If your baby was born early, this very drowsy time might last longer; if your baby was born past the expected date of delivery, the drowsy period might be brief or nonexistent.)

A few days later, babies begin to wake up more. This increased wakefulness reflects the normal maturation of your baby's nervous system. I tell families that the brain wakes up after three or four days, just in time to catch the breast milk that is now available in ample amounts. The baby looks around more with wider eyes and is able to suck with more strength and for longer periods. Within days, the weight loss stops and a dramatic growth in weight, height, and head circumference begins. Also, slightly longer periods of wakefulness begin to appear after a few days. Although your baby is intently interested in you and is quickly able to recognize your face and voice, he is not yet curious about objects such as toys or mobiles. He does not appear to care about the general buzz or noises, colors, or other activities surrounding him, and therefore he falls asleep almost anywhere. The extremely fussy/colicky baby is not like this and appears to have difficulty falling asleep and staying asleep even at only several days of age. All babies gradually seem to become more aware of action, motion, voices, noises, vibrations, lights, wind, and so forth as they become more curious. At that point they often do not "sleep like a baby."

During the day, your baby will have a one- to two-hour "window" of wakefulness, and then become drowsy and want to go to sleep. Some parents mistakenly think that you must always keep baby up for one to two hours before putting her to sleep. Remember, the one- to two-hour guideline is a ceiling, not a floor.

I discovered this window during my research on naps. Because most naps are quite brief, your baby may need to go back to sleep after being up for only thirty to ninety minutes. Other children might have long naps and can comfortably be up for an hour to two hours. Respect your baby's need to nap and avoid keeping her up too long.

Watch your baby closely for drowsy signs. If you soothe your baby during the beginning of drowsiness, most likely he will easily fall asleep. The exception is the extremely fussy/colicky baby, who might fall asleep, but not easily; these babies need longer and more complex soothing efforts to help them fall asleep. The other exception is during the evening fussy periods and especially around 6 weeks of age.

Here are some ways to note that your baby is becoming drowsy. Watch for the signs of drowsiness—quieting of activity, less movement of the arms and legs, eyes that are not as sparkling, eyelids that droop a little, less intense staring at you, and sucking that may be weaker or slower (see page 113). If your baby is over 6 weeks old, you may notice less socially responsive smiling, or your baby may be less engaging. This is the time to begin soothing to sleep. All babies become this way within one to two hours of waking.

You might miss signs of drowsiness if you are digitally distracted. If the intervals of wakefulness are too long because grandparents keep the new baby up too long or you run too many errands with her, then she gets keyed up (a second wind) and has difficulty self-soothing to sleep. Instead of thinking of overstimulation as very intense or active play, think of it as an interval of wakefulness that is too long. Don't beat yourself up if real-life circumstances occasionally or frequently interfere with brief intervals of wakefulness. It is a fact of modern life that day care and nanny care have become more common. Thus, older infants and children are experiencing more missed naps, brief naps, or naps not in sync with circadian rhythms. What can be done about this? An extra-early bedtime partially compensates for poor-quality naps, and being vigilant about good-quality sleep on weekends helps keep your child well rested.

What happens if you miss this window of drowsiness? Your baby will become overtired if she cannot fall asleep because of too much stimulation around her. When you or your baby becomes overtired, the body is stressed. Chemical changes then occur to fight the fatigue, and this interferes with the ability to easily fall asleep and stay asleep—that is, the baby gets a second wind. Babies vary in their ability to self-soothe and deal with this stress, and parents vary in their ability to soothe their babies. Not all babies go bonkers if they are kept up a little too long. But you will have a more peaceful and better-sleeping baby if you respect his need to sleep again within one to two hours after waking. I consider this to be the beginning of teaching self-soothing for babies.

Teaching self-soothing starts with developing a sense of timing, so that you are trying to soothe your baby at the time when your baby is naturally getting drowsy before falling asleep. Some young babies will need dark and quiet environments to sleep well, and others will appear to be less sensitive to what is going on around them. Respect your baby's individuality and do not try to force him to meet your lifestyle. I like the analogy with feeding: We do not withhold food when our baby is hungry. We try to anticipate when he will be hungry, so that we will be somewhere calm where we can feed him. We do not feed him on the run. The same applies for sleeping.

If your newborn does not fall asleep, continue trying to soothe. Do not let him cry or ignore him. A mother's report of allowing her 4-week-old to cry is described on page 126. Elsewhere, I advise letting infants cry in order to teach them self-soothing skills, but newly born infants are a different matter. You cannot spoil a newborn. You cannot teach a newborn a crying habit.

Bedtime Routines

Just as soothing helps your child feel safe and secure, bedtime routines help all children calm down before falling asleep, because both are associated with the natural state of relaxed drowsiness. As with soothing, bedtime routines should be started early, before sleepy signs change into overtired fussy signs. Older children and more regular babies will develop predictable sleep times, and these children might be "slept by the clock." Pick and choose from the following list based on your child's age and your personal preference. Try to follow the same sequence at all sleep times, because a consistent bedtime routine has been found to be a predictor of better sleep, including, specifically, fewer night wakings. Follow any routine that you feel comfortable with and stick with it. Don't worry if Mom and Dad have different routines. Your baby will learn to associate each routine with each parent.

BEDTIME ROUTINES
Before sleep times, reduce stimulation: less noise, dimmer lights, less handling, less playing, lower levels of activity

Bedroom should be quiet, dark (use room-darkening shades), and warm, but not too warm

Bathe

Massage after bath with smooth, gentle motions

Dress for sleep

Swaddle if it comforts and relaxes your baby; use a blanket warm from the clothes dryer

Lullaby, quiet singing, listening to music, or humming words, sounds, or phrases

Rock

Cuddle

Feed, but do not rush in to feed again at the first sound your baby makes

May put down drowsy but awake, but do not deliberately awaken before sleeping (this often fails for colicky babies and all 6-week-olds in the evening)

Read books to the baby

Quiet play

Say prayers

Brush teeth

In addition to being consistent in your bedtime routines, try to cultivate patience, because it may take time for your child to get the message that this is not playtime. I would also add that, except for premature babies and trying to correct a sleep problem, you should never wake a sleeping baby.

Breast-feeding Versus Formula, and Family Bed Versus Crib

Because breast-feeding and a family bed often go together, the topics of how to feed your baby and where to put your baby to sleep are linked.

How you feed your baby and where you sleep with your baby might depend on many factors, including whether the baby is easy or difficult to soothe and whether you and your baby are well rested or not. Ask yourself these questions:

1. Do you spend a total of more than three hours per day soothing your baby to prevent crying? That is, when you add up the total amount of minutes spent walking, rocking, driving around in the car, swaddling, singing, humming, running water, offering the breast or bottle even when not hungry, using a pacifier, and so forth, does the total exceed three hours?
2. Do you behave this way more than three days per week?
3. Have you been doing this for more than three weeks?

If you answered yes to all three questions, then your baby has colic. Because of your soothing efforts, there may be no crying, just endless fussing. Or she might sometimes cry anyway despite your soothing efforts. Please stop here and skip ahead to Chapter 5 to better understand the challenges you will be up against.

If you answered no to some of the questions but your baby fusses often, especially in the evening and especially around 6 weeks of age, then your baby has common fussiness.

BREAST-FEEDING VERSUS FORMULA

Breast-feeding is considered best for baby and mother. The mother's decision on how to feed her baby may be influenced by the support or lack thereof from her husband, her mother, or other family members, along with other issues such as prematurity, twins, or perinatal complications. However, many babies are formula-fed because of adoption, prematurity, or medical problems with the baby or mother. Bottles can contain expressed breast milk or formula, so "bottle-feeding" may include feeding breast milk or formula. Formula-fed babies grow up to be just as healthy as breast-fed babies. Many studies have shown that breast-feeding does not prevent extreme fussiness/colic, and does not prevent or cause sleep problems. At night, breast-fed babies are often fed more frequently than formula-fed babies, but it is not known whether this is caused by the breast-feeding mother responding more promptly to her baby's quiet sounds or whether breast milk is digested faster, causing the baby to wake up more often. In general, research has shown that sleep/wake rhythms evolve at the same pace whether the baby is breast-fed or formula-fed, whether the baby is demand-fed or schedule-fed, or whether cereal is given in the bottle or by spoon. Some babies with a birth defect of the digestive system are fed continuously by vein or tube in the stomach. Because of the constant feeding, they are never hungry. These babies develop the same sleep/wake rhythms as all other babies. This is why I tell parents that "sleep comes from the brain, not the stomach." Although there are rare medical exceptions, changing formulas will not reduce fussiness/crying or promote better sleeping.

How Do You Know if Your Child Is Getting Enough Food?

Your baby's pediatrician will check her weight at each office visit, and seeing that weight gain will reassure you that your baby is getting enough food overall. But sometimes you might not be sure on a particular night or at a particular feeding whether she is really hungry. She will suck at the breast or bottle when she is just fussy but not hungry, because sucking is soothing. There are three ways to tell if your baby is truly hungry at night:

1. *Pay attention to the suck-swallow pattern.* A hungry baby sucks, fills up her mouth, and swallows, so the pattern is suck-swallow, suck-swallow, suck-swallow, and so forth. A swallow usually follows almost every suck. A fussy baby in the middle of the night will have a different pattern: suck-suck-suck-swallow, suck-suck-suck-swallow. There will be many more sucks before each swallow.

2. *Offer a bottle immediately after breast-feeding in the middle of the night.* The well-fed breast-fed baby will not take much from the bottle. If your baby takes a small volume slowly, this tells you that you have sufficient breast milk and your baby is not hungry even though the baby wants to suck more at the breast. If your baby takes a large volume quickly, this tells you that your breast milk supply is low. An exception might be a colicky baby who does rapidly suck down more (for soothing, not hunger) and then spits up.

3. *Once, have Dad offer a bottle instead of Mom breast-feeding in the middle of the night.* If your baby is truly hungry or thirsty, she will take a large volume quickly. If not, this tells you that your baby is up at night but not hungry.

The reason it is important to resist the temptation to always feed your baby whenever he vocalizes at night is because this particular behavior partially or fully awakens your baby. This may cause fragmented sleep or encourage a night crying habit whereby your baby learns to cry more frequently and louder at night for the pleasure of your company, not because he is hungry. This might not occur when the breast-feeding mother is bed sharing, because both she and her baby may be more asleep than awake at these frequent feedings (please see Chapter 1 for why bed sharing is discouraged).

Of course, if your baby is not being fed enough, then she might be too hungry and fuss/cry or not sleep well. In this situation, the child will not be gaining weight, and some help will be needed to establish a better breast milk supply or evaluation for medical problems that are causing poor weight gain. In my practice, I encourage first-time mothers to give a bottle of expressed breast milk or formula once per twenty-four hours beginning when their baby is 2 to 3 weeks old. This allows fathers and other family members to have the pleasure of feeding the baby, as well as giving the mother a mini-break once a day to rest and allow for the healing of cracked or painful nipples. It also gives the parents the chance to have a date to recharge their energy. Fathers can be more helpful during fussy/crying periods or middle-of-the-night feedings to allow mothers a little more sleep. Some experienced mothers, who have previously breast-fed successfully, give the single bottle sooner. They have confidence in their ability to breast-feed and either give formula in the hospital or start pumping sooner. They know that the single bottle does not confuse the child or interfere with breast-feeding. The reason the bottle is given every twenty-four hours is to keep the baby adapted to taking the bottle. Some babies do well with less frequent bottles, but others will reject all bottles if days go by without having had one.

FAMILY BED VERSUS CRIB

Our goal is a well-rested family, and a family bed—sometimes described as co-sleeping or bed sharing—may be something you have considered (again, please see Chapter 1 for why co-sleeping is discouraged). The decision to sleep with your baby might be made before the child is born, because this is what you want for your family. You might decide that unrestricted breast-feeding day and night, always caring for your baby, and sleeping with your baby at night, or day and night, will promote a tighter or more sensitive bond between you and your baby. Parents then begin the practice of co-sleeping as soon as the baby is born. Researchers use the term "early co-sleepers" to describe these children. Alternatively, you might not have thought about or not really wanted to have a family bed, but you discovered that because your baby was so fussy/colicky, or when your child was older and not sleeping well, that the only way anyone got any rest was to sleep with your baby in your bed. Researchers use the term "reactive co-sleepers" to describe these children. Scientific studies have shown that co-sleeping in infancy is often associated with the later development of sleep problems. I suspect that the majority of these problems occur among former reactive co-sleepers. In other words, some parents find that the family bed is a short-term and partial solution to sleep problems, and the sleep problem continues long after the child has been moved to his own crib or bed because the child was not given the opportunity to learn self-soothing skills.

Many families frequently sleep together in a family bed for all or part of the night. By itself, this is neither good nor bad. Studies in the United States suggest that the family bed might encourage or lead to a variety of emotional stresses within the child; opposite results were found in studies conducted in Sweden. This probably reflects differences in social attitudes toward nudity, bathing, and sexuality. Think of it as a family style, one that does not necessarily reflect or cause emotional or psychological problems in parents and children.

But when someone is not getting enough sleep, either parent or child, the family bed can cause potential problems. I suspect this often develops in older toddlers, because by the age of 1 to 2 years, sleeping together is often associated with night waking. Once there is a well-established habit, the child is unwilling to go to or return to his own bed.

So if you want to enjoy a family bed, fine. But understand that your cuddling in bed together may make any future changes in sleep arrangements difficult to execute. Remember, while it sounds like an easy solution to baby's sleep problems, you may wind up with a twenty-four-hour child even when he gets older.

In contrast, many families use a family bed overnight only during the first few months, then shift the baby to her own crib for overnight sleep. Then at 5:00 or 6:00 a.m., parents might bring their older infant or child into their bed for a limited period of warm cuddling.

Sleeping with your baby might include both day and night or just night, and all night or part of the night, in your bed or using a small crib attached to your bed, with other children in your bed or other children in your bedroom but not in your bed. All of these variations are collectively called "family bed." In many cultures, families sleep together because of tradition or a limited number of bedrooms. It is rare in Japan or in traditional or tribal societies for children to sleep apart from their parents. There is a great appeal for sleeping together. A powerful word to describe soothing is "nestling," and this easily brings forth the image of creating a nest for your baby in your bed.

However, it is important to note that both the U.S. Consumer Product Safety Commission and the American Academy of Pediatrics actively discourage the family bed because of the risk of entrapment between the mattress and the structures of the bed (headboard, footboard, side rails, and frame), the wall, or adjacent furniture. There is the hazard of suffocation or overlying by an adult who is in an unusually deep sleep caused by alcohol, mind-altering drugs, or a medical condition. Also, soft surfaces or loose covers can cause suffocation. They point out that there is no evidence that bed sharing protects against sudden infant death syndrome. Nor is there any evidence that bed sharing prevents extreme fussiness/colic.

So if you want to use a family bed, try to make it a safe environment by not drinking or taking drugs at night and by making sure your baby is always sleeping on his back. Also, fill in the spaces between the bed and any walls or furniture and eliminate loose bedding.

SOLID FOODS AND FEEDING HABITS

Big meals make us sleepy, so shouldn't solids make babies sleep better? Wrong. Feeding rhythms do not alter the pattern of waking and sleeping.

Sleeping for long periods at night is not related to the method of feeding, whether it be breast or bottle. The studies I think are the most convincing involve comparing the development of sleep/wake rhythms of infants fed on demand with those who are continuously fed intravenously because of birth defects involving their stomachs or intestines. The babies who were fed on demand cycled between being hungry and being full. The other babies were never allowed to become hungry. Objective recordings in sleep laboratories show that there were no sleep differences between these groups of infants. Other studies involve the introduction of solid foods; they all show that solid food, such as cereal, does not influence nighttime sleeping patterns. No published studies have ever shown that the method of feeding (breast milk versus formula, or scheduled feedings versus demand feedings) or the introduction of solids affects sleep.

Some studies, however, do indicate that formula-feeding is more popular than breast-feeding among mothers who are more restrictive. Mothers who feed their babies formula tend to be more interested in controlling their infant's behavior and like being able to see the number of ounces of formula given at each feeding. These parents are more likely to perceive night waking in a problem/solution framework and consider the social wants of the child instead of nutritional needs. In contrast, the nursing mother, perhaps more sensitive to the health benefits of nursing, might respond to night waking more often or more rapidly because she perceives herself as primarily responding to her infant's need for nourishment. After a while, of course, the child learns to enjoy this nocturnal social contact. Over time, the baby learns to expect attention when he awakens.

This explains why there is no difference in night waking between breast- and formula-fed infants at 4 months, but by 6 to 12 months night waking is more of an issue among breast-fed babies.

The bottom line is that cereal does not make babies sleep better. Formula may appear thicker than breast milk, but both contain the same twenty calories per ounce. Giving formula to breast-fed babies or weaning them also will not directly cause longer sleeping at night, although it is possible that attitudes toward breast-feeding may indirectly foster a night-waking habit. Here is one mother's account of how breast-feeding led to a night-waking habit.

Maren was born July 18, 1984, after an uneventful pregnancy and an easy Lamaze delivery, three days past term.

We were committed to breast-feeding, with no preconceived expectations of its duration. Maren behaved as a normal infant for about two weeks, at which point persistent crying jags began to occur daily. Though we were assured real colic was worse, we came to refer to these spells as "Maren's colic." We endured the inconsolable crying without much complaint. Although her crying mostly lasted one to two hours, the worst individual days would include unabated crying spells lasting for eight to ten hours. Various experiments were tried to ease the colic suffering, including having Maren sleep with us, having her sleep on a hot-water bottle, et cetera. Predictably, none worked. At 2 months, the colic ended relatively abruptly.

From 2 months on, a very happy, trusting relationship developed between Maren and me. For about 7 months, Maren was fed virtually exclusively on breast milk. From 7 to 10 months, increasing amounts of solid food were introduced at breakfast and lunch. Maren has always been a happy, bubbly, joyful child. The breast-feeding seemed to contribute to this sunny disposition.

Maren's nap patterns were completely normal. Generally, I would sleep with her in the morning. Part of the feeding ritual for these 10 months included twice-nightly breast-feedings for Maren, interrupting my sleep.

Massive campaigns were mounted by both sets of grandparents to convince me that breast-feeding needed to end. These began at 2 months and reached fever pitch around 7 months. We listened politely. Except for a brief experimental period at around 8 months, I didn't attempt to pump my breasts to permit me extra sleep. This was a conscious decision; direct feeding was easier and more satisfying for both of us. But after nearly a year without a full night's sleep, I began to reach a whole new level of fatigue, and I realized it was time to wean Maren to a bottle.

Maren didn't like the plan much. She obviously disliked formula as much as I disliked feeding it to her. For nearly a week she rejected cow's milk. I ended the midmorning nap breast-feeding ritual first. Juices (orange, apple, pear) in the morning or during car rides helped to improve Maren's familiarity with bottles. They also allowed my husband, Larry, to feed her while I rested later in the mornings. Putting cow's milk in a special bottle (formed and painted to look like a dog) allowed this unpleasant white stuff to become gradually more acceptable. After a few days, Maren started to respond more favorably to her "pooch juice" and the games I created and associated with it.

Maren was fully weaned at 11 months. The last feeding to change over was at bedtime. But even if she was given milk at bedtime, Maren continued to wake up once or twice per evening, crying to be fed. The next step was to get her to sleep through the night. We were repeatedly advised to let her cry herself to sleep. The phrase "even for five or six hours" was used, a reminder of colic days. We considered this proposition but continued to feed Maren warm milk, sing lullabies, and rock her to sleep, once or twice per night. The big question: what was waking her up?

We decided it was mostly habit, and that she just wanted the comfort of our company. A new go-to-sleep ritual was introduced: after much playing and affection, Maren was put to bed with her favorite doll, not rocked to sleep. If she woke, warm milk was provided, but Maren was purposely not picked up. Maren cried ten minutes when left alone the first night, then rested her head on top of her favorite doll and drifted off to sleep. After expecting possibly an hour or more of crying, this was an unbelievable, almost anticlimactic relief to us. After two or three nights of feeding without picking her up, Maren began sleeping through the night.

At the end of month eleven, the go-to-sleep is routine. Maren rarely cries at all. Key elements: a big dinner, a bath, gentle play, eight ounces of warm milk, hugs, and her favorite doll. Even a babysitter can do it. At 1 year, Maren had finally learned to sleep eight hours straight. In retrospect, maybe I should have made the switch to a bottle sooner, and not waited so long before we tried to put her to sleep alone. Our parents continuously warned us we were being too indulgent. They may have been right. But then, first-time parents are like that.

Earlier Bedtime Around 6 Weeks Old

Around 6 weeks after the due date, a baby's brain develops the capacity for specific social smiling, more calmness in the evening, longer blocks of sleep at night (four to six hours), and an earlier bedtime. All of these wonderful changes will occur independent of parenting. Six weeks is the time when moms start to get more night sleep and maybe get their sanity back! So hang in there.

After 6 weeks of age, it is possible to inadvertently put your baby to sleep past the time of her biological drowsiness, with the unwanted consequences of accumulating a sleep deficit. The biological bedtime is based on a night-sleep circadian rhythm and is signaled by changes in the baby's mood and behavior late in the afternoon and early evening. Watching her is more important than watching a clock. Synchronize your soothing to sleep with her emerging drowsy cues. Catch the wave. Digital distraction might cause you to miss her emerging subtle drowsy cues. A parent returning home from work might *mask* the baby's drowsy signs with intense social stimulation. So watch her carefully when she is more on her own. Her bedtime is not a fixed clock time, because of her variability in daytime sleep. Occasionally keeping your baby up late for special events is fine, but if her behavior suffers the next day, please ask yourself whether it was worth it. If she is frequently allowed to stay up too late, the ill effects of cumulative sleep loss will definitely appear.

I have had many sleep consults with parents of children around 3 or 4 months of age in which I am told that their child slept well until about 6 to 8 weeks. Thereafter, the child had trouble falling asleep or staying asleep at night. I always ask these parents to remember how their child looked in the evening before bedtime, before the sleep problem began, around 2 months of age. I ask them: "Do you think your child could have gone to sleep a little bit earlier?" The answer is always yes.

One parent put it this way: "The early bedtime is a nonnegotiable component of healthy sleep training. If you want your child to sleep soundly, wake up well rested, you have to marry the idea of an early bedtime."

Naturally, all parents want to spend time with their children in the evening. But I encourage families to try to avoid a bedtime that is chronically too late and instead focus on morning activities with their baby: bathing, changing, feeding, and playing. Parents are also encouraged to go to bed earlier themselves so they feel less rushed in the morning. Sadly, this means that some parents will not see their baby when they return home from work. But they will have the opportunity to thoroughly enjoy their calm baby every morning. And because the family is well rested during the week, weekends are relaxed and fun.

An early bedtime might be resisted by parents because they do not appreciate the power of healthy sleep or that sleep problems are directly caused by a too-late bedtime. Therefore, I would tell both parents that one possible benefit of an earlier bedtime was that their child might grow taller due to increased exposure to growth hormone, which is secreted only during sleep and especially before midnight.

My impression is that sleep problems caused by bedtimes that are too late are now more common than colic-related sleep problems. Some modern reasons for a bedtime that is too late include more dual-career parents returning home late and more parents who do not notice the baby's drowsiness in the early evening because they are distracted by digital devices.

For 80 percent of parents, sleep training is a process of helping your baby learn to sleep that never requires you to let your baby cry. But for 20 percent of all parents, their colicky baby needs constant soothing during the first few months to prevent crying and to encourage some sleeping. For these colicky babies, the phrase "start as you mean to go on" does not make sense.

Do not worry during the colicky phase if, despite your best efforts, you think your baby is not getting enough sleep. Do whatever works to maximize sleep and minimize crying for the first few months, even though she may later be described as parent-soothed and lacking in self-soothing skills. It is extremely important for parents of colicky babies to get help and take breaks without guilt. Around 3 to 4 months of age, parents of colicky babies should begin to change gears and employ methods such as check and console, graduated extinction, or extinction to allow their baby to learn self-soothing skills (see Chapter 4). The well-rested post-colic baby may make this transition with little or no crying, as described in my book *Your Fussy Baby*. The somewhat sleep-deprived post-colic baby may cry during this transition. Crying is hard, but sleepless-ness is harder.

Colicky babies who fail to make this transition from parent-soothed to learning self-soothing at 3 to 4 months are at risk of accumulating a sleep debt and becoming chronically sleep deprived. If you think that your post-colic child is short on sleep, try to fix his sleep problem around or soon after 3 to 4 months of age.

On the other hand, even for the colicky baby, there is nothing wrong with trying an earlier bedtime around 6 weeks of age. This is tricky because the colicky baby might not show drowsy signs. So if you want to try this, start on a Saturday when both parents are home to support each other and you are able to try a really early bedtime. Label his last nap as the sleep period that starts between 4:00 and 5:00 p.m. When he wakes up from this nap, depending on its duration, plan for a bedtime thirty to ninety minutes later. Then attempt to put him to sleep drowsy but awake even though he may be much more drowsy than awake! If he cries hard, pick him up im-mediately; otherwise you might decide to leave him alone for a short period of time to see if he nods off. Repeat this plan on Sunday night, and based on what happens and your own feelings, you might decide to abandon this effort completely and wait it out until he is 3 to 4 months of age or you might want to try again after a couple of weeks.

WHEN THE BEDTIME IS TOO LATE

What occurs when children are allowed to fall asleep too late at night? They wake up short of sleep in the morning in a state of higher neurological arousal that in turn makes it harder or even impossible for them to nap well. The consequences of not napping well are that by the end of the day a child's sleep tank is empty (the "witching hour") and he is in an even higher state of arousal, which makes it even more difficult for him to easily fall asleep and stay asleep at night. A vicious cycle is generated. In contrast, an early bedtime permits long naps to occur because the child awakens in a lower state of neurological arousal. It is easier for parents to catch the wave of drowsy signs, and there is no witching hour. It becomes a *virtuous* cycle: sleep begets sleep.

Parents might not appreciate that bedtime battles, long latency to sleep (time needed to fall asleep), or night waking result from a bedtime that is chronically too late. Of course, the child eventually crashes late at night. But this bedtime is preceded by an unhealthy state for the child, stressful interactions with him, stressful interactions as a couple, and stress for each parent as an individual.

Sometimes naps are very long and late (e.g., 1:00–4:00 p.m.) because the bedtime is too late; this makes a witching hour less likely but also makes a reasonably early bedtime difficult to achieve. Also, the child's sleep deprivation at the end of the day may be masked by parents returning home from work and playing with the child. Some parents do not believe that their child's bedtime is too late, because when they moved the late bedtime from 9:00 p.m. to 8:00 p.m., they saw no benefit; but what these parents fail to appreciate is that their baby was starting to get drowsy around 7:00 p.m., so a second wind had already developed by 8:00. Obviously, watching your child closely for drowsy signs in the late afternoon and early evening is more valuable than watching the clock. If this is impossible due to the parents' work schedule, have a trustworthy caretaker look for the signs, or the parents themselves can do it on weekends, where there is more time.

Protect Naps Around 3–4 Months of Age

As your baby becomes more aware of her environment, she is less likely to sleep well in brightly lit or noisy places in the stroller. A goal is to use her emerging nap rhythms as an aid to obtain long periods of deep day sleep. Nap rhythms begin to emerge around 3–4 months of age. Now parents have the opportunity to "catch the wave" of developing drowsiness and synchronize their soothing to a drowsy-but-awake state with the wave before it crashes into a second wind. The midmorning nap becomes more regular before the midday nap. Typically, the approximate times are around 9:00 a.m. and between 12:00 and 2:00 p.m. An additional nap or naps occur in the late afternoon or early evening. The midmorning and midday naps may be brief at first, but between 4 and 6 months of age they become more predictable and longer, so that each one is one to two hours long. Often there is one late afternoon nap that may not occur every day and is usually less than the midmorning and midday naps.

After 3 to 6 months of age, it is possible to inadvertently put your baby to sleep for a nap before or past the time of her biological drowsiness, with the unwanted consequence of accumulating a sleep deficit from no naps or poor-quality naps. Please remember that good-quality naps are those that occur during the biologic rhythm of daytime drowsiness, and naps while you are outside and in motion might be less restorative than motionless naps at home or in a quiet park.

One parent wrote, "My 4-month-old is still getting the kinks out of cycles, and so I am starting to go by the clock more for his midday nap. But I am still going by sleep cues for the midmorning nap."

No Television or Other Digital Media Devices in the Bedroom

Having a television in your child's bedroom is an invitation for sleep problems. A 2007 nationally representative survey showed that

18 percent of children under 2 years of age had a television in their bedroom. This number rose to 43 percent for 3- and 4-year-olds and to a whopping 75 percent for 5- and 6-year-olds. If these statistics are true, and there is little reason to doubt them, an entire generation of children is at risk of the serious developmental and other health-related problems that cluster around the failure to learn proper sleep habits at a young age. Much attention has been focused recently on the subject of childhood obesity, and rightly so, but our modern lifestyle is contributing to another epidemic, one less visible, perhaps, than obesity, but no less pernicious in the long run.

Prevention Versus Treatment of Sleep Problems

There sometimes appears to be a contradiction about whether or not to let your child cry. For the 80 percent of babies who have common fussiness, if the parents have ample resources for soothing, sleep solutions that involve *no crying*—such as starting early to teach self-soothing, utilizing many hands (that is, enlisting the help of the father and others), putting the baby down drowsy but awake, providing the opportunity for many naps, feeding only at night when hungry, instituting bedtime routines, starting an earlier bedtime around 6 weeks of age, and protecting naps around 3 to 4 months of age—should work to *prevent* sleep problems. A few of this group of common fussy babies (5 percent, or four out of a hundred babies) do become very overtired 4-month-olds. When you try to treat or correct the sleep problem, some crying might occur. However, in this group, improvement in sleep patterns and improvement in the child is often dramatic and rapid.

For the 20 percent of babies with extreme fussiness or colic, however, if the parents have enormous resources for soothing, sleep solutions that involve no crying—such as always holding your baby, always promptly responding, and soothing your baby as long as needed to induce sleep—might work to *prevent* sleep problems. But about 27 percent of these twenty extremely fussy/colicky babies (or five out of a hundred babies) do become very overtired 4-month-olds. *Treatment* to correct the sleep problem might involve more crying, and improvement in sleep patterns and improvement in the child are often slow and not dramatic. This is especially hard for parents because they have already endured 4 months of sleep deprivation associated with the child's constant fussiness, crying, and not sleeping.

Some parents allow their child to cry to help him sleep before 4 months of age (see page 126, and Chapters 4–6). Perhaps they started to encourage self-soothing when their baby was several weeks old, saw improvement, and wanted to quickly end the sleep deprivation that they and their child have experienced. Another example is the mother who has to return to work and desperately wants to see if her child will sleep better at night with less attention. Another example is the exhausted and overwhelmed mother who is becoming depressed or getting angry or resentful toward her baby. Under these and similar circumstances, I usually try to enlist the assistance of the father to help his wife put the baby to sleep, to feed and soothe the baby at night, and to try to give the mother a well-earned break by making her go somewhere for several hours or a night to get some uninterrupted sleep. Obviously, these suggestions are impractical for some families. Nevertheless, the instructions are to give the child less attention at night, perhaps feeding only twice at night, and ignoring crying for either brief or long periods of time, and to do this for only four or five nights. Sometimes the crying quickly diminishes, especially in the child who had common fussiness. Sometimes the crying does not decrease, especially in the child who had extreme fussiness or colic, and the plan is abandoned. Parents then resort to whatever method maximizes sleep and minimizes crying until the child is older.

Parent Issues or Barriers That May Make Prevention or Treatment of Sleep Problems More Challenging

Parents can prevent sleep problems in their children by encouraging them to learn self-soothing skills. Some parents find this endeavor to be fairly straightforward, especially if their child has an easy temperament. Other parents struggle to accomplish this, especially if their child has a more difficult temperament. Putting aside the issue of infant temperament for now (see Chapter 7), you might ask why it is that some parents appear to find the teaching of self-soothing fairly manageable, while others find it an ongoing, frustrating challenge. In fact, sometimes allowing their child to learn self-soothing skills is simply too tough for some parents, and they give up completely. The short answer is that parents vary enormously in their ability to restore a calm balance to their lives after the baby is born, assuming that their lives were reasonably stable beforehand.

Imagine an idealized family in which there were no complications around the delivery for baby and mother. The marriage is strong, both parents are actively involved in parenting and agree on how to care for their child, there is no postpartum depression or baby blues, there is only the one child, breast-feeding is easy, there are no medical problems in the family, extra bedrooms are available for the child and those relatives and friends who want to help, there is adequate housekeeping and child care assistance, and the mother is under no financial pressure to return to work soon. In this lucky family, one might say that the parents have many resources to support them in their effort to teach self-soothing skills to their baby. Of course, most of us are not so fortunate! But even these parents might find themselves faced with unanticipated real-life challenges that would interfere with their ability to teach their child self-soothing skills. Job pressures, family emergencies, distractions large and small: all these and more can cause parents to overlook the subtle signs of drowsiness in their baby, and thus miss the window of opportunity to reinforce the baby's natural sleep rhythms.

But not to worry. We all can muddle through in our efforts to help our baby learn self-soothing skills, and most of us usually do, even though there may be some setbacks. Take heart! It might be three steps forward and one step back, but with patience and reasonable consistency, the reward of a well-rested family is within reach.

The greater your resources to soothe your baby during the first few months, and the better you are able to become attuned to your baby's changing sleep needs, the more likely your baby will sleep well during the first 4 months. That, in turn, will help you *prevent* sleep problems from developing after 4 months.

Now, if you are like most parents, you do not have an ideal soothing support system, so there are likely to be moments during the first few months when your child might become more irritable and fussy and cry more because, despite your best efforts, he or she becomes overtired. Don't let these frustrating occasions get you down. Stick with the overall plan. Perseverance pays off in the long run, but if you give up, your infant will not learn the self-soothing skills essential to preventing later sleep problems from emerging.

If you have the misfortune to be dealing with a colicky infant, who appears to have less ability to soothe him- or herself, your infant is likely to become mostly parent-soothed during the first few months. That is inevitable, and there is no reason to beat yourself up because of it. But after 4 months, even the colicky baby will more easily learn how to independently fall asleep and stay asleep. That is the time to start teaching self-soothing skills.

Parenting is the hardest work there is because there is no instruction manual that applies to all families. Not only that, but again and again, just when you think you've got the hang of it, your child changes and you have to start all over again. But if your baby sleeps well, you sleep well. Then not only will you be better able to figure out a plan that is a good fit for your family, you will be more adaptable to making changes in that plan as your baby changes.

Treatment of a sleep problem is more difficult when parents lack the resources that would have otherwise helped them teach self-soothing skills to their baby in the first few months. But sometimes there are parent issues or barriers that may make prevention and treatment of sleep problems more challenging. They make the hard work of parenting even harder. Some of these issues might be sensitive or highly personal matters that really could get in the way of your ability to do what is best for your child. Sometimes these barriers are only speed bumps that slow down the process of helping your child sleep better. However, if they are major roadblocks, then, before working on your child's sleep problem, consider professional counseling. In such cases, you cannot help your baby until you help yourself.

What do I mean by speed bumps or roadblocks? Here are some examples.

Parents lack information or tools. Your child does not come with a parenting manual. Starting in infancy or early childhood, parents may have unrealistic expectations or misunderstandings regarding age-appropriate sleep needs and sleep schedules. Or parents do not appreciate the benefits of healthy sleep and the harm caused by sleep deprivation in their children. Parents may be misguided or unaware regarding how to set limits, discipline, or socialize their children. Even if they have the right attitude, they may lack the proper techniques or tools and so become paralyzed or inconsistent.

Working parents' guilt, exhaustion, or absence. Parents may feel guilty because they are not available or do not want to be available to their child. So they give in to whatever their child wants. Or, selfishly, they feel that their child has to adapt to their work schedule and stay up late at night. A parent might truly believe that it is more important for the child to spend time late at night with his mother or father than it is for him to get more sleep from an earlier bedtime. Keeping a child up too late is more common with a parent who works outside the home, because he or she is not present to see the overtired child of late afternoon but instead sees only the child running on the fumes of a second wind. Sheer exhaustion from the demands of work may prevent the parent from being persistent and consistent. Too often, because of fatigue from work, the parent simply surrenders whenever the child cries. Sometimes the problem is neither guilt nor exhaustion but simply absence. Many modern parents do not do a lot of parenting. Because they spend so much time at work, they heavily rely on day care or nannies. They are in denial or do not see the seriousness of the problem. Fathers especially, who are often less involved in child care than mothers, tend to say dismissively, "He'll outgrow it" or "It's not a big deal."

Bad marriage. Three themes frequently occur here. The first is that one parent wants the child for support and love and thus becomes overly permissive in order to keep the child allied with him or her. This alliance maintains the parent's self-esteem. In the extreme version, one parent seeks the child's exclusive love as a means of expressing resentment or anger toward his or her spouse; in these cases, the child becomes a pawn in a struggle between mother and father. The second recurring theme is a control issue. A parent arrogantly asserts that he or she is right no matter what and knows best, end of story. There is no compromise in child raising. No shared philosophy. Just "my way or the highway." The third theme is lack of communication. The parents are unable to communicate effectively with each other to develop a practical plan that they can consistently implement. Thus they are constantly at loggerheads.

Parent has abandonment issues. Because they had bad relations with their own parents, new parents might desperately want their child to like them. New parents might feel that their parents were not in tune with their feelings as a child, so they want to be very sensitive to and always address their child's feelings. They want to be their child's best friend. They do not want their child to feel hurt as they did when they were children. This leads to giving in to their child's every demand. A variation is that the parent does not want to break his child's spirit or damage his self-esteem. In these cases, parents are projecting onto their child, seeing their child less as a unique individual than as a "do-over" for unresolved issues from their own childhoods.

Parent has authority issues. Some parents do not feel comfortable enforcing rules and communicating authority. This could be for a variety of reasons. They are not comfortable with telling anyone what to do; they would rather ask for help. They might have a "live and let live" philosophy and do not want to enforce rules. Or they behave as if rules do not apply to them; because they act irresponsibly and cannot say no to themselves (with illicit drug use, for example), they cannot say no to their child. In the extreme version, a parent wants to be rebellious but cannot, and so the parent gets some gratification in seeing their child being rebellious.

Family stress issues. Parents facing money worries, job pressures and responsibilities, the illness of a loved ones, or other sources of stress often do not have the energy to establish routines, plan events, or create schedules such as sleep times. In such cases, family life is chaotic, lurching from crisis to crisis. The parents are reactive instead of proactive; they respond emotionally instead of thoughtfully. These parents are not necessarily overindulgent; instead, they are overly inconsistent.

Parent has undiagnosed anxiety disorder, depression, attention deficit hyperactivity disorder (ADHD), bipolar disorder, or other mental health problem. Anxiety disorders occur in 18 percent of U.S. adults, depression in 5 percent, ADHD in 4 percent, and bipolar disorder in 1 percent. When a person is sleep deprived, the symptoms associated with these conditions can worsen. In this setting, education and coaching to help solve a sleep problem may fail because of the parent's significant unrecognized or untreated mental health issues. Adult ADHD occurs equally in mothers and fathers. But problems regarding parenting are especially prominent if the mother is affected, because she is the one who is usually expected to organize schedules and routines such as regular bedtimes and naps.

In a study of more than seven thousand children between 1 and 2 years of age, researchers compared those who frequently woke during the night with those who slept through the night (see "Injuries," Chapter 11). Among those who frequently woke during the night, the parents, usually mothers, were more likely, compared to the parents of infants who slept through the night, to *immediately go to their child when they heard a cry in order to prevent further crying.* These mothers were more likely to describe themselves as more irritable in general and "out of control." A sign of family tension was that these mothers were unable to confide in their husbands. Two additional studies on night-sleep awakenings focused on the role of maternal depression.

An extensive study by Dr. Marsha Weinraub of risk factors for nighttime sleep awakenings between 6 and 36 months of age was published in 2012. The study identified the following risk factors: being a boy, having a more difficult temperament, being breast-fed (being nursed to sleep), having a more depressed mother, and greater maternal sensitivity. Maternal sensitivity was measured by videotaping mother-child interactions in a semistructured play activity. Maternal sensitivity means that, in Dr. Weinraub's words, "rather than allow infants to self-soothe and return to sleep on their own, parents who respond to awakenings with attempts to comfort or feed may interfere with their infant's growing ability to self-soothe and return to sleep independently. Parent responsiveness to infant night awakening may reinforce infants' signaling behavior following awakening and teach them to expect parental interventions. Alternatively, a lack of parental responsiveness can eventually . . . extinguish the signaling behaviors. Findings support this notion. *Feeding after awakening* [even when the child was not hungry] *was the factor most strongly associated with infants not sleeping through the night* at 5 months, and parental presence until sleep onset was the factor most strongly associated with sleep awakening at 17 and 29 months" (emphasis added). The lead researcher in the study said, "The best advice is to put infants to bed at a regular time every night, allow them to fall asleep on their own [that is, put them down drowsy but awake] and *resist the urge to respond right away to awakenings*" (emphasis added). Contrary to what was seen in other studies, "infant-mother attachment measures were not related to these sleep awakenings . . . despite our attempt to use measures of attachment security and separation distress." These identical results of unnecessary attending to their child at night were found in another study of maternal depression.

A study by Dr. Douglas Teti investigated the relationship between maternal depressive symptoms and their children's sleep issues. Because these researchers discovered the maternal behavior by which maternal *depressive symptoms* affect infant sleep, I wish to present this study in detail. The researchers documented what the mother was actually doing and not doing by placing multiple cameras in the home and child's bedroom:

> In the context of infant sleep, mothers who harbor cognitions that their infant will feel abandoned if they are not by the infant's side during the night or that their infant will go hungry if not fed (even when the infant is not distressed) may be more likely to spend more time with their infants at bedtime and at night and in turn awaken their infant more frequently or keep them awake longer than mothers who do not harbor such cognitions. . . . Mothers reporting higher depressive symptoms [were much more likely to] not have a calming bedtime routine for their infant. Prior to the infants' bedtime, these mothers had the television on, allowed older children to play rough/make loud noises near the infant, appeared insensitive to the infant's needs (e.g., hunger), and kept their infants awake after the infant appeared ready for sleep. . . . [They] were observed responding very quickly to infant vocalizations. For example, a mother of a 12-month-old infant appeared to be hyperattentive to her infant during the night. She responded to nondistressed vocalizations very quickly throughout the night. . . . Two other mothers were observed waking their sleeping infants unexpectedly during the night. Consider the mother of a 1-month-old

infant who woke her nondistressed, sleeping infant during the night (i.e., not for the purposes of feeding) and brought the baby to the parents' bed for the rest of the night. *This behavior was only observed among mothers reporting higher symptoms of depression.* A final behavior observed included mothers' inability to set appropriate limits with their children after bedtime and during the night, especially among older children. . . . The most striking example of this included a mother who appeared unable to structure bedtime for her 24-month-old infant. As the rest of the family went to sleep, this infant remained awake until 2:00 a.m. with a TV that remained on in the bedroom, occasionally wandering out of the bedroom to other areas of the home. This mother eventually brought her infant close to her and held her until she fell asleep. (Emphasis added.)

The researchers concluded:

Mothers with elevated depressive symptoms and worries about infant nighttime needs were more likely . . . to be hyperresponsive to nondistressed infant vocalizations (i.e., babbling or cooing that did not appear to function as a signal for parental assistance), to pick up and nurse the infants even when it appeared that the infants were not in need of nursing, to go to their soundly sleeping infants and move them from their cribs to the parents' bed to sleep (and in the process, wake their infant up), and to poorly structure bedtimes that in turn led to prolonged infant wakefulness. We suspect that mothers who *worry excessively* about their infants' well-being at night may be motivated to seek out and intervene with their infants, regardless of whether the infants require intervention or not, in order to alleviate *mothers' anxieties* about whether their infants are hungry, thirsty, uncomfortable, and so on. We suspect that mothers with elevated *depressive symptoms* may be motivated to spend time with their infant at night in order to satisfy mothers' emotional needs. (Emphasis added.)

In a nutshell, both studies observed that among mothers with *depressive* symptoms, the mothers' behavior at nighttime was associated with infant night waking because they incorrectly believed ("dysfunctional cognition") that they had to attend to their nondistressed infants and feed them even if they had just been fed.

This research emphasizes a mother-driven path of influence (see Chapter 5) whereby the mother's depressive symptoms and dysfunctional cognition about infant sleep behavior causes maternal nighttime behavior that causes infant night waking. The other direction, or an infant-driven path of influence, is also possible. Here, infant night waking (a baby with colic) causes maternal night behavior that causes both mother's depressive symptoms and mother's dysfunctional cognitions about infant sleep behavior. This second path appeared to be a contributing factor in the research by Dr. Teti discussed above: "It is very possible that both mother- and infant-driven influences are at play in terms of linkages between maternal depressive symptoms and infant night waking." So the directionality of effects probably goes both ways.

The good news is that parents with depressive symptoms can be helped! Education about sleep helps parents: A 2014 paper titled "Preventing early infant sleep and crying problems and postnatal depression: A randomized trial" showed that "Education about sleep and cry behavior at about 4 weeks caused caregivers to attend to infant night feeding less." And another paper concluded that prevention is successful when "Once the baby is 3 weeks old, healthy, and putting on weight normally, they can begin to delay feedings when baby wakes at night, in order to dissociate waking from feeding. This is done gradually, using [diaper] changing or handling to introduce a delay, and does not involve leaving babies to cry."

Therapist failure

Sometimes a therapist has preconceived ideas that he or she attempts to shoehorn onto every family. Such therapists do not listen to parents and will often press them to try something experience has shown not to work for that particular family. Or the therapist gives good advice but fails to make clear to the parents that they must work every day to permanently prevent the problem from resurfacing. I see this time and time again in my patients. For example, after working hard to successfully correct a sleep problem caused by a bedtime that was too late, the parent asks me if he can now keep his child up later at night, since everyone is sleeping better!

Successful therapists such as Dr. Karen Pierce, a child psychiatrist, often start by asking a fundamental question: "There are many barriers to change. Is it the child, is it the parent, is it the couple, is it the larger family, or outside stress issues?" She emphasizes the importance of locating the particular barrier that prevents particular parents from solving problems. Identifying and dealing with the barrier allows the family to focus their energy on the solution to the child's sleep issue.

Dr. Robert Daniels, a child psychologist, often starts with questions such as: "What is the desired behavior you want from your child? What is the desired outcome? What is the endpoint of treatment? What would you like to see happen?" Both parents need to agree on what the goal is and how to achieve the goal before beginning a treatment plan. The failure to agree on a goal makes it difficult for parents to cooperate with each other to achieve success. Dr. Daniels observes that most parents agree on the goal but not necessarily on the path to accomplish the goal.

Child psychologist Dr. Vicki Lavigne emphasizes that parents have to see the connection between what they do and the effect it will have on the behavior of the child. Parents have to be more focused on their behavior than worrying that their child has a problem or peculiar trait. For example, focusing on "He has a strong will" instead of your own behavior interferes with success.

Dr. John Bates, another child psychologist, encourages families to cast a wide net and seek support by talking to relatives and close friends, community mental health groups, parenting groups, or religious leaders, because resources and substantial support may be available but not known to new parents.

It is important for parents to try to figure out a way to separate their marriage issues from bedtime issues, compartmentalize other barriers, restructure their priorities, or seek professional counseling in order to heavily invest in soothing their newborn during the first few months. By gathering up all their resources for soothing during the first few months, parents are more likely to *prevent* sleep problems in the future.

Some parents may need professional help to establish reasonable, orderly home routines, to iron out conflicts between parents, or to help an older child with a well-established sleep problem. To maintain healthy sleep for your young child, you need the courage to be firm without feeling guilt or fear that she will resent you or love you less. In fact, the best prescription I can offer for a loving home is a well-rested child and well-rested parents.

THE MOST IMPORTANT POINT

If some of these speed bumps or roadblocks occur in your family, then work extra hard with what resources you have available to teach self-soothing during the first 4 months in order to *prevent* sleep problems from ever arising in the first place.

Summary and Action Plan for Exhausted Parents

1. *Teach self-soothing.* Learning self-soothing does not mean that your child will necessarily cry. Patience and perseverance will pay off.

Start early. It is never too late to start, but the earlier you start the easier it might be.

Many hands. Get Dad and others on board.

Put your child down drowsy but awake. Trial and error is needed to get it right.

2. *Soothing.* Find out what works for *your* baby. Don't compare babies. See page 116 for different ways to soothe your baby. To find out what works best for your baby, see page 397.

3. *Many naps.* After a brief interval of wakefulness, put your child down for a nap based on drowsy signs (see page 113) or clock time. This prevents a second wind. Sleep begets sleep!

Start early, right when you come home from the hospital, to put your child down, drowsy but awake, for a nap within one to two hours of waking up.

4. *Bedtime routines.* Consistency helps signal to your child, just like the yellow traffic light at the intersection, what will happen next. (See page 132).

5. *Breast-feeding versus formula, family bed versus crib.* These are decisions that should fit your family and not what someone else claims is best. The American Academy of Pediatrics discourages the family bed because of sudden infant death syndrome (see Chapter 3).

6. *Earlier bedtime around 6 weeks old.* Once your baby is older, go ahead and experiment with an earlier bedtime.

7. *Protect naps around 3–4 months of age.* Establishing good naps and an early bedtime may be socially limiting, but it is liberating to have a well-rested child.

8. *No screens in the bedroom. All* screen-based media in the bedroom at bedtime will interfere with healthy sleep.

9. *Prevention versus treatment of sleep problems.* Expect no crying with successful prevention of sleep problems; crying may occur to treat sleep problems that you created or when you help a post-colic baby learn self-soothing.

10. *Parent issues or barriers that may make prevention or treatment of sleep problems more challenging.* When certain parent issues (see page 150) are present, sleep problems are more likely to occur and persist. Recognition of these issues might lead to making a family plan of action, even before the baby is born, to help your baby sleep well, including, if necessary, seeking professional assistance.

CHAPTER 4

Sleep Solutions

The previous chapter, "Preventing Sleep Problems," could just as well have been titled "How to Establish Healthy Sleep Habits." Parents teach healthy habits such as hand washing, tooth brushing, wearing helmets when riding bikes, and wearing seat belts throughout their child's life. It's the same for healthy sleep habits. It's an ongoing process. This chapter, "Sleep Solutions," may also be an ongoing process—not a onetime cure like a penicillin shot for strep throat—because of natural disruptions of sleep schedules. Because sleep schedules often may get derailed, think of helping your child return to a healthy sleep schedule more as an ongoing regimen of *care* and not as a onetime *cure*.

All parents want their child to sleep well so they themselves can have more calm private time and get more sleep. Some parents do not fully appreciate how powerfully the beneficial effects of sleep directly help their child (Chapter 2) or, because of their own issues (including sleep deprivation), they find it difficult to make the lifestyle changes that are necessary to help their child sleep better (Chapter 3). Because changing lifestyle habits is hard for everyone and even harder if you are sleep deprived, I am presenting more facts in this chapter than you might think necessary. But I believe that more information is empowering and will encourage and enable you to make changes. Also, because you may be struggling with your own sleep deprivation, some points are deliberately repeated here and elsewhere so the message will really sink in.

An important first step in actually doing something to achieve healthy sleep is knowing for certain that your child's sleep is impaired. For a moment, focus on the following five behaviors that might indicate your child is not getting healthy sleep. These are some of the target behaviors we want to reduce or eliminate.

IS MY CHILD GETTING HEALTHY SLEEP?

After 3-4 months of age, you can tell that your child is not getting healthy sleep if these are present:

1. Witching hour behavior
2. Sleep inertia and/or wakes up crying (see Chapter 1)
3. Fatigue signs or a second wind before naps (see Chapters 1 and 3)
4. Often easily falls asleep in the afternoon in a moving stroller in public or in a car
5. Difficulty getting out of bed and/or headaches in the morning

Children who often show these behaviors are *short on sleep* (SOS). Think of SOS behaviors as a distress signal: "Help me, I need sleep!"

Here are a few typical questions and answers:

Q: *I don't believe in this kind of unnatural programming.*

A: Healthy sleep habits are learned, not innate. Unless you want your child to suffer the "natural" effects of chronic sleep fragmentation, you will have to help her learn how to sleep.

Q: *I've heard that if I nurse my baby to sleep, I'll create a night-waking problem.*

A: The issue isn't whether nursing to sleep is good or not, but rather whether nursing too frequently or nighttime nursing is part of a night-waking problem. Please include nursing, if you wish, in nap or bedtime rituals, but after you finish nursing, whether the child is asleep or awake, put her down, kiss her cheek, say good night, walk away, turn the lights off, and close the door.

Q: *I've heard that because my baby learns to associate my breast with falling asleep, she will be unable to return to sleep later in the night if my breast is not present.*

A: Nonsense! Almost all the mothers in my practice nurse their babies to sleep at bedtime, and at night, when the baby is hungry, either the mother nurses or the father bottle-feeds the child. Usually the babies are drowsy but not in a deep sleep when they are put down. I believe it is perfectly natural to nurse a baby to sleep, and by itself this act does not cause sleep disturbances. Older children can be very discriminating; they can learn to expect dessert after dinner, if that is the family custom, but not after breakfast. I think babies can also become very discriminating; they can learn to expect to be fed when they are hungry but not to be fed when they are not hungry in the middle of the night.

Q: *Once I let my child cry a long time and she vomited. Won't I be trading one problem for another?*

A: Consider other sleep strategies that involve less crying. However, if the vomiting always occurs, I think you will want to always go in to clean her promptly and then leave her again.

Q: *Won't my baby simply outgrow this habit?*

A: Believe it or not, 18-year-old college freshmen who don't sleep well had difficulties sleeping as infants, according to their mothers, as reported in one study. It seems that if the child doesn't have the early opportunity to practice falling asleep by herself, she'll never learn to fall asleep easily.

Q: *Even if she won't outgrow this habit, what's really wrong with my still going to her at night?*

A: Consider your own feelings. Good studies at Yale University show that all mothers eventually become anxious, develop angry feelings toward their child, and feel guilt about maintaining their child's poor sleep habits. These feelings may persist for years. If going to your child at night fragments her sleep, then eventually a cumulative sleep deficit will develop.

Sleep Solutions

TEACH SELF-SOOTHING

Self-soothing skills are the foundation upon which any successful sleep solution rests. Understanding how to teach self-soothing skills and the related subjects (bedtime routines, early bedtimes, protecting naps, and parent issues) will give you a perspective on what you wish to accomplish with any sleep solution that you choose. Please review these subjects in Chapter 3 and remember that all sleep solutions will not work or will not work quickly if your child gets a second wind at night from not napping well or from a bedtime that is too late.

When treating a sleep problem, the improvement in sleeping is *sequential,* not *simultaneous.* First, improvement will be seen for night sleep, then for the midmorning nap, and lastly for the midday nap. Improvement in night sleep may take only a few days, but improvement in naps may take longer.

EXTINCTION (OR UNMODIFIED EXTINCTION)

Extinction, sometimes called unmodified extinction, means that after your child is put to bed, he is ignored, except for feedings, without time limit until morning to allow him to develop self-soothing skills. Of course, parents practicing extinction are mindful of and monitor issues of safety and illness. If you think your child might be ill, rush to your child, feel the forehead for fever and take the temperature if needed, and look for signs of distress such as vomiting or difficulty breathing. But if when you arrive he smiles at you with a look of "Gotcha!" or appears well, turn around and leave without social interaction or soothing.

Going in to soothe sometimes and not going in at other times is called "intermittent reinforcement." Intermittent reinforcement is a powerful way to teach your child to cry louder, longer, and more frequently at night, because he is sometimes rewarded by his effort to enjoy the pleasure of your company. This will occur even if your curtain calls involve minimal soothing such as only shushing or soft stroking. For your baby, even minimal social contact is a very powerful motivator. For extinction to work, there should consistently be no social contact except for the feeding that you have chosen.

After initial success, several days or weeks later, expect a *response burst:* a reappearance of crying or calling out for attention. Because it is now out of character, rush to your child to make sure he is healthy. Most likely he will stop crying and smile at you when you arrive. Maintain silence, kiss him, and leave. No soothing. Your child is testing to see whether he can return to the old style. This is frustrating for parents because they misinterpret it as a failure or a setback. No, it is to be expected. Stay the course.

Night-sleep rhythms emerge around 6 weeks of age, so extinction might be used after 6 weeks of age to get night sleep in sync with sleep rhythms, but most commonly extinction is used after a few months of age. Nevertheless, it can work earlier: parents' reports of success in helping babies, even with colic, sleep better starting at *3–4 weeks* are described in Chapters 3 and 5.

For children over 3–4 months of age, when nap rhythms emerge, extinction might be used for only one hour at nap times.

Not responding to your child at night is most difficult for parents. It may not always be clear if your baby is hungry or not. Between 6–8 weeks and 4 months, some but not all babies might be hungry and need to be bottle-fed two or three times a night, but after 4 months, only once or twice, and after 9 months, not at all. The idea is to respond if you think your child is hungry but not at other times. This determination may be harder for a mother who is breast-feeding, because of uncertainty regarding her breast milk supply. When breast-feeding, if every suck is followed by a swallow, he is probably hungry. If you really think he is hungry, feed him. The middle-of-the night feeding is done lovingly but silently and without lots of social interaction. After the feeding, the child is put back in bed with a single kiss or brief hug, but the return to sleep is not associated with prolonged soothing.

If your full-term child is several weeks old and needs to be fed at night, then the parents may choose to wait at least four hours after the last feeding, because babies this age can go without a feeding for four hours. For example, if your baby is fed at a 7:00 p.m. bedtime, do not attend to your child or go to feed before 11:00 p.m. Also, in the middle of the night (around 11:00 p.m. to midnight), your baby might vigorously suck during this first feeding and suck more leisurely a few hours later (for example, at 2:00–3:00 a.m.) and again appear to be hungry at 4:00–5:00 a.m. If this pattern occurs, always attend to your child for the strong feeding in the middle of the night and in the morning around 4:00–5:00 a.m. but ignore the feeding in between (2:00–3:00 a.m.). A common pattern is to feed only twice overnight.

Fathers may give a bottle of expressed breast milk or formula to help clarify whether the baby is hungry or not. Having Dad give a bottle at different times and watching how much and how fast your baby feeds might make it clear when he is really hungry. Whenever a bottle is given, watch your child's behavior and do not count ounces: when he really slows down in his sucking, end the feeding. Otherwise, the time spent trying to "top him off," with the misguided idea that he will sleep longer, is lost deep sleep for your child and for you.

When parents avoid unnecessary feedings at night and remove

themselves as reinforcers of crying at bedtime or nighttime, crying decreases and then disappears. Giving your child less attention at night allows the sleep process to surface and lull her to sleep. Because night sleep and social smiling develop around 6 weeks of age, it is possible after this point that parents' attempts to soothe at night might be more socially stimulating than soothing. Too much middle-of-the-night soothing will interfere with the naturally evolving sleep wave, teaching the child to fight sleep in order to enjoy more parental contact.

If your baby is hungry at night, feed your baby at night. If your baby is sleepy at night, let your baby sleep at night.

Extinction with a Cap
Some parents might wish to put a cap on the number of minutes of ignoring their child so they know they are not committing to endless crying. They fear that the crying will persist for hours. I recommend a cap of forty-five minutes. This cap may give you the peace of mind of knowing that you are not committing to ignoring crying forever and may enable you to have the confidence to try extinction. A much briefer cap might allow your child to learn to cry to the time limit and be rewarded by parental soothing. Crying for more than forty-five minutes typically occurs only when your child is extremely fatigued from not napping well or a bedtime is too late.

Extinction with Parental Presence
Some parents feel more comfortable using extinction if they remain in the room until their child falls asleep. Extinction with parental presence is based on the unproven assumption that sleep problems are due to separation anxiety. The parent remains in the room during the extinction procedure and can incorporate "fading out," whereby the parent gradually leaves the bedroom. This approach often takes at least seven nights to achieve results.

Crying is hard, but sleeplessness is harder.

Q: *With extinction, how long will my child cry?*

A: If, and only if, all the elements of self-soothing are in place (these elements, including enlisting many hands for help, putting your baby down drowsy but awake, and allowing many naps, as discussed in Chapter 3), the bedtime is not too late, and a child who is older than 4 months of age is napping well, the process usually takes only three to five nights. In children who are short on sleep, there may be multiple bouts of crying of forty-five to fifty-five minutes the first night; the crying bouts on the second night are usually a little more or a little less. The reason there may be more crying on the second night, especially for older children, is that your child is trying harder to get your attention. The third night is much better (bouts of twenty to forty minutes), and by the fourth or fifth night there is no crying. Your baby will likely cry less at sleep onset if Dad is putting the baby down after soothing and Mom has left the house. This process might take longer for an older and for a post-colic child. For children under 4 months of age without colic, there may be less crying.

Parents who do not see a rapid improvement usually do not have all the elements of self-soothing in place, and/or the bedtime is too late, and/or naps are not going well, and/or there is some other inconsistency in their approach to sleep.

In my research for *Healthy Sleep Habits, Happy Twins*, I found that many parents quickly became extremely sleep deprived because of double-duty feeding at night and consequently did extinction when the twins were younger than 4 months old (counting from the due date). For twins who have an early bedtime and naps in place, extinction usually takes three to five nights. In general, the first night was associated with thirty to forty-five minutes of crying, the second night ten to thirty minutes, and the third night up to ten minutes. This suggests that *there is less crying associated with extinction when performed earlier than 4 months of age.*

I think there may be circumstances when a trial of extinction or extinction with a cap is warranted *at night* shortly after 6 weeks of age (counting from the due date), because night sleep is becoming organized around this time. I hesitate to list the exact circumstances because my list could not cover all the possible variables that might go into making this decision. Briefly, when the parents are extremely stressed, the child's sleep is worsening or not improving despite the parents' heroic efforts, and other methods are not working or are considered by the parents to be unlikely to help, I think a five-night trial of extinction or extinction with a cap may be considered. Ideally, you try to maximize daytime sleep and minimize daytime crying by whatever soothing method works (for example, swings). And you might temporarily abandon attempts at putting your child down drowsy but awake. But it is necessary that you start the night sleep before your baby gets a second wind (put the baby to bed at 6:00–8:00 p.m., or earlier if needed). Practically, this might be started on a Saturday when both parents are available to work together as a team. Feed your baby at night whenever you think she is truly hungry, even more than twice if needed. If after the fifth night there is no clear improvement in night sleep, I would give it up, do whatever works to maximize night sleep, and consider trying again in a couple of weeks. Discuss your situation with your pediatrician, so that you can feel sure that your child is healthy and gaining weight well.

I know that this will help some babies shortly after 6 weeks to sleep better at night. When this fails, I do not know whether the lack of success resides in issues involving the baby (such as colic), the parents (such as inconsistency), or parent-child interactions (too many or unnecessary feedings). The most common reason for failure is a bedtime that is too late, so that your child develops a second wind.

Seeing is believing, so here are some reports from parents who successfully used extinction.

We did extinction around 8 weeks for my first two children. The first was colicky, and I was at my wits' end. The second was one of those kids whose sleep was worsening. After she got out of the "sleep around the clock" phase, around 6 weeks she started sleeping less and less at night—up for hours at midnight or 2:00 a.m. I was depressed, and my husband was the hero, sleeping with her in the living room so it didn't disturb me. Oh, and we had an 18-month-old at the time, too! By the third night, both babies were falling asleep, on their own, at a good time, and sleeping all night (with a couple of feeds). While I sometimes feel guilty about doing it so early, and wonder if I could have just stuck it out, I don't really regret it. We did do full-on extinction. My first, the colicky one, was much worse off when we tried checking and leaving. With my second, we just saw how well it had worked with the first and did it. I went in on the first night after she had cried for two hours, nursed, and she went to sleep, but it didn't hurt progress at all.

I used extinction for my first two children at around 2 months. Both were still being swaddled at the time, and we kept them swaddled through extinction. They did not use pacifiers and did not suck fingers or thumb (though both started around 5 months). So it is entirely possible to do extinction with a swaddled baby (we started unswaddling them around 4 or 5 months with no problem at all). But if you know your son likes to suck on his fingers or thumb, then you can unswaddle him, too. A lot of parents decide to just do it all at once.

When Ron and I interviewed and selected our pediatrician before David was born, we left his office comfortable with the care we felt our child would receive. Although we knew the doctor had a special interest in sleep disorders, we never dreamed we would be faced with a baby whose internal clock thought day was night and night was day.

Oh, it didn't happen right away. In fact, the first few weeks were spent nursing and changing diapers in between. At the same time, I was beginning to relax and feel, yes, everything is going along normally. David became more alert; Ron and I knew it was a great step in his development. We looked forward to his periods of wakefulness as a time to interact with him. But a pattern began to develop: David didn't want to go to bed at night.

The doctor listened to what we were going through and assured us that, first of all, this was normal for some babies. David was really too young to go through sleep training at 6 weeks. So Ron and I resigned ourselves to some more of the same.

When David was 2 months old I began to panic. My maternity leave would soon be over. I could barely stand up most of the time, I was so tired. I also wanted to continue to nurse David whenever I was home. I knew we had to do something before I went back to work. So we called Dr. Weissbluth and made an appointment to see him.

First, the doctor checked David's physical condition. He was in perfect health. Then we talked. Dr. Weissbluth explained that we would have to make some changes in the way we handled David's sleep periods. David was to have a quiet, darkened room when sleeping. No more night-light, music, et cetera. Naps should last at least forty-five minutes to an hour. If David got up sooner, we were to leave him there until he got the rest he needed. Instead of letting David stay up late, we were told to put him to bed between 7:00 and 9:00 p.m. No rides in cars, strollers, or swings, where sleep occurred for a short time.

We decided to start that next Monday, since Sunday was Mother's Day. I nursed David at 9:00 p.m., and by 9:30 p.m.

he was asleep in my arms. I tiptoed him into bed and crept back to the living room and turned on the intercom. It was quiet until 9:45, when I heard David sucking his fingers. I thought, "Okay, he'll get back to sleep soon," but by ten o'clock the crying began. David cried until twelve-thirty—two and a half hours. For every cry I heard I shared his frustration, anger, and seeming pain. And I was angry—at David, the doctor, Ron, and myself. Finally, David fell asleep, and he slept until 6:45 the next morning, when I woke him to nurse.

The morning wake-up was planned and agreed to with Dr. Weissbluth. The idea was to get David to wake before I left for work so that I could nurse him. David seemed fine. I was exhausted.

Tuesday I let David wake himself up. That day he took naps ranging between two and three and a half hours, but his schedule was rather loose. At 8:30 that night, when he woke up, I fed, bathed, and played with him until he had one last nursing and I put him to bed, although he was not asleep, at 10:50 p.m.—this was later than Dr. Weissbluth had recommended. This time he cried from 10:50 until 11:15. Only twenty-five minutes? Could it be this easy? I was very encouraged. Weeks of David's inability to get to sleep at night seemed to be at an end. Once again he slept through the night.

Although we were still unsuccessful at getting David to bed early, the periods of crying himself to sleep were getting shorter. On day three he cried for twenty-one minutes and then didn't let out another peep until the next morning.

Just when Ron and I began to let out our breaths, David put us back in our places. On day four David cried for nearly an hour and a half. My spirits dropped. Was this just a temporary setback, or had the last three days been a fluke?

We found that if we responded to him quickly, assuming

he wanted to nurse, he became irritable and difficult to feed. Those were the nights the crying seemed to go on forever.

At the end of our third week of sleep training, David, Ron, and I really had our acts together. Ron and I could tell when David was ready to call it a day, and we didn't push him to stay up any later than he wanted.

My son, who was 11 weeks at the time, was extremely colicky. Having experienced colic in the past with my daughter (different type of colic, with more constant fussing and less crying), I felt that there might be the possibility of sleep training now rather than waiting until he was post-colic, around 4 months old. Not only was it for his sake, but in all honesty it was for us as a family also. We are so worn out and my poor little guy is so sleep deprived. We started putting him down at 5:30 p.m. and did complete extinction. Within four or so days he started doing much longer stretches at night and better, not great, but definitely better sleep during the day as well. He still has days that seem more colicky than others, but our bedtime routine and early bedtime have made a world of difference for him.

I started sleep-training my first at 10 weeks and my second at 12 weeks. My oldest was an extremely fussy baby who was insanely sleep deprived, and waiting until he was 16 weeks old to sleep-train him seemed impossible! While I was ready for him to sleep, I wasn't nearly as ready as I thought I was to hear all of the crying while training him! Regardless, he was ready, even if he didn't know it, because he needed sleep! We went from co-sleeping to putting him in his crib, so it was a significant difference for him. While he did cry, after the first couple of nights he fell asleep very quickly on his own in his crib. Soon thereafter, he began going to sleep at 5:00 p.m. to make up for all of his lost sleep and waking up at 7:00 a.m. He did wake to eat, but would go back to sleep on his own. Our second, who is much easier than our first, already could soothe himself to sleep pretty well. After the first two nights of sleep training, he made immense leaps and bounds. I found that it was more me who was not ready to sleep-train, less the kids, but once I sucked it up (and had my husband hold me back from going in to check on them when they cry) they became happier kids, and I became a happier, less tense mom. You need to keep reminding yourself about the big picture, and one day you'll thank yourself for doing what seemed impossible and heart-wrenching.

We just utilized the total extinction method for our 3-month-old (13 weeks) son. It took three or four days (the first two days of which were quite difficult) but has been unbelievably successful and a lifesaver for our family and our son. At least in our case, 3 months old was the right time for him. Essentially he would only sleep tightly swaddled in his car seat with a pacifier. We had to constantly reinsert his pacifier every 15 minutes or he would cry and wake. It was exhausting for both us and him as his sleep was terribly choppy. We tried graduated extinction at various times from 8 to 12 weeks—waiting ten, fifteen, or twenty minutes before going in to soothe—but he would always outlast us. Last week at 3 months old we decided to utilize total extinction, and while extremely difficult emotionally, it has been an unbelievable success. The process took three or four days. The first night we put him to sleep at 6:30 p.m. and he cried almost ninety minutes—he had a second wind. It was heartbreaking, as most parents experience. He then slept until his normal feeding time of 1:00 a.m. but had several night wakings where we allowed him to cry. The second night he cried approximately sixty minutes. He woke only for his two feedings. Next we moved his bedtime up half an hour to 6:00 p.m.

He cried for just five minutes and then woke only for his feed-ings. Last night he did not cry at all when he was put down! He slept his longest stretch of sleep ever—eight hours—then woke to eat. He had one second night waking to eat and then slept until 7:30 a.m. rather than the 6:00 a.m. waking he has been having. His naps are also now falling into place, and he is finally sleeping on his own, in his crib without a swaddle, taking three or four naps a day of one to three hours each. He goes down for a nap after an hour to an hour and a half of wake time. He is now going to sleep for naps and nighttime without any crying, and waking up coo-ing and smiling in his crib rather than crying. While it took several days and was emotionally very difficult (and perhaps not over yet), his overall crying has gone from constant to very infrequent, and he is sleeping wonderfully. When he is awake he is alert, smiling, and interactive. I am sure we will have to continue to reinstitute the technique as he grows, but it has been so worthwhile.

We had success with my 4-month-old son (he's now 2 years old). We decided on extinction because it seemed to be likely to cause everyone, including my son, the least amount of stress. Our plan was to get him to a sleepy state and make sure all of his needs were met, and then put him down to bed awake. The first night, he cried for 35 minutes, and I cried, too. But then he slept seven hours! He woke once and went back to sleep for four more hours! I thought I'd died and gone to heaven. He was in a much better mood the next day, and his napping was much better as well. I began to wonder if this was really my son! The next night, he cried for twenty minutes and then slept for nine hours straight before waking. He was even more content and had even better naps the next day. I'll never forget how he had his first night without waking on Labor Day, a few days after starting the extinction method. I told everyone that it felt like a gift for all of my motherly labors. After a few days, he no longer cried when I put him down. My husband and I are such believers that babies/children (and parents!) need sleep to function well. We call what we did for him "sleep empowerment."

An important element for success is an early bedtime that prevents a second wind from developing. In general, using extinction past 4 months of age may be more difficult for the parents because everyone is more stressed from sleep deprivation and habits are more ingrained. But it still works quickly!

At 6 months of age, Stephen was strong, happy, and healthy in every respect but one—he didn't sleep well. He did all his daytime napping in the car, the stroller, or our arms. If we put him in his crib, he awoke immediately and cried until we picked him up. His nighttime pattern was different but equally exhausting. He went to sleep in his crib promptly at 8:00 p.m. but usually awoke within the first hour for a brief comforting, and two or three times between 11:00 p.m. and 5:00 a.m. for a feeding.

This routine was taking its toll. I was almost as tired as when Stephen was a newborn, and I had no emotional re- serve for handling everyday problems. I was sharp with the rest of the family and got angry if my husband was even ten minutes late getting home from work. We needed to make a change. We had the weekend ahead of us, when my hus- band would be around for support, so we decided to start that night.

We put the baby to bed at 8:00 p.m., and he awoke for the first time around nine-thirty. We didn't go in to him, and he cried for twenty minutes before going back to sleep. He awoke again around 2:00 and 4:00 a.m. and cried about twenty minutes each time. When he cried at 6:00 a.m., I rushed into his room, anxious to hold him and be sure he was the same healthy, happy baby I had put down the night before.

Over the next few days it was amazing to see how quickly he fell into the schedule we had set up for him. He cried ten to fifteen minutes several times, but never again for an hour. Now he naps regularly and sleeps all night, occasionally crying for one or two minutes during the night as he puts himself back to sleep.

Letting my baby cry was one of the hardest things I've ever had to do. Now that the experience is behind us, however, I have no doubt at all that it was right. It gave me more confidence in my abilities to handle tough issues as a parent.

I read that you should always take your baby everywhere and "wear" your baby like the Native Americans did. I carried him around in a Bjorn baby carrier on walks and to do errands. By the time he was 10 months old, his nighttime routine was established. I would nurse him to sleep at 8:00 p.m., put him in his crib, and he would wake up at 10:00 p.m. and cry. I would change him and nurse him back to sleep, and carefully, oh so carefully, put him back in his crib, and repeat this process all night every two or so hours. Sometimes he would wake up when I put him back in bed and I would have to start all over again. As the night progressed, and he became more and more exhausted, he was more likely to wake up when I put him down, and it took longer to soothe him back to sleep. By 6:00 a.m. he was up for the day, napping occasionally and only briefly. Sometimes I couldn't even put him down long enough to eat dinner. I held him while I ate. One night I went to him when he cried and nursing did not soothe him. He could not stop cry-

ing no matter what I did. I realized at that moment that he didn't need me so much as he needed to sleep. We were all exhausted.

We had heard about "crying it out" before, and I thought it sounded cruel. But my husband wanted to do it, and it was clear that we had to change our methods, because although I was perfectly willing to deprive myself of sleep on his behalf, Ares was clearly suffering from sleep deprivation. Ares had all the symptoms of an overtired child. He was easily startled, and cried uncontrollably at sudden or loud noises. He was unable to go to sleep on his own, and unable to stay asleep once he did. The book explained that in going to Ares every time he cried at night, I was stimulating him and keeping him awake, not soothing him and reassuring him as I had thought. All that stuff I had read about "nighttime parenting" and "attachment parenting" was not only not helping, it was hurting Ares. We decided to try extinction.

The first night I put Ares to bed at 8:00 p.m. as usual, but when ten o'clock came and he cried, I didn't go to him. It was one of the hardest things I have ever done, but I wanted to give it a try for his sake. He cried for forty-five minutes. I thought I would die. My nervous system went haywire. I cried, my whole body got hot, I was shaking and sweating, and my heart pounded. "He's going to think I abandoned him," I thought. "He will never trust me again." But once he stopped crying he slept all night long. Ares had never slept for more than four hours in a row. I thought for sure he had died. But he woke up the next morning happy and rested and then fell back to sleep a couple of hours later on his play rug, another first. Ares had never in his life fallen asleep without nursing.

We worked to make sure Ares got the sleep he needed. At night we developed a sleep ritual of bath time, reading to him, and nursing him at 6:00 p.m., and putting him down sleepy but awake. He took two naps a day, following a slightly abbreviated sleep ritual, and slept for two hours in the morning and one hour in the early afternoon. For some reason he didn't cry at nap time, he just went quietly to sleep. At night, however, for several weeks he still cried for forty-five minutes when I put him down. This was extremely difficult, even painful. But once he fell asleep he stayed asleep for twelve hours, which was incredible to me, and he was so much happier during the day that we stuck with it. In the daytime, he was so much calmer; he even seemed sleepier for the first few weeks. He almost never cried anymore, and his attention span was longer. Eventually Ares went to sleep without crying, and he still sleeps every night all night long, for at least twelve hours a night.

When I am doing a sleep consult, during the first two or three days mothers often call me, worried because there is still crying at night. Upon questioning, though, they might also describe a six-hour block of night sleep or a midmorning nap of two to three hours. When I ask if these events have ever occurred in the past, the answer is invariably "Never." Recognizing that a new, better sleeping event has occurred helps you accept the crying as a means to an end.

Here is an account that was published in a professional journal for psychologists, so please forgive the dry style of writing, which clearly describes that extinction is not harmful:

Case Report: The Elimination of Tantrum Behavior

Carl D. Williams

This paper reports the successful treatment of tyrantlike tantrum behavior in a male child by the removal of reinforcement. The subject child was approximately 21 months old. He had been seriously ill much of the first 18 months of his life. His health then improved considerably, and he gained weight and vigor. The child now demanded the special care and attention that had been given him over the many critical months. He enforced some of his wishes, especially at bedtime, by unleashing tantrum behavior to control the actions of his parents.

The parents and an aunt took turns in putting him to bed both at night and for the child's afternoon nap. If the parent left the bedroom after putting the child in his bed, the child would scream and fuss until the parent returned to the room. As a result, the parent was unable to leave the bedroom until after the child went to sleep. If the parent began to read while in the bedroom, the child would cry until the reading material was put down. The parents felt that the child enjoyed his control over them and that he fought off going to sleep as long as he could. In any event, a parent was spending from one-half to two hours each bedtime just waiting in the bedroom until the child went to sleep.

Following medical reassurance regarding the child's physical condition, it was decided to remove the reinforcement of this tyrantlike tantrum behavior. Consistent with the learning principle that, in general, behavior that is not reinforced will be extinguished, a parent or the aunt put the child to bed in a leisurely and relaxed fashion. After bedtime pleasantries, the parent left the bedroom and closed the door. The child screamed and raged, but the parent did not reenter the room. The duration of screaming and crying was measured from the time the door was closed.

The child continued screaming for forty-five minutes the first time he was put to bed. The child did not cry at all the second time he was put to bed. This is perhaps attributable to his fatigue from crying. By the tenth occasion, the child no longer whimpered, fussed, or cried when the parent left the room. Rather, he smiled as they left. The parents felt that he made happy sounds until he dropped off to sleep.

About a week later, the child screamed and fussed after the

aunt put him to bed, probably reflecting spontaneous recovery of the tantrum behavior by returning to the child's bedroom and remaining there until he went to sleep. It was necessary to extinguish this behavior a second time.

No further tantrums at bedtime were reported during the next two years.

It should be emphasized that the treatment in this case did not involve aversive punishment. All that was done was to remove the reinforcement. Extinction of the tyrantlike tantrum behavior then occurred.

No unfortunate side- or after-effects of this treatment were observed. At three and three-quarters years of age, the child appears to be a friendly, expressive, outgoing child. (Emphasis added.)

My daughter Chelsea is almost 3 years old. Putting her to bed has always been an ordeal. At 18 months of age she started to climb out of her crib anywhere from seventy-five to a hundred times a night. The problem seemed to be solved with the advent of a "big bed." She now sleeps through the night. However, having her stay in bed and fall asleep is still an ordeal.

I have yelled and screamed. I have used gates and locks on her door to physically keep her in her room. I have used treats as an incentive for positive reinforcement of desired behavior. Unfortunately, the only consistent behavior has been my inconsistency.

If Chelsea knows that I will put a gate on her bedroom door if she leaves her room, even once, then she will gradually conform and stay in her room. But there is a catch! She eventually will start to challenge my inconsistent behavior. One night she will appear in the living room and say, "Mom, I need a hug and kiss good night." As a parent, do you deny your child such a loving request and lock her in her room? So you give her a hug and kiss and send her off to bed again. Then the next night she wants water, and before long she's out of bed three or four times a night for hugs and kisses, water, Band-Aids, scary noises—you name it! Within a week, saying good night and falling asleep takes an hour or more. Then we have to start over. Webster's dictionary defines the word "consistent" as "free from self-contradiction; in harmony with." I long for the night when I'm in harmony with Chelsea.

As this mother said, "Unfortunately, the only consistent behavior has been my inconsistency." In other words, when a behavioral approach fails with older children, it almost always is not a failure of the method but rather a failure of the parents' resolve to implement it consistently

A father told me that it was painful for him and his wife to admit that what they had been doing was wrong and not good for their child. What were they doing? The child was several months of age, and they were going in about every two hours, every time the child cried a little. He said that it would have been much easier to blame or get angry with someone like me who said that too much attention at night was not good for their baby, and accuse me of giving bad advice, than it was to recognize that they were the ones responsible for her continued night wakings and irritability during the day. Another mother said that the reason some mothers and fathers have such strong emotional rejection of my advice is quite simple: parental guilt. Since they spend so little time with their child because they are both working, they feel bad and try to spend more time after work in the evening playing with their child. They cannot consider that the bedtime is too late for the child's health, so they conclude that my advice regarding early bedtimes must be incorrect. Some parents think that even if it is not incorrect, it must be harmful in the long run.

When parents stop reinforcing a child's night waking, the habit can be eliminated quickly. In fact, psychologists have shown that the more continuous or regular you are in reinforcing the night waking during the first few months, the more likely it will rapidly be reduced simply by stopping the reinforcing behavior. The advantages of ending the habit by not going to your baby at night are that the instructions are simple and easily remembered, and the whole process usually takes only a few days. But the seeming disadvantage is that a few nights of crying are unbearable for many parents. This procedure strikes many people as too harsh, too abrupt, or cruel. Those are personal value judgments, but bear in mind that this procedure is effective and safe. It works.

Please remember that providing minimal soothing in the middle of the night will sabotage your effort, and your child will cry longer and harder with the hope of receiving a major soothing intervention. Therefore, if you have decided to "rip the Band-Aid off" with extinction, then do not go to your child at all except for a feeding.

> Small soothing efforts such as kissing the forehead, rearranging the blankets, comforting, and patting appear trivial to parents, but they can interfere enormously with learning to fall asleep unassisted.

One parent described extinction as follows: "Extinction is intended to be a carefully monitored, intentional method of refraining from further stimulating overstimulated and overtired babies in order to allow them to fulfill their need for sleep."

Q: *I don't think I can do nothing when my baby cries for me at night.*

A: Letting your baby cry is not doing nothing. You are actively encouraging the development of independence, providing opportunities for her to learn how to sleep alone, and showing respect for her ability to change her behavior.

Q: *How long do I let my baby cry?*

A: To establish regular naps, no more than one hour, but to establish consolidated night sleep, there is no time limit at night if your child is not hungry or ill. If we place an arbitrary small limit on the duration of crying at night, we might train the child to cry to that predetermined time. When it is open-ended, the child learns to stop protesting and to fall asleep.

Q: *Why is it good for my child to cry? Why not delay sleep training until he is older and more reasonable?*

A: Crying is not the real issue. We are leaving the child alone to learn to sleep. We are leaving him alone to forget the expectation that he will be picked up. We *allow* him to cry; we are not *making* him cry in the sense that we are hurting him. When he is older and still not sleeping, it will be harder for him to learn how to sleep well. Plus, losing sleep is physically unhealthy, just as is too little iron or too few vitamins in his diet.

Q: *Isn't crying harmful?*

A: Not necessarily. In fact, studies have proven that *crying produces accelerated forgetting of a learned response.* So when a child cries, she may more quickly unlearn to expect to be picked up. When trying to stop an unhealthy habit, crying may have some benefit, because crying acts as an amnesic agent.

Graduated Extinction

Graduated extinction means that you let your baby fuss or cry for a predetermined brief period, say five minutes. Then you pick up your baby, talk to him, feed him, and do whatever is necessary to calm him down. A progressive (graduated) checking schedule means that you leave your baby for five minutes the first time he cries; when he next cries, you leave him for ten minutes, and the next time for fifteen minutes. This sequence continues with an additional five minutes of ignoring before repeating the soothing process. The hope is that during one of these delays, your child learns to fall asleep unassisted because he is developing self-soothing skills. The major problem with a progressive checking schedule is that because you are likely to be sleep deprived yourself and have to remember how long the new delay interval is, often the child outlasts the parents' resolve.

Your baby will likely cry less at sleep onset using this method if Dad is the one putting her down after soothing and Mom has left the house. This is for two reasons. First, your baby knows that Dad cannot nurse, so what is the point of crying? Second, moms are usually more sleep deprived and therefore likely to be inconsistent with the schedule. Mom might go for a walk, get a cup of coffee, or hang out with friends until Dad calls to tell her that the baby is asleep. Some mothers leave not just at bedtime but spend the entire first night away at a friend's or at a hotel to get some much-needed rest and sleep. If affordable, one night of pampering self-maintenance at a spa hotel is a smart idea for the family and not selfish. Other mothers cannot bear the thought of being away from their baby, and that is fine, too.

Research has shown that graduated extinction takes about *four to nine nights*. Parents who do not see a rapid improvement usually do not have all the elements of self-soothing in place, and/or the bedtime is too late, and/or naps are not going well, and/or there is inconsistency in the approach to sleep. A common pitfall is to "just once" pick up your baby, bring her back to your bed, and nurse her back to sleep.

This method appears less harsh than extinction to many parents and works well for many children. However, graduated extinction may take longer than extinction, and if you are using a progressive checking schedule, it requires you to keep track of the delays. Because extinction is simpler and may succeed faster, when a natural sleep disruption inevitably occurs in the future, redoing extinction may be easier for the parents than redoing graduated extinction.

It is my impression that for extremely fussy/colicky babies and for babies much older than 4 months of age, because parents are so worn down from sleep deprivation and the child is way overtired, graduated extinction often fails or takes a long time because the child's crying outlasts the parents' resolve to be consistent. In these situations, extinction is more likely to succeed and produce results sooner.

POSITIVE ROUTINES PLUS FADED BEDTIME WITH RESPONSE COST

With this method, parents minimize bedtime resistance by allowing their child to go to sleep as late as the child wishes. By employing prolonged, calming, and pleasurable bedtime routines, the child's second wind is minimized or masked. If, upon being put to bed, the child protests, he is immediately removed from the bed (response cost); later, when the child is settled again, the soothing bedtime routine is restarted. The process of falling asleep for the child is associated with parent soothing (positive routines), not with protest crying or unpleasant associations, and he begins to associate his bed with falling asleep. The association between being in bed and falling asleep is called "stimulus control" and is described in more detail below. After the child is falling asleep without protest, the bedtime is moved earlier (faded).

My experience with this method is that real-life issues with some parents make it difficult for them to remain calmly attentive to their overtired child late at night; they wish to hurry along the process to get their child asleep so they will have some time for themselves. This impatience interferes with their ability to remain calm late at night for prolonged soothing. Although this method and scheduled awakenings (described below) work in a structured research environment, parents may not find them acceptable or practical in the real world.

SCHEDULED AWAKENINGS

With this method, parents note the approximate times when their child wakes up at night and then awaken him before those expected times, so that the child does not cry out. If needed, the child is fed and changed, and then the child is soothed back to sleep. Research by Dr. Jodi Mindell has shown that extinction works much faster than scheduled awakenings, but that scheduled awakenings do work.

My observation is that most parents hate to awaken a young child for scheduled awakenings because sleep is so precious for themselves and their child.

A recent report by Dr. Timothy Morgenthaler examined many publications on the four sleep solutions above by looking at the designs of the study and the strengths of evidence. Each study was analyzed for the quality of the study. For example, a prospective randomized study on a large number of children is superior to a retrospective nonrandomized study on a small number of children. Studies of superior quality support a "standard" recommendation of a sleep solution, indicating that there is very strong evidence to support the sleep solution's effectiveness, and studies of lesser quality support a "guideline" recommendation, indicating that the sleep solution may or may not be effective.

The only standard recommendation for effectiveness is extinction. "It should be noted that, although generally found to be effective, unmodified extinction has limited parental acceptance. Some parents find extinction with parental presence, which involves a similar structure except that the parents remain in the child's room at bedtime during the extinction procedure, more acceptable." In other words, extinction has the strongest empirical support but seems too harsh to some parents.

The guideline recommendations include graduated extinction, positive routines plus faded bedtime with response cost, and scheduled awakening, but "studies suggest that [scheduled awakenings] may be less acceptable to parents and may have less utility in very young children."

While extinction may appear harsh, it is my impression that the total amount of crying with this method is less than with graduated extinction because success occurs faster. Some parents feel comfortable with either method, while other parents feel more uneasy about extinction.

Other research comparing extinction with graduated extinction showed that parents using extinction reported less stress in parenting. This supports my observation that parents who are less stressed about normal disruptions in sleep are more willing and able to employ extinction repeatedly following changes of sleep routines during special events such as birthdays, holidays, or illnesses. These repeat extinction events usually take only one night and are called "resets" (described below). If you can muster the courage to try extinction once, when it is needed in the future you will be more able to do it again, and the old sleep problems will be a thing of the past. In contrast, because graduated extinction often takes longer, those parents employing it, who are already experiencing more stress regarding parenting, are less willing to repeat the procedure when changes of sleep routines cause the child to become overtired, because the idea of adding more stress to an already stressful situation is unbearable. So the old sleep problems return.

Another observation is that for older babies or children, where there is less uncertainty regarding hunger at night, extinction is simpler to execute and parents can therefore be more consistent. In contrast, graduated extinction requires a detailed plan of action to be modified gradually but consistently over several days or longer. I think simpler is better.

CHECK AND CONSOLE

Responding to your child at night is less difficult than ignoring cries. The process of "check and console" means that when your baby cries at night you immediately go to her and try to minimally soothe her back to sleep by stroking, petting, making shushing sounds, or gently rocking the crib or bassinet. Because your response is immediate, your child is not fully awake nor crying at full force, so minimal soothing is attempted, unlike in graduated extinction. You quietly enter whenever your baby first cries to see that she is all right and gently soothe her in darkness, but you try to not pick her up. Instead, you rub her tummy, stroke her hair, or gently rock the crib. You do the least amount of rocking, singing, and, if necessary, nursing needed in order to soothe her back to a calm, sleepy state. This method appeals to those who practice attachment parenting (discussed in more detail below), because they believe that it provides *emotional security* to the child. When the child learns that her cries will not go unanswered, she learns to trust her mother, and in turn does *not feel abandoned*.

However, there is no evidence that babies are harmed when they are allowed to cry with extinction or graduated extinction. Furthermore, this method could teach some babies to cry more frequently and longer in order to receive more soothing. In addition, it is very hard to only partially soothe a crying baby at night. On the other hand, if your baby is well rested and did not have extreme fussiness/colic, this method might work well. The hope is that this minimal parental attention allows your baby to begin to learn some self-soothing skills. This method works best if it is Dad who is doing all the curtain calls. A common pitfall is to "just once" pick the baby up, bring him to your bed, and nurse him back to sleep.

Parents who do not see rapid improvement usually do not have all the elements of self-soothing in place, and/or the bedtime is too late, and/or naps are not going well, and/or the parents are inconsistent.

The "check and console" method is less likely to be successful in an infant 6 months of age or older because your soothing attempt is more likely to stimulate your baby and cause her to cry harder in the hope that you will pick her up and play with her.

Also, if your child is a post-colic child who became completely parent-soothed, or if the child is very sleep-deficient, then success might be elusive.

SOUND MACHINES

Continuous sounds help reduce the signal intensity of intermittent sounds. Tabletop fans or music may work well to partially drown out street noises. Sound machines should be on their lowest setting and farthest from the baby for safety.

FADING

A gradual approach to reducing the number of night wakings until the baby can return to sleep independently is called "fading." Over a period of time you gradually reduce your efforts at night, so that your child takes over for himself and falls asleep or returns to sleep by himself. This is like teaching an older child how to ride a bike. You first provide balance and support or training wheels and then gradually withdraw assistance as the child gains confidence and skill. Here is an example of a fade sequence in an older child to eliminate night wakings.

Respond promptly; spend as much time as needed
Father gives bottle or mother doesn't nurse
Change from milk to juice
Dilute juice to only water
No bottle
No picking up
No singing, talking, verbal communication
Minimal contact, patting, or hand-holding
No eye contact; sober, unresponsive face
No physical contact; sit next to child
Move chair away from crib toward door, slowly over several days

Reduce time with child
Delay response

At every stage of reduction of parental attention, expect the problem to get worse before improvement begins, because the child will put forth extra effort to cling to the old style.

Fading has also been called the "chair method" when done with an older child in a bed because you are slowly moving the chair farther from your child until you are just outside the door.

In an English study of children about 3 years of age, psychiatrists examined children who displayed difficulty in going to bed, night waking, or both. Parents were counseled to keep a sleep diary for a week and establish goals for the child that included sleeping in his own bed, remaining in his bed throughout the night, and not disturbing his parents during the night. The treatment consisted of identifying the factors that reinforced the child's sleep problem and then gradually withdrawing them or temporarily substituting less potent rewards. It was a fade strategy, not a "cold turkey" approach. Here is an example of how parents in this study gradually reduced reinforcement: (1) father reads story to child in bed for fifteen minutes; (2) father reads newspaper in child's bedroom until child falls asleep; (3) child is placed back in bed with minimal interaction; (4) father gradually withdraws from bedroom before child is asleep. In another example: (1) parents alternate, but respond to child; (2) parent gives no drinks but provides holding and comforting until crying stops; (3) parent only sits by the bedside until child is asleep; (4) parent provides less physical contact at bedtime.

In this study, 84 percent of the children improved. Not surprisingly, *the two factors that most likely predicted success were both parental: the absence of marital discord and the attendance of both parents at the consultation sessions.* Also, when one problem such as resistance in going to sleep was reduced or resolved, other problems such as night waking rapidly disappeared. And although half of the mothers in this study had current psychiatric problems requiring treatment, this did *not* make failure more likely.

This study points out the importance of working with professionals who can provide guidance that is directed toward changing the child's behavior. Of course issues such as marital discord or maternal depression have to be considered and do affect treatment success, but the focus is on the child's behavior.

Another study from England included children who took at least an hour to go to bed, who woke at least three times a night or for more than twenty minutes at a time, or who went into their parents' bed. Treatment started with the parents recording the present sleep pattern in a sleep diary. A therapist worked with the parents to develop a program of treatment based on *fading* by gradually reducing or removing parental attention, adding positive reinforcement for the desired behavior, making bedtime earlier, and developing a bedtime ritual. Target behaviors were identified, and an individual treatment program was developed for each child. Also, mothers were evaluated for psychiatric problems. Mothers who showed psychiatric problems were more likely to terminate treatment, which again points out how stressful treatment can be. But for those families who completed four or five treatment sessions, 90 percent showed improvement. The authors concluded:

> The evidence that children's nighttime behavior could thus change so radically, often within a surprisingly short time, suggests *that parental responses were extremely important in maintaining waking behavior.* . . . A rapid achievement of improved sleep pattern with reduced parental attention would be unlikely if *anxiety in the child or lack of parental attention were causing the sleep difficulty.* . . . Parents needed help in analyzing goal behavior into graded steps so they could achieve successes. Once some success was obtained, *the morale and confidence of the parents rose,* and they were rein-

forced in their determination to persist by the more peaceful nights (emphasis added).

This improvement in the parents after a fade solution has also been documented with extinction in several studies, described below.

MAJOR POINT

The rapid improvement of sleep patterns produced by reduced parental attention tells us that neither lack of parental attention nor anxiety in the child was causing the sleep difficulty.

I have seen this over and over again: when you see even partial improvement, you gain confidence and you no longer feel guilty or rejecting when you are firm with your child. It is precisely this increased morale and confidence in parents who see some success when they start with graduated extinction that emboldens them to switch to extinction. In doing so, they are more able to redo extinction when a natural sleep disruption occurs.

Often it appears that older children are listening to the treatment plan in the office, because they often sleep better that very night, as if they knew something was going to be different. I think they are responding to the calm resolve and firm but gentle manner in their parents, which tells them that things are going to change.

The apparent advantage of gradually weaning the child from prolonged, complex contact (fading) is its seeming gentleness. A disadvantage for many parents is that it takes several days or weeks, during which many brief crying spells may occur. The major reasons this approach usually succeeds only partially, or fails completely, are (1) unpredictable, real-life events interfere with parents' best plans and schedules; (2) parents do not appreciate the enormous power of intermittent positive reinforcement to maintain a behavior ("I'll just nurse him this one time"); and (3) parents' resolve weakens from their own fatigue and sometimes from impatience.

As mentioned, it is common for parents to start with a gradual approach (fading or graduated extinction) and then, because of either frustration, exhaustion, or partial success, try extinction. The most important thing is to start early with any approach to see how it goes.

SWINGS

Swings might be used to soothe a baby into a deep sleep: they may be the only way to get a nap for a baby with colic; they may be used by a parent with other children to have more time to be with them; or perhaps their use evolved out of simple habit. But regular use of swings for soothing may interfere with the ability of your child to learn self-soothing. After your child falls asleep, he may stay in the swing for an entire nap or be transferred to a crib for a nap. Eventually, all children will need to be transitioned to a crib and acquire some self-soothing skills. But the acquisition of self-soothing skills as you transfer from a swing to a crib might not be an all-or-none event, and there might be a messy month before your child gets better at self-soothing and accepts the crib without protest.

During the transition from sleeping in the swing to sleeping in the crib, parents should be mindful that other factors will help, such as putting the baby down drowsy but awake and instituting a bedtime that is early enough to prevent a second wind, especially around 6 weeks of age, when early bedtimes develop. Another item that will help are brief intervals of wakefulness between naps before 3–4 months of age and synchronizing the soothing-to-sleep process with nap rhythms after 3–4 months of age, when nap rhythms emerge. After 6 months of age, when babies are more able to protest longer and louder, it will be necessary to ignore more protest crying.

To make the transition from swing sleep to crib sleep, your general plan is to allow your baby to fall asleep in the moving swing and, once in a deep sleep, turn it off and leave him in it so he gets used to sleeping without the rocking. The next step is to transition him when in a deep sleep from the stationary swing to his crib. The next step is to not use the swing in the first place.

If your child is younger than 6 weeks of age and is not colicky, skip the swing and practice putting your baby down in the crib drowsy but awake after only one hour of wakefulness *in the morning* and maybe accept some low-level crying for several minutes in the crib. The reason for doing this in the morning and after only one hour of wakefulness is because he is best rested from night sleep and you avoid a second wind.

If your child is 6 weeks of age or older, also consider allowing some self-soothing skills to develop *at bedtime* by skipping the swing at bedtime and putting him down drowsy but awake, or by having the father do the soothing at bedtime. Here also, if there is some low-level fussiness when placing your baby in the crib, try to ignore it for several minutes to see if he will drift off to sleep. But if there is loud crying, pick him up and try again another day.

If loud crying frequently occurs when you try to transition your child from the swing to the crib, consider leaving him in the swing (moving or stationary) for a longer period of time. If you are successful in making the transition from the swing to the crib but initially the naps are shorter in the crib, temporarily move the bedtime earlier. Later, when the naps in the crib lengthen, the bedtime may be moved later.

Accept that this entire process will involve some trial and error and that there will be a trend toward success punctuated with frustrating setbacks. But if you stick to the age-appropriate plan and consider all sleep elements (bedtime, consolidated night sleep, and timing of naps), you will succeed.

NAP DRILL

Biological nap rhythms begin to develop between 3 and 4 months of age and are well established by 6 months of age. So beginning around 3–4 months of age, you want to try to harmonize the onset of soothing to a drowsy but awake state with the onset of the biological nap rhythm. The midmorning nap develops first. Initially naps tend to be regular but brief. The nap drill may be attempted anytime between 3 and 6 months when you think your baby is ready, and certainly anytime after 6 months of age. But the nap drill may fail in babies younger than 6 months because nap rhythms might be too weak. However, there is no harm in trying it for several days. Some young children, especially if they are post-colic, nap best in a very dark and quiet room, while others do not appear to be so sensitive. Experiment with different rooms in your home; one family living on a noisy street temporarily used a very large walk-in closet with the door open, because it was so dark and quiet. In addition to too much light or noise, the nap drill may fail at any age because the quality of night sleep is poor.

Here is the nap drill. Put your child down to sleep, after soothing, drowsy but awake around 9:00 a.m. or as close to this time as you can if she wakes up very early in the morning. There are three scenarios in which the nap is substantially less than one hour:

1. When you put her down, she might cry at this time and never fall asleep. Totally ignore her for one hour. This represents your attempt to get a midmorning nap. If she does not fall asleep, pick her up after one hour and actively play with her. This may be thought of as extinction with a one-hour cap. Graduated extinction and check and console will not work for naps because the expected nap duration is not long.

2. When you put your baby down, she might fall asleep then or sometime during the hour of being alone, but after she falls asleep, the sleep duration is *less than 30 minutes*. Then you have two choices:

   A. Try to extend the nap by quickly doing minimal and brief soothing such as feeding, rocking, shushing, patting, or stroking, and then leave her. If this fails to extend the nap and she cries, you might decide to end the nap opportunity or you might decide to ignore her for thirty minutes to see if she will return to sleep. If she has not fallen asleep after thirty minutes, pick her up and actively play with her.

B. Ignore her for an additional thirty minutes to see if she will return to sleep unassisted. If, at the end of that time, she is still awake, pick her up and actively play with her.

If your attempts to extend the nap or to ignore your baby for thirty additional minutes rarely work, then abandon them. Neither method is likely to work around or after 6 months of age.

3. When you put your baby down, she might fall asleep then or during the hour of being alone, but after she falls asleep, the sleep duration is *thirty minutes or longer* yet substantially less than one hour. In this case, you might try to extend the nap by quickly doing minimal soothing such as feeding, rocking, shushing, patting, or stroking. Because the longer the nap, the less successful you will be in extending the nap, you might decide to end the nap and pick your child up and have fun together. But do not ignore her for an additional thirty minutes to see if she will return to sleep unassisted.

For babies a little younger than 6 months of age, in all three scenarios, after you pick her up, enjoy her company and try to keep her up as long as possible for a midday nap. Your goal is to reach 12:00–1:00 p.m., but you might only get to 10:00–11:00 a.m. if there is no midmorning nap or the midmorning nap is brief. Alternatively, especially for babies substantially younger than 6 months of age, for the rest of the day you might do whatever you can to maximize sleep and minimize crying, but focus on maintaining brief intervals of wakefulness, putting the baby down drowsy but awake, getting Dad and others on board, and enabling good-quality night sleep. For these babies younger than 6 months of age, the midmorning nap usually falls in place several days after night sleep is going well.

The *midmorning* nap develops before the *midday* nap. Just as night sleep lays the foundation for the midmorning nap, the midmorning nap lays the foundation for the midday nap. So you probably want to work on the midmorning nap first and wait until it is well established before tackling the midday nap for infants less than 6 months.

If your baby is 6 months of age or older, because two major nap rhythms are well developed, definitely try for a midday nap as follows. Once a midmorning nap pattern is established, try putting your baby down drowsy but awake around 12:00 to 1:00 p.m., or earlier if needed, because the midmorning nap is regular but brief. Or you may wish to work on both naps at the same time. The three scenarios described above also constitute the nap drill for the midday nap.

Some babies take a third nap in the late afternoon, but this nap may be brief, and the time when it occurs is irregular. Other babies do not take this third nap. If you attempt a third nap and your baby cries, immediately pick her up. This is a "no-cry nap," meaning if she cries upon being put down or shortly thereafter, she is picked up immediately and you do not try to extend the nap by soothing or ignoring. In general, if this third nap starts too late in the afternoon or is too long, it will interfere with a reasonably early bedtime. A guideline is that if your child is allowed to sleep past 4:00 p.m. from a third nap, you may have difficulties with a bedtime that is in sync with her early night-sleep rhythm.

As previously mentioned, establishing naps often works best when Dad puts the baby down for a nap and Mom leaves the house. By smell, babies know that Mom is gone, and they seem to protest less when Dad does the soothing to sleep. So consider starting the nap drill on a weekend, when Dad is available.

Night Sleep Is Fine; Why Are Naps a Problem?

There are three main determinants regarding your child's naps (and night sleep):

1. *What parents do.* Naps that take place while the parent is doing errands or socializing might be brief or have less restorative deep sleep.

2. *Innate traits in the child.* For example, some children have a temperament trait called "regularity." It appears that sleep rhythms are more regular for these children and more irregular for others. So some parents with an "irregular" child are naturally going to feel a bit frustrated because there is more variation in their child's sleep patterns compared to those of other, more "regular" children. Because temperament is mostly inherited, trying to mimic the sleep schedule that worked for a parent of a "regular" child to get more predictable sleep in your "irregular" child will not work. Also, the "irregular" child might need more regular and consistent parental efforts to keep on schedule. Another trait is "sensitivity," which means the amount of external stimulation required to have the child respond. Some children are much more sensitive than others; they have a lower sensitivity threshold and are much more easily stimulated by light, noise, and vibrations. Also, there is individual genetic variation in the duration of naps. Some children during the first 18 months take long naps, while others take short naps. Any or all three of these factors might affect naps more than night sleep.

3. *The child's environment.* Light, noise, and vibrations might affect naps but be absent at night.

Parents have more influence over night sleep than naps for three reasons:

1. Parents are tired themselves at the end of the day and really want their child to sleep, not only for the child's benefit but also so that the parents can have some private time for themselves. Parents are more able to have consistent bedtime routines.

2. The night-sleep rhythm is a powerful and predictable wave within the child, developing at and after about 6 weeks of age.

3. It is more dark and quiet at night, and the child is home in the crib for night sleep.

Parents have less influence over naps for three reasons:

1. Parents are sometimes conflicted between naps and errands, scheduled events, visitors, and the needs of their other children during the day. There may be time pressure to do other things, so nap time routines may not be consistent. Day care, nanny care, or grandparents may introduce more variables regarding naps. Digital distractions interfere with noticing subtle drowsy signs, so the timing of naps may be off. Dual-career parents may have a bedtime that is too late, or an oversolicitous nanny or night nurse might interfere with self-soothing at night, producing poor-quality night sleep that leads to problematic naps.

2. Nap rhythms develop around 3 to 4 months and naps become more predictable and longer around 6 months of age. So between 6 weeks and 6 months, night sleep might be highly predictable . . . but not so for naps. Naps change over time; as your child gets older, she has fewer and then no naps. This lack of regularity and the transitions to fewer naps may make it difficult to catch the wave of emerging drowsiness. The congenital temperament features of sensitivity to environmental

stimuli and regularity of nap rhythms create much nap variability between children of the same age. As previously mentioned, some children are born to take long naps and some children are born to take short naps, adding to the variability among children of the same age.

3. It is more light and noisy during the day, and your child may be outside or moving about in a carrier or stroller during nap time.

When attempting to get naps in place around 9:00 a.m. and 12:00–2:00 p.m., it is important to *not let your baby sleep at other times* or he will never get on this nap schedule.

CONTROL THE WAKE-UP TIME

If the bedtime is too late, there may be bedtime resistance or night wakings. Because of the late bedtime or fragmented night sleep, the wake-up time might also be late and mess up naps. A simple solution to help achieve an earlier bedtime is for the parents to awaken the child early in the morning, say around 6:00–7:00 a.m. This helps shift the circadian night-sleep rhythm to an earlier hour, especially if the child is exposed to bright sunlight after awakening. In other words, the child's night-sleep rhythm now starts earlier. This makes it easier for parents to establish an earlier bedtime. Published results showed that this simple change may dramatically and swiftly reduce night wakings without the parents doing anything else differently. This strongly supports the idea that the time when your child falls asleep is especially important.

When to Start the Day

When using extinction, graduated extinction, check and console, or some other sleep solution, your child may often start the day around 6:00 a.m. This is an approximate time: 5:30 a.m. or 6:30 a.m. might be the time for now. A mistake is to start the day much earlier, at 4:00 or 4:30 a.m., because your child awoke then and has difficulty returning to sleep. The reason starting the day too early is a problem is because your child will be sleepy around 8:00 a.m. and you will never be able to get naps in place around 9:00 a.m. and 12:00–1:00 p.m. Depending on your child's age, you might need to quietly feed the baby early in the morning, around 4:00–5:00 a.m., change her quickly, and then leave her, ignoring subsequent crying. Or you can try not going in at all if your child is not hungry.

When the Wake-up Time Is Too Early

After a few months of age, when night and nap rhythms are in place, some very *well-rested* children wake up too early for the parents. They are ready to start the day around 5:00–5:30 a.m. I want to emphasize that I am now talking about *well-rested* babies who have an early bedtime, consolidated night sleep, and great naps. For these babies, I do not know how to make them sleep later in the morning. The logic of keeping them up later so that they will sleep in later appeals to many parents, but it rarely works during the first few months of life, when children need two or three naps per day. And keeping them up later often backfires because you create bedtime battles or night awakenings. But feel free to try it; move the bedtime later gradually. If bedtime battles emerge, abandon the effort. For older children who need only one nap, it sometimes works and sometimes does not work, and depending on your circumstances you might want to try this for several weeks, as long as bedtime battles do not emerge. Moving the bedtime later in well-rested older children who are not napping often works, but it may take several weeks to see the desired result. The reason it may take a long time to see improvement is because the slightly later bedtime is only slowly creating pressure to shift the wake-up time later.

In the long run, these *well-rested* babies eventually begin to sleep later on their own, but this may occur anytime between 4 and 12 months of age. Meanwhile, I urge parents to go to bed earlier themselves to better tolerate the early morning wake-ups of their babies.

Sometimes a parent innocently helps create or perpetuate too-early wake-up times in the morning. Imagine a 3-year-old getting up around 5:00 a.m. and the parents turn on a video for their child so they can get more sleep. After a while, the child might learn to fight the early morning light sleep and force himself awake or refuse to return to sleep unassisted at earlier times (4:00–5:00 a.m.) in order to have the pleasure of watching the video. In my experience, when the parents stop the video and ignore the protests, eventually the child begins to sleep later. I am not sure whether highly pleasurable parental interaction early in the morning with younger children or babies might have a similar effect on the "wake-up time." I have advised some parents whose babies used to get up around 5:00–5:30 a.m. but were now getting up earlier (these babies were completely well rested and had an early bedtime) to go to them around 5:30 but to try to not be highly stimulating. This means that you would change and feed your baby and be pleasant, but in a quiet way in dim light, instead of giving her your customary loud, bright, and enthusiastic greeting to start the day. The hope is that the baby does not fight the very early morning light sleep to have the pleasure of playing with parents.

In *overtired* children, moving the bedtime later only makes matters worse. Overtired children, in contrast with well-rested children, are in a state of higher neurological arousal near the end of the day, so they may have more difficulty falling asleep or staying asleep either in the middle of the night or in the early morning during light sleep. This is especially true if they lack self-soothing skills. In fact, for many of these children, moving the bedtime earlier helps erase the sleep debt, and the child is better rested at 4:00–5:00 a.m., so he is able to return to sleep unassisted more easily and thus sleeps later! To help solve the problem of a too-early wake-up time in these children, all elements of healthy sleep have to be dealt with.

A common problem associated with these overtired children who get up too early is that they are at an age when they should be taking a single midday nap but are instead taking an early nap (because they got up too early). This causes them to not be tired between 12:00 and 2:00 p.m. (when they should be napping); instead, they take a late nap (between 2:00 and 3:00 p.m.), which interferes with an early bedtime, thus pushing the bedtime later and causing the wake-up time to be too early. To correct this vicious cycle, because your goal is to encourage the naps to be in harmony with nap rhythms, try hard to get a single midday nap. There will be a rough patch late in the morning because the wake-up time was too early. This overtired state around 10 a.m.–12 p.m. is fairly easy to deal with because both parent and child are better rested in the morning from night sleep. In contrast, if you allow the single nap to occur before midday, you will have a much rougher patch between 4:00 and 5:00 p.m. because both parent and child are less well rested near the end of the day. The now earlier single nap will allow an earlier bedtime, which is likely to erase the too-early wake-up. Sleep begets sleep.

PARENT-SET BEDTIMES

Data show that children's bedtimes have become later since the 1970s. In children 6 months to 5 years, a statistically significant trend toward later bedtimes was reported by Dr. Igo Iglowstein in three birth cohorts: 1974–78, 1979–85, and 1986–93. For example, for 2-year-olds in the first cohort, the bedtime was 7:08 p.m., and in the third cohort it was 8:30 p.m. This trend toward later bedtimes preceded the trend of having a television in the bedroom, which has been previously mentioned and is described in more detail below. For 10-year-olds and 14-year-olds, the bedtimes in the first and third cohort were 8:45 to 8:59 p.m. and 9:43 to 10:02 p.m., respectively; these differences were not statistically significantly different.

However, the *nineteen-minute difference* for 14-year-olds may be important! Different research, by Michelle Short, shows that teenagers with parent-set bedtimes on weekdays have earlier bedtimes, obtain more sleep, and experience improved daytime wakefulness and less fatigue during the day. The teens in the study went to bed twenty-three minutes earlier than teens without parent-set weekday bedtimes and obtained, on average, nineteen minutes of extra sleep. She concluded, "While the 19 *extra minutes* of sleep per night . . . may seem small, the *cumulative effect* of this extra sleep was associated with improved daytime functioning and may have further reaching effects in terms of improved emotional regulation and reduced risk of psychopathology (emphasis added)." As discussed in Chapter 1, small changes can make big differences when it comes to sleep!

As little as *nineteen extra minutes* of sleep may benefit your child.

Additionally, the children last studied by Dr. Iglowstein were born in 1993, and, as discussed below, the trend toward using more screen-based electronic media in the bedroom at night has dramatically increased, contributing to even later bedtimes in children of all ages.

Temporary 5:30 Bedtime

A temporary 5:30 p.m. bedtime is useful to repay a sleep debt that accumulates because of brief naps, naps out of sync with biological nap rhythms, a too-late bedtime, or fragmented night sleep, or during the transition to fewer naps or no naps. How long does it take to see improvement with a 5:30 p.m. bedtime? It depends on many variables, such as whether there was an acute sleep disruption in a well-rested child or chronic sleep problems, the presence or absence of colic, your child's self-soothing skills, whether his night sleep is fragmented or consolidated, how well he naps, and the presence or absence of day care. Older children with more sleep deprivation probably take longer to settle in. Do not always expect overnight improvement (but this can occur). Work on all the sleep issues at the same time, but do not expect a 5:30 p.m. bedtime to be a miracle cure if other sleep issues are ignored. It may take five to seven days or longer to be certain that a change was or was not helpful. Sometimes parents make a change to see if their child sleeps better, but do not allow several days to see whether there is improvement before they reverse course or make a different change. This results in too many changes occurring too quickly, and the parents get frustrated because none seems to help.

How do you know if a temporary 5:30 p.m. bedtime might be useful? The answer is based on how your baby looks between 4:00 and 5:00 p.m. If he appears slightly out of sorts, short-fused, frazzled, rough around the edges, clingy, whiny, or crisp, then his sleep tank is going dry and he needs a temporary 5:30 p.m. bedtime, or a slightly earlier bedtime in general. Sometimes these signs of sleep deprivation are masked by placing your child in front of a television or DVD. If he appears socially animated, engaged, calm, focused, or independent, then he probably is fine with the current bedtime.

Some parents use the 5:30 p.m. bedtime for only one night after an acute sleep disruption. This is called a reset (discussed below).

Reset

If your child has been a good sleeper but develops cumulative sleepiness or sleep inertia, then repay the sleep debt quickly with a *reset* before major sleep problems develop. A reset is simply an extremely early bedtime that is strictly enforced for only one night to repay an accumulated sleep debt. Ignore all protests and excuses (extinction). Get him back in the good-sleep groove quickly. A reset might be done just a few times a year in some families, but in other families it may be necessary many times a year. Here are some parent reports:

I would consider a five-thirty reset once a month to be a completely normal variation. I have three kids, and one of them (my oldest) is like that. The other two make up the missed sleep from a cold or trip themselves. My oldest does not! About the only thing that gets him extra sleep is an earlier bedtime. We do travel a lot (we live at least five hours from all family) and have visitors a lot (one or the other at least once a month). If you are using the reset because of illness, travel, etc., you are just doing your job.

We do this when our son skips a nap or when his naps are way too short (thirty minutes) and he is getting overtired. Last week he went to bed at 5:15 p.m. and woke up at 6:30 a.m. the next morning, with two or three night feeds. We have noticed that this reset seems to work but with a delayed effect. His naps get longer the morning after the early bedtime, but they are out of sync (8:00 a.m., 11:00 a.m., 2:00 p.m.). It usually takes one more day of a 6:00 p.m. bedtime for him to be on the proper schedule (9:00 a.m., noon). Then we go back to our regular schedule, with bedtime between 6:00 and 7:00 p.m., depending on if he gets a third nap. No matter when bedtime is, he wakes up at 6:20 a.m. on the dot. Knowing he won't wake up earlier (or later, for that matter) encourages us to put him to bed early for his sake.

By temporarily getting more sleep at the front end, the hope is that your child will become better rested at night and a sleep debt will be repaid. This should enhance nap quality, and the subsequent improvement in naps will lead to a later bedtime—for example, 6:30–7:00 p.m. in young children. But after you see improvement, if the move to a later bedtime produces bedtime battles or night awakenings, try 6:00 p.m. Choosing an earlier bedtime to help your child sleep better may involve trial and error.

How to Choose an Earlier Bedtime

Move the Bedtime *Slightly* Earlier

Parents coming home from work late or picking their child up from day care want to play with their child in the evening. This is understandably very important for them, and they fundamentally do not want to reduce the duration of this interaction. Such parents might try moving the bedtime earlier in small increments of fifteen to twenty minutes. If the sleep-deprived child does not show much improvement—evidenced in bedtime battles, long latency to sleep (time needed to fall asleep), night waking, daytime behavioral or developmental problems, and brief naps—then the bedtime is still too late. Do not become frustrated and declare the "treatment" a failure! Instead, after four or five nights incrementally move the bedtime an additional fifteen to twenty minutes earlier. Repeat this process until you reach a bedtime where the child calmly goes to bed. If you reach a point where he does not seem sleepy and calmly lies in bed but does not easily fall asleep, then simply reverse course and let him stay up an additional fifteen to twenty minutes.

Still, the above plan may be impractical for some parents who return home late from work. How are they to get their child down to sleep at night? The reality, as with so much of parenting, is that you do the best you can. Your baby might need a 7:00 p.m. bedtime, but the best you can do is 8:00 p.m. This is still better than 9:00 p.m.! Life isn't perfect, so don't beat yourself up. Simply try for the earliest possible bedtime. Have your child already bathed, fed, and dressed for sleep by the caretaker. Do minimal soothing to sleep and get the earliest bedtime you can for your child. Go to bed earlier yourself so you can enjoy morning time with your child. If you are not rushed, mornings may be filled with joy with your child: bathing, dressing, feeding, and playing together. Be rigidly strict with nap schedules because the better rested he is from good-quality naps, the more likely he will be able to stay up comfortably later at night. On weekends, protect naps and an early bedtime so his sleep battery is recharged. I have dual-career parents in my practice who do not see their baby when they come home from work late but spend joyful time with their baby every morning and on weekends. Because everyone is always well rested, they accept this trade-off.

Move the Bedtime *Much* Earlier

Some parents are desperate to improve their child's sleep either because they are sleep deprived themselves or they recognize that their child is suffering from sleep deprivation or both. These parents, eager for relief, choose a much earlier new bedtime, perhaps as much as *an hour or more* earlier. It may be that this much earlier bedtime is in sync with circadian rhythms and thus produces better-quality sleep and a better-rested child. But if the new bedtime is way too early, it may backfire, because although your child now might get up in the morning better rested, the wake-up time is too early, which makes for a napping problem. Although the parents might benefit in the short term by experiencing no bedtime battles or night waking in their child, the price they pay will be getting up earlier themselves or nap problems that will keep the child from showing any improvement during the day. The solution here is the same as above: by trial and error, find a sweet spot somewhere between the original too-late bedtime and the new too-early bedtime.

With either plan, remember that if you choose an earlier bedtime and your child falls asleep at this new earlier bedtime, then you have after-the-fact confirmation that the old later bedtime was too late. Choosing an earlier bedtime takes time, and the earlier bedtime should *vary* based on the child's mood and behavior around 4:00–5:00 p.m. In turn, the child's mood and behavior around that time might *vary* based on naps and outdoor exercise or play. If you do not see your child during the week in the late afternoon, be very attentive on weekends to observe your child's mood and behavior closely around 4:00–5:00 p.m. to determine the optimal bedtime. If your child is in day care and there is a big difference between nap duration in day care and nap duration at home, then the bedtime has to vary in order to reflect this difference.

Of course, parents might not see the deterioration of mood and behavior at 4:00–5:00 p.m. because they are at work. Furthermore, upon arrival home, the joy and pleasure of parent-child interaction, with games, stories, and comforting, might mask the child's sleep-deprived state. These parents are skeptical that an earlier bedtime will help. Also, some parents fear that an earlier bedtime will always cause an earlier wake-up time, and this inhibits them from trying an earlier bedtime.

The early bedtime allows the child to wake up better rested. Thus, he takes better naps. When naps improve, parents can move the bedtime a little later. If he is now well rested but early morning wake-ups still occur, consider moving the bedtime a little later. I've said this before, but it really bears repeating: a big part of finding the right bedtime for your child is trial and error. It can be a matter of hitting a moving target. But be cautious in pushing back the bedtime, because if you push it back too far, your child will once again start accumulating a sleep debt.

During the transition from three to two naps, or from two naps to one nap, some families temporarily move the bedtime earlier (5:30 p.m.) because of less day sleep. But again, this super-early bedtime might backfire and cause your child to wake up too early, with the result that he now has difficulty getting to his first 9:00 a.m. nap or his only midday nap because he is drowsy much earlier. This throws the entire day off kilter for naps, so that by 4:00–5:00 p.m. the child is exhausted and wants to fall asleep at 5:30 p.m. In this case, the early bedtime has created a problem—a too-early wake-up time. Yet when parents attempt to correct the problem by moving the bedtime later, the child gets a second wind, leading to bedtime battles. Many parents have described this dilemma to me as "being stuck in the 5:30 p.m. bedtime rut!"

The 5:30 Bedtime Rut

We have seen how well-meaning parents, attempting to secure sleep for themselves and their child, can wind up trapped in the 5:30 bedtime rut, seemingly with no way to get back out. For a *young child,* here is the solution to the 5:30 bedtime rut.

If your child is going from three naps to two, try to *keep him up for his first nap,* or else the rest of the day's naps will be off kilter. It is more tolerable to deal with early morning fussing as you struggle to get to a 9:00 a.m. nap than it would be to let him nap around 7:30–8:00 a.m. and then have an off midday nap and a miserable late afternoon when his sleep tank goes dry.

Similarly, if your child is going from two naps to one, though you do have to temporarily maintain an early bedtime even when he wakes up too early, you can try to *push his single nap toward midday.* This will be difficult, and the going will be slow and rough in the late morning. But if you give in and allow a single nap early in the morning, you and your child will pay for it with a much more difficult fussy time in the late afternoon.

Often these nap transitions are messy because the child develops a second wind, so go slowly. It may take about a month, and during that time you may feel stuck with a too-early bedtime. But trust me: it will not last forever. The best way to transition smoothly is to ensure that your child is well rested at the outset. Then the nap transition will be easier for everyone. In contrast, children who are borderline short on sleep have much more difficulty when they drop a nap.

As stated earlier, by getting more sleep at the front end, the hope is that your child eventually becomes better rested at night or a sleep debt is repaid. This improved night sleep should enhance nap quality and eventually lead to a later bedtime, for example 6:30–7:00 p.m. in young children or later in older children. Sometimes parents find it frustratingly difficult to find the right bedtime. If the bedtime is too often just a little too late or a little too early, like Goldilocks tasting porridge, then the child may cycle in and out of good sleep.

Here is one parent's story:

With our 24-month-old, particularly over the last six months, we found that with super-early bedtimes (6:00–6:30 p.m.), we were getting waking in the 5:00–5:15 a.m. range. So we took the plunge and went to 7:00 p.m. We are full-on Weissbluth Method parents, so this was a big step for us! And the 7:00 p.m. change was successful... for about 4 weeks. Then her mood began to tank between 4:00 and 6:00 p.m. Next came a fragmented nap quickly followed by one night with some waking. We knew she had sleep debt, so we went back to the 6:00–6:30 time, which is where we are presently. And the corresponding wake-ups are early (always between 5:00 and 5:30 a.m.).

So we have a dilemma: If we put our child to bed super early, she gets up super early. If we put her to bed later, she accumulates a sleep debt over a period of time, even if it helps with the wake-up. It would seem the options are (a) keep the earlier bedtimes and accept early wake-ups, or (b) put "pressure" on her to sleep later with a later bedtime, but deal with periods of fallout. Frankly, neither option is attractive. My question is: while children are still napping, is it normal to be varying the bedtime constantly? It seems to us that we have never found a bedtime that works for any significant period of time. After a few weeks, every bedtime seems too early or too late.

Note that for this child, a "super-early bedtime" was 6:00–6:30 p.m. Maybe there would be success if that bedtime was more regular, with a temporary 5:30 p.m. bedtime, or if the bedtime was always a little earlier, for example, 5:45–6:15 p.m. instead of 6:00–6:30 p.m. But even with sufficiently early bedtimes, naps will vary and the bedtime will vary.

For some *older, persistent children,* I have temporarily pushed the bedtime to a very late hour, and it caused them to sleep later. They receive lavish praise and token rewards (such as a small treat, stickers, or stars) for sleeping later. Then the bedtime is slowly and gradually moved to an earlier time, but the later wake-up time is preserved because the child continues to receive the praise and rewards. See also "Positive Routines Plus Faded Bedtime with Response Cost," page 188.

Regular Bedtimes

Dr. John Bates and associates directly evaluated the interaction between family stress, family management, disrupted child sleep patterns (variability in amounts of sleep, variability in bedtime, and lateness of bedtime), and adjustment in preschool in children about 5 years old. Children with disrupted sleep did not adjust well in preschool. In the researchers' analysis, disrupted sleep directly caused the behavior problems. They did not find any evidence that family stress or family management problems caused both disrupted sleep and behavior problems. Dr. Bates concluded that "sleep irregularity accounted for variation in [behavioral] adjustment independently of variation in family stress and family management."

Research on 7-year-old children with irregular bedtimes or bedtimes later than 9:00 p.m. showed that they had more behavioral difficulties than children who had regular, earlier bedtimes. The effects of not having regular bedtimes appear to be reversible.

Bedtime Routines

Bedtime routines like those described in Chapter 3 help children sleep better. My wife used to remind one of our sons about the "dolphin story" as part of his bedtime routine. She explained how a dolphin swims deep in the water and sleeps in the water but sometimes has to come up for air before returning to a deep sleep. Then she told our son to pretend that he was a dolphin at night and that it was perfectly all right to come up from sleep, but that he had to go back down by himself. It worked.

SLEEP LOG

The sleep log is a graph to help you see how your baby is sleeping—or not sleeping. Online sleep log graphs are available, or you can make your own. A sleep log is a series of bar graphs showing the times each day when your child was awake, asleep, quiet in bed or crib, and crying in bed or crib. A sleep log is superior to a diary because a detailed diary, in which parents keep a minute-by-minute daily record of all the times their child is awake and asleep, is so focused on the small details that it becomes hard for parents to see the forest for the trees. A sleep log shows the forest at a glance.

Here's how to make a sleep log. Each twenty-four-hour day is shown as a separate bar on a graph with the horizontal axis as the day of the week and the vertical axis the time of day. Each bar is color-coded for sleep times and wake times. Other times, such as crying times, feedings, periods in crib awake, periods in crib asleep, or periods asleep in a parent's arms, may also be included. Studying the sleep log allows you to pay closer attention to the timing of these events over several days and even weeks. The baseline data in these logs enable parents to compare interventions such as an earlier bedtime. Spotting trends such as less crying or longer naps is often easier when they are represented graphically. And if there is a setback amid success, the motivation to persist despite some crying or inconvenience is right there before your eyes.

For twins and triplets, instead of a single bar for each day on separate graphs for each child, put two or three bars, one for each child, next to each other for a given day on the same graph so you can see for any period of days whether one sibling's schedule can be slightly modified to help synchronize the entire group.

CRIB TENTS, GATES, AND LOCKING THE DOOR

One- or 2-year-olds who climb out of their bed may receive too much social interaction from parents and therefore continue the behavior because they are curious and social. To protect their sleep and prevent the development of sleep problems, consider buying a crib tent.

In 2012, the United States Consumer Product Safety Commission recalled all crib tents from a specific manufacturer because of the hazard of entrapment and strangulation. Since then, newer and allegedly safe crib tents, bed tents, and crib canopies became available, and they might encourage your toddler to stay in the crib. A crib tent will usually prevent your child from getting out of the crib, and it allows you to remove yourself from his protest crying without fear that an injury might occur. Sometimes duct tape is needed to cover the zipper because your clever child otherwise figures out how to escape. Don't worry about some theoretical sense of failure if the child has to return to the crib with a crib tent. Many children fall in love with their crib tent as if it were their personal hideaway—they seem to view it like a personal teepee or fort. They do not appear sad or angry. The crib tent is useful for families who know that they are unable or unwilling to do the silent-return-to-sleep routine when their child climbs out of the crib. For a minority of children, moving them to a bed solves the problem; they want to sleep in a bed and they will stay put to enjoy it. But in most young children, moving to a bed simply means it is now easier to go visit Mom and Dad.

Some parents feel that the crib tent "locks their child in the crib like an animal caged in the zoo" and prefer to place a gate at the door or lock the door instead. But if you stand at the door preventing your child from leaving the room, your child will fight sleep all the more because he is getting attention from you. Most families find the crib tent more acceptable and effective, but let's talk about gates and locking the door.

To me, this is absolutely the last thing a desperate family might want to try, and because it sounds so extreme I want to share with you my observations in some detail. The reality is that not all marriages are made in heaven, not all jobs allow parents to spend much time with their children, not everyone can begin sleep training early and prevent sleep problems, and, to be perfectly honest, it is difficult and inconvenient to be consistent in handling sleep routines. Circumstances beyond your control, such as twins in a one-bedroom apartment, sick relatives who need your attention, or medical problems like frequent ear infections, conspire to rob children of healthy sleep. So what are we to do when all else fails and the entire family is stressed from sleep loss?

For younger children, around age 2, some parents place gates at the child's bedroom so he cannot leave his room, or, alternatively, safety gates are in place and the parent's bedroom is locked. Either way, the child is safe but receives no social stimulation from the parents at night. Usually everything begins to turn around within one to two nights. You may need earplugs in order to ignore the banging, crying, or yelling. You may or may not place the child back in his crib or bed after he falls asleep. Definitely praise him well when he eventually stays asleep in his own room.

For children about 3 years or older, perhaps you have already tried other sleep strategies, patient reasoning, threats, and criticisms. Perhaps you've even tried spanking, which of course never works by itself, but all methods have failed. Maybe the answer is a stiff door hook that, when locked, holds the door in a slightly open position but prevents opening or completely closing. The door is held locked in a slightly open position to protect the child's fingers from a crush injury. Completely closing and locking the door may be an overwhelming degree of separation for either you or the child.

Take your child with you to the store when you purchase the lock, and make your child watch or help you install the lock on the door. Often this installation of the lock alone will cause a change in your child's behavior. Your child is told that if he leaves the room, he will be put back in and the door will be locked. Almost all the time, the child picks up on her parents' serious demeanor and does not even attempt to leave the room in the first place. This is so important, I want to restate it: many families desperate to get their well-rested child back never actually have to use the newly installed lock, because their child knows on the first night that this is the beginning of a new routine.

Buying and installing the lock establishes the unambiguous message that leaving the room after a certain time is unacceptable. The child learns that you mean business. You avoid the repeated prolonged stresses of trying to physically separate from a child who is clinging to you, or of trying to keep the door closed while your child is in the room on the other side trying to pull it open.

If, however, the child tests the rules and leaves the room, and the parents place her back into the room and lock the door, although there may be loud and long protest crying, it is usually only for one night, because the child is now highly motivated to prevent the door being locked the next night.

Simply locking the door solves nothing, however, if your child is going to bed too late, getting up too late or too early, not getting the nap he needs, taking a nap too late in the afternoon, or having a very irregular bedtime, or if you talk to your child through the closed door. You will still have an overtired child. No quick fix, whether a locked door, or, worse, drugs to make your child sleep, will make an overtired child less tired.

SLEEP RULES AND SILENT RETURN TO SLEEP

It's quite natural for 2- and 3-year-olds to climb out of the crib or bed to check out the interesting things they think their parents are up to. Or maybe they just want to watch the late late movie or have a bite to eat. Of course, what they like to do most is to come visit with their parents and perhaps get into their bed. This not only disrupts their parents' sleep but also fragments the child's sleep.

Sleep Rules are a strategy I created that works well for children over 2½. The first step is to make a Sleep Rules poster and tape or pin it to the wall in your child's bedroom. Just talking about what to do without the poster is much less effective. The poster is essential because it serves as a constant reminder for your child. It encourages behaviors compatible with sleep and discourages behaviors incompatible with sleep (such as singing, calling, and running around). Decorate the poster with art, markers, and stickers, and let your child help make the poster. The more colorful and dramatic it is, the more motivational it will be. Insert your child's first name before the title so that John will listen carefully when a parent recites "John's Sleep Rules" every time he is put to sleep. At every bedtime and nap time, recite the rules and explain the consequences. Sleep Rules should be implemented for both naps and nighttime sleep in order to be consistent. At nap time, if the child follows the Sleep Rules for one hour but does not sleep, he is rewarded for a good-faith effort. For success, the bedtime must be early enough to prevent a second wind. You simply say, "John, remember your Sleep Rules. One, stay in bed; two, stay very quiet; three, close your eyes and keep them closed; and four, try to sleep."

_____'S SLEEP RULES
(insert your child's name)

1. Stay in bed.
2. Be quiet.
3. Keep your eyes closed.
4. Try to sleep.

In general, perfect consistency is the preserve of robots, not human beings. When it comes to parenting, if you are 80 percent consistent, then you should consider yourself as close to perfect as is humanly possible. But if you embark on Sleep Rules with silent return to sleep, try to be 100 percent consistent for five to seven days to convince your child that you are serious. Expect to see sequential improvement, first for night sleep and later for naps.

To indicate when the Sleep Rules are over in the morning, use a clock radio with very quiet classical music, a digital clock with a picture of the morning wake-up time, or a color-changing light that is set at the wake-up time you choose. If your child sleeps through this time, do not wake him. But explain to your child later that Sleep Rules are in place until he hears the music or sees the color change on the light or the digital clock looks like the picture. At that point, he can call out for you, and you will immediately go to him. Rewards and privileges are an important component of this plan.

Reward your child in the morning for compliance at night and immediately after a nap: a piece of candy, a cookie, wholesome snack foods, stickers, small toys, special events or trips, or more screen time (use a timer) in addition to hugs, kisses, and praise. After you recite the Sleep Rules at night, tell your child what the reward will be in the morning if he cooperates. If you use something like candy, place the treats in a glass jar above the refrigerator where they are visible to the child; this will enhance motivation. One mother rewarded cooperation by placing a piece of candy under a special doll after her child had gone to sleep; part of the motivation was the excitement of discovery in the morning when the child looked for her treat. Give an immediate reward in the morning and after a nap for compliance. In general, even if there is no problem around naps, for the sake of consistency, also give the reward after the nap. Also, use stickers or stars on a calendar so that three or four stickers equal a bigger reward. This way, there is both immediate and delayed gratification. After several weeks of smooth sleeping, instead of giving the child the treats immediately, they can be placed in a "treat bowl" to be given to the child after dinner. This delayed gratification helps the child to substitute heightened self-esteem for the treats. Later, forget the reward but continue with the hugs, kisses, and praise. Of course, this method is guaranteed to fail if the rewards are insufficiently motivational or if the rewards are stopped or inconsistently applied before new sleep habits are well established.

Let's take a moment to look more closely at the difference between rewards and bribes. I am sensitive to the fact that some people will claim that it is wrong to give something to a child to make a behavior occur—that it is like a bribe, which is given *before* the desired behavior. The simple answer is that we smile, hug, and praise our children *after* they perform in a socially desirable way. This is how a child learns to share toys and develop manners and desirable social habits. But our social rewards simply aren't powerful enough to change the behavior of a strong-willed 2- or 3-year-old who is dead set on fighting sleep for the pleasure of your company. Opponents to giving rewards come up with theoretical objections, but the fact remains that when rewards are used in the context in which I am describing them, they work.

If your child is very young and you are not sure he understands the concept that actions have consequences, use the rewards alone and do not restrict privileges. But if your child is older and does understand, then *restrict privileges* for noncompliance: less light on in the bedroom, bedroom door is less open, less screen time, remove toys, and remove stuffed toys or other bed items. You might close the door in a progressive fashion every time he gets out of bed. You can put three or four white tape marks on the floor, and after each time he gets out of bed, the door is closed a little more until it is barely open. If he stays in the bed, the door is left open to the first tape mark. A similar progressive strategy could be used with brighter or dimmer night-lights.

After you recite the Sleep Rules and remind your child of the rewards he will receive in the morning for cooperation, tell him what privileges will be restricted for noncooperation. Remember, rewards are only half the story here. Think of what your child loves to do around the house and label it a privilege. Never restrict outdoor play and creative activities such as reading, painting, art, or building things. Rather, think of somewhat passive things, such as watching DVDs or television, playing video games on the computer, or perhaps playing with some favorite dolls or trucks. Choose one activity to be the privilege. So, after you recite the Sleep Rules, you say, "John, remember to follow the Sleep Rules so that when you wake up you can choose a treat and play with your trucks." All the trucks are put in a box in the closet. If he follows the rules, after he wakes up you say, "Thank you for following the Sleep Rules. Here, choose a treat. And here are your trucks to play with." Or if he did not abide by the rules, say, "You did not follow the Sleep Rules, so no treat and no trucks to play with until you follow the rules." Alternatively, the restriction of privilege means that noncompliance causes one or a few trucks to be taken away each time and removed from play so that the child sees his truck supply dwindling. If he has a hundred trucks, remove ten at a time. The same number of trucks is taken from the locked garage each time and returned to him for compliance. If John decides he doesn't care about his trucks, then restrict some other privilege next time in addition to the trucks. Sequentially restrict additional privileges. Some families with older children do only the rewards but not the restriction of privileges, and the method fails.

> **Consider rewarding even partial cooperation: small rewards for some cooperation, bigger rewards for more cooperation.**
> **Rewards are best given in the morning after awakening or immediately following a nap.**

Silent return to sleep means that if your child leaves her room, you gently pick her up and place her back in bed. Every time you determine that she is out of her crib or bed, or discover her in your bed, gently place her back in her bed. Put a bell on her doorknob so you know right away when she is leaving her room. The signal makes her aware of what she's doing, and it helps you to be consistent. If you hear the bell at night, by prior agreement one parent intercepts the child as she leaves her room. You are not sweet or stern; you are bland and silent.

> **Do not underestimate the enormous power of partial or intermittent reinforcement to ruin your efforts to overcome your baby's habit of getting out of the crib. If you are not *silent* and you discuss getting out of bed when it is occurring, your social**

behavior undercuts your words and reinforces getting out of the crib.

Silence when you take your baby back to bed is important, because if you are sweet or stern while trying to explain why everyone needs sleep, the verbal attention will reinforce your child's desire to get out of bed to get more attention. Attending to the problem in this way will cause the problem to occur more often. Many parents do not understand that negative attention—even yelling or getting angry—is still attention, and it will encourage your child to continue the behavior.

Be *silent* and unemotional; appear disinterested or mechanical. No social contact at night.

After you recite the Sleep Rules to your child, you might add: "I love you very much, but you need your sleep and I need my sleep, and if you leave your room, I am not going to start a conversation with you." Plan to not get much sleep the first two nights, as your child may try many, many times to get back to her old style. Parents might want to alternate nights so that at least someone gets some sleep. Do not take turns on the same night, because the child might think one parent will behave differently. When silent return to sleep is practiced consistently, children learn quickly that there's no benefit in getting out of bed, so they stay there and sleep through the night. In short, every time your child gets out of bed, she should encounter a silent, unemotional parent who gently picks her up and returns her to bed.

When your child refuses to comply with Sleep Rules, either at night or for one hour during the day when a nap should be taking place, employ the silent-return-to-sleep strategy. When you employ Sleep Rules and silent return to sleep, do not be surprised if your child's behavior gets worse for a short time. It's as if she is putting forth more effort to get back to the old way. But patience pays off.

Many children become proud of their accomplishments and brag about how they are following their Sleep Rules. One very cute and bright girl ripped up three Sleep Rules posters before she got the message. Then she started to tell her friends, with great pride, that she now sleeps by the rules. Be optimistic!

Problems may get worse before they get better during a retraining phase.

We know from many studies that when parents think they have finally solved a sleep problem, it may resurface sooner or later. This is known as a "response burst," and it occurs either because the child is testing to see if the rules still apply or because the parents have slipped a little regarding consistency in enforcing the rules or maintaining a healthy sleep pattern. Parents have another name for it: a "train wreck." Knowing that train wrecks occur is no reason for despair. On the contrary, it should give you confidence to stay the course and not give up in frustration by convincing yourself that you are back to square one. Don't be dismayed at these temporary if often striking setbacks. Stick to what worked, and usually the problem will subside for good.

Keeping track of progress with a sleep log will strengthen your resolve to continue even though you may be frustrated by many curtain calls. Once you have achieved success, feel free to occasionally skip naps and early bedtimes and enjoy special occasions maybe once or twice a month—but not once or twice a week. Do not be a slave to your child's sleep schedule. Well-rested children can tolerate occasional breaks in routine without going bonkers. However, even after you achieve success, there may be a few times a year when sleep gets seriously off track and you will want to use this method again as a reset with a super-early bedtime.

Now let us consider the fifth Sleep Rule, for older children in a bed.

SLEEP RULE #5

Do not leave your room until you hear the music (or hear the birds, or hear the alarm, or see the color change in the lamp).

This rule is for older children who like to get up too early, leave their room, and bother their brother, sister, or parents. Again, set a clock radio, a CD or MP3 player on a timer, or an alarm clock—placed under a pillow to muffle the loud noise—to the time it is okay for your child to leave her room. Or use a programmed light or bunny that changes color at a set time in the morning.

Some children who have never slept well and have just turned 3 might completely disregard all Sleep Rules and trash their room or simply stay up late playing in their room with the lights on. These children might need extra reinforcement. For example, they may have to be placed in a crib with a crib tent for a while, or the light-bulbs will have to be removed to keep the room dark, or a lock will need to be placed on the bedroom door. Whatever restriction you choose, compliance with Sleep Rules is rewarded by the removal of the crib tent, the return of the light, or no lock.

Expect Sleep Rules and the silent return to sleep to reduce or eliminate the getting-out-of-bed routine within three to four days. All you have to do is remove the previous nighttime social interaction (whether pleasant or unpleasant) as a reinforcer to your child's habit of getting out of his crib.

Here are some typical questions and answers about this strategy.

Q: *My child is scared at night, and I don't want to leave her alone.*
A: Try to spend extra time soothing her to sleep, buy a dream catcher or guardian angel to protect her, or go around the room catching all the monsters and put them in a bag that you take out of the room. Maybe give her a bell that she can ring on one occasion, and only one, at night when she is scared, to which you will respond promptly. This will give her a sense of security, knowing that you will come promptly once in the middle of the

night. When you respond, consider using a timer, placed under a pillow to quiet it, for a measured amount of middle-of-the-night soothing. Controlling the duration of soothing creates expectations and a routine that both a parent and child will accept. If the duration of soothing is open-ended, sometimes the parent will have the ability to stay for a long time and sometime for a short time, and this irregularity might cause your child to learn to protest for more and more soothing. Tell your child that when the timer buzzes or the alarm goes off, you will kiss her and leave and not come back until morning. After a while, your child will learn to associate the sound of the timer with your departure and will return to sleep without protest, knowing not to expect any curtain calls. In fact, this could be a sixth Sleep Rule: "If you are scared, ring the bell and I will come, but I will come only once." Tell your child not to abuse ringing the bell. Ringing the bell on more than one occasion would violate this Sleep Rule and be a cause for some restriction of privileges that you should also make clear at bedtime. Alternatively, for older children, a pass system (described below) might help your child sleep better.

Q: *Won't my child hurt himself when he climbs or falls out of his crib?*

A: This is a common worry and often used as an excuse to go to your child or buy a big-kid bed. But the truth is that serious injuries rarely occur when the child bumps on the floor as he lets himself down.

Q: *Can the plan fail?*

A: Yes, when both parents aren't committed, so that one partner passively or actively sabotages the program. One father in my practice loved to sneak a bottle of formula to his baby once or twice a night. This caused the baby to suffer excessive wetness and a severe, persistent, and painful diaper rash. Only in the course of trying to eradicate the rash did the father's behavior come to light. Failures also sometimes occur when the child is still chronically fatigued from too late a bedtime hour or nap deprivation.

Q: *What if he stays in his crib but cries?*
A: Letting your child cry when he protests going to sleep or staying in his crib is not the same as making your child cry as if you were hurting him. Leave him alone (extinction) or try graduated extinction.

One family instituted this five-step program when their daughter, Nicole, was 26 months old—after 26 months of poor sleeping. She had always had difficulty falling asleep and difficulty staying asleep. Nicole always wanted to, and did, get out of her bed and go into her parents' bed. After the birth of Daniel, her brother, her parents decided this had to stop.

Their record showed the following results:

Night 1: Between 8:13 and 9:45 p.m.—*69* return trips to bed. Slept until 8:30 a.m. with one brief awakening at 2:15 a.m.
Night 2: Between 8:20 and 10:30 p.m.—*145* return trips to bed. Slept until 7:20 a.m. with one brief awakening at 2:15 a.m.
Night 3: After 9:14 p.m. (bedtime)—*0* return trips to bed! Slept until 7:40 a.m., awakening once at 3:20 a.m.

That's it!

An important point to note is that almost all of Nicole's getting out of bed occurred within the first hour or two of the night. Many children follow this pattern, so don't expect that you will necessarily lose a complete night of sleep during this training period. I suggest that you sit near your child's room for an hour or so at bedtime for three or four nights when you do silent return to sleep.

After the third night of Nicole's program, the curtain calls at bedtime ceased. Furthermore, at naps her mother would now leave after fifteen or twenty minutes of reading, whereas before she had stayed in the room until Nicole fell asleep. The parents described Nicole as easier in many ways: less resistant in dressing, less argumentative, more charming, and better able to be by herself. It is possible that Nicole's bedtime, shown above, was too late and contributed to the development and maintenance of her poor sleeping.

PASS SYSTEM

In one study, 3- to 6-year-old children exhibiting bedtime resistance were given a card exchangeable for one parental visit or excused departure from the room after bedtime, with parents ignoring subsequent bids for attention. They left their rooms and called and cried out significantly less than control children who were not given a card. A variant of the pass system, discussed above, is placing a bell by the child's bed with the rule that the parents will respond promptly once, and only once, if the child rings the bell. Once the child learns that he can have his parents come to him at any time—but only once—he will use this power with restraint.

DAY CORRECTION OF BEDTIME PROBLEMS*

Another sleep strategy appropriate for 3-year-old or older children is called "Day Correction of Bedtime Problems." The idea here, developed by Dr. Edward Christophersen, a prominent child psychologist, is that because everyone is tired and less able to cope with the stress of bedtime battles or night-waking problems at the end of the day, daytime behavior should be tackled first. The following instruc-

* From *Beyond Discipline: Parenting That Lasts a Lifetime*, 2nd ed., by E. R. Christophersen (Shawnee Mission, KS: Overland Press, 1998), 127–128. Copyright 1998 by Edward R. Christophersen. Reprinted with permission.

tions explain this strategy in detail. Under item number 3, "Relaxed," Dr. Christophersen says, "Perhaps the easiest way to teach self-quieting, during the day, is by allowing your child to self-quiet during naturally occurring times of frustration." ("Self-quieting" is Dr. Christophersen's term for what I call "self-soothing.") In a conversation with Dr. Christophersen, he clarified this statement by explaining that you do not always rush to help a child struggling with a puzzle or accomplishing some task. When there is something that is slightly bothering your child, it is sometimes better to leave her alone to learn to deal with it. Dr. Christophersen's observation is that some mothers need to be taught to disengage or to ignore some of their child's low-level distress. He does not mean you should ignore your child when she comes home from school crying or has had a very frightening experience! In one study, when children learned how to cope with frustration during the day, they were observed to settle themselves better at bedtime and later at night when they awoke. I will let Dr. Christophersen speak for himself:

> There are three important components to getting a child to go to sleep at night. The child must be:
>
> 1. Tired
> 2. Quiet
> 3. Relaxed
>
> When these three components are in place, children who have adequate "self-quieting skills" will be able to go to sleep rather easily.
>
> 1. *Tired.* The easiest way to make sure that your child will be tired when he or she goes to bed is by getting him or her up at the same time every day and by getting him or her an adequate amount of exercise during the day—vigorous exercise that requires a good deal of energy. For an infant, include several

long periods of time when he or she is on the floor and can see what you are doing, but the infant must hold his or her head up in order to really see much. For almost any child, twenty minutes of good exercise each day, after a nap, is usually adequate.

2. *Quiet*. You can elect to either quiet down the entire house or quiet down your child's room. Quieting down your child's room by closing the door and keeping it closed is probably the easiest. . . . You might need to turn on the furnace or air-conditioning fan as a masking noise for the first few nights.

3. *Relaxed*. Children can relax only if they have learned self-quieting skills. Self-quieting skills refer to a child's ability to calm himself or herself, with no help from an adult, when the child is unhappy, angry, or frustrated. Whereas older children (at least age 6 years) can be taught relaxation procedures [see below], infants and toddlers need to practice self-quieting skills in order to know what works for them. Perhaps the easiest way to teach self-quieting during the day is by allowing your child to self-quiet during naturally occurring times of frustration.

Self-quieting behaviors. The baby who goes to sleep with help from one of his or her parents by nursing, rocking, or holding learns only adult transition skills and needs an adult present in order to fall asleep. The baby or toddler who goes to sleep alone cuddling a stuffed animal, holding his or her favorite blanket, or sucking his or her thumb learns valuable self-quieting skills that can be used for many years to come.

How they feel. Children who go to bed easily and sleep through the night uninterrupted get a good night's sleep. They will feel better during the day, just as the adults in their household will feel better during the day. It may take from several nights to one week to teach a child the skills he or she needs for going to sleep alone, but this is one behavior that the child will be able to use for the rest of his or her life.

These three components described here have the added advantage that they can be taught during the day, which removes many of the fears parents have about handling behavior problems at bedtime. Even parents who choose co-sleeping can allow their infant or toddler the opportunity to fall asleep on their own, with the parent joining the child at the parents' regular time for retiring. In this way, the infant or toddler gets the perceived advantages of co-sleeping and the known advantages of learning self-quieting skills.

REMOVE TELEVISION AND ALL OTHER SCREEN-BASED MEDIA FROM THE BEDROOM

Having a television or other electronic screen-based media in the bedroom is associated with a variety of sleep problems and short sleep durations. Removal of all electronic media by the parents at a parent-set lights-off time may be a powerful solution (see Chapter 10). I view this as an underappreciated public health problem that has quietly developed over the last thirty years. Data I collected around 1980 showed no strong correlation between more television viewing and less sleep, but at that time television was uncommon in children's bedrooms. Shortly thereafter the presence of a television in the bedroom became much more common. In 1988, 10 percent of 3- to 10-year-old children had a television in their bedroom. In 1999 it was 26 percent, and more sleep problems occurred in children who watched more television. By 2005 it was 40 percent; even among children under 2 years old, 18 percent had a television in their bedroom! In 2013, more television viewing, computer use, mobile telephone use, and video gaming were associated with later bedtimes and less sleep in children ages 10 to 18 years. By 2014, more television viewing was associated with less sleep in younger children ages 2, 4, 6, and 9 years.

RELAXATION TRAINING

Let's look at the two major areas of concern for older children: falling asleep and maintaining a healthy sleep schedule. In treating these sleep problems, we attempt to break the self-perpetuating sequence in which sleep disturbances cause hyperarousal, which further interferes with sleeping well. Working with a therapist, older children can learn to sleep better through relaxation training techniques similar to those used by adults. The attempt is to reduce the level of pre-sleep arousal, thereby permitting the sleep process to surface. Here are a few techniques:

1. *Progressive relaxation* is a method whereby you tense individual skeletal muscle groups, release the tension, and focus on the resulting feeling of relaxation.

2. *Biofeedback* involves focusing on a visual or auditory stimulus that changes in proportion to the tension within skeletal muscles. Both progressive relaxation and biofeedback techniques can help reduce muscle tension and thus make it easier to fall asleep.

3. *Self-suggestion* to produce relaxation involves repeating suggestions that your arms and legs feel heavy and warm.

4. *Paradoxical intention* is based on the idea that trying hard to spontaneously fall asleep might create a vicious circle, which can be broken by focusing on staying awake.

5. *Meditative relaxation* procedures vary, but simple instructions to focus on the physical sensation of breathing seem to help some people fall asleep.

STIMULUS CONTROL AND TEMPORAL CONTROL

Stimulus-control treatment tries to make the bedroom environment function as a cue for sleep. Spending lots of time in bed watching television, reading, or eating directly competes with sleeping, and therefore these activities must be discontinued. *Temporal control* means establishing a regular and healthy sleep schedule.

Richard R. Bootzin, a psychologist specializing in insomnia, incorporates the elements of stimulus control in the following instructions he developed:

Stimulus-Control Instructions

1. Lie down intending to go to sleep *only* when you are sleepy.

2. Do not use your bed for anything except sleep—that is, do not do homework, read, watch television, eat, or worry in bed.

3. If you find yourself unable to fall asleep, get up and go into another room. Although you should not watch the clock, you should get out of bed if you do not fall asleep within about ten minutes. Stay up as long as you wish, engaged in a focused activity (reading is best), but no screen-based media, and when feeling sleepy return to the bedroom to sleep. Remember, the goal is to associate your bed with falling asleep *quickly*! If you are in bed for more than ten minutes without falling asleep and have not gotten up, you are not following this instruction. You want to avoid being in bed feeling upset or frustrated that you can't fall asleep.

4. If you still cannot fall asleep, repeat step 3. Do this as often as necessary throughout the night.

5. Set your alarm and get up at the same time every morning, irrespective of how much sleep you got during the night. This will help your body acquire a consistent sleep rhythm.

6. Do not nap during the day.

Dr. Rosalind Cartwright, a pioneer adult-sleep researcher, teaches a variation of Bootzin's stimulus control that has helped some older children fall asleep more easily.

1. Before bedtime, do something that is pleasurable for a limited amount of time, using a timer set for fifteen to twenty minutes. Do anything you want, but not in your bedroom.

2. Take the hottest lavender bubble bath you can tolerate for fifteen to twenty minutes. This is for relaxation, so don't read a book or listen to music while you're in the tub. The bath helps prevent the storm of thoughts and worries that strikes the brain like a meteor shower when the protective shield of activity, sports, or homework is down.

3. After the bubble bath, immediately get into bed. Don't start any other activities—no books, no music, no telephone calls. Close your eyes and try to sleep.

If these instructions do not provide help, consider encouraging your child to get involved in sports programs in order to increase the amount of physical exercise he gets during the day. If this fails and your child still can't sleep well and appears exhausted, too tired, and not interested in outside activities, ask yourself whether the cause might be a medical problem or depression.

Children do get depressed, and some crazy, risk-taking "accidents" in overtired teenagers are really deliberate suicide attempts. If this is a concern of yours, seek outside help immediately. Start with school social workers, your physician, or local suicide prevention centers.

MEDICATION

Dr. Judith Owens wrote in a recent review of medications used to help children sleep better that "in almost all cases, medication [including melatonin] is neither the first treatment choice nor the sole treatment strategy for children with insomnia. . . . Nonpharmacological treatments have been shown to have more long-lasting effects (i.e., persistent after medication has been discontinued)." More than thirty years ago, I incorrectly thought that an antihistamine that induces drowsiness might be used temporarily to help a child sleep so the exhausted parents could get more sleep and be better able to change their child's sleep routines. But instead, after only a few attempts, it became clear to me that the parents who desperately wanted medication were the same parents who were most unwilling to make the changes necessary to help their child sleep better. I have not prescribed medications for sleeping since then.

> **WARNING**
> When your overtired child first starts to sleep better during a retraining period, he may appear, in the beginning, to be more tired than before! You are unmasking the underlying fatigue that had previously been present but was hidden by the turned-on, hyperalert state.

Choose a Sleep Solution

Happily, if a sleep problem exists, it usually can be corrected. If your child is not sleeping well, the goal is to have parents impose upon him an age-appropriate, biologically healthy sleep schedule within the context of the family. This approach is no different from when parents choose a healthy selection of foods at meals. Parents' responsibility in teaching sleep habits is the same as teaching other health habits such as hand-washing, tooth-brushing, or wearing a helmet when riding a bike. But there is no one-size-fits-all approach to helping children sleep well, because all families are different.

There are many ways to help your child sleep. You should choose the solution that works best for you and your child. Some do not work well for the extremely fussy or colicky baby, some will be difficult to use because of limited resources for soothing, and some are appropriate only for older children. Also, one method may be more powerful in the hands of some families than in others. Often I will refer to ignoring all crying or extinction as the preferred solution to help your child sleep better, because I think this works best for the 20 percent of babies who have extreme fussiness/colic; after 4 months of age, I think they represent the largest group of children with sleep problems or have more severe sleep problems. However, I understand that this is probably the hardest sleep solution for parents, and you should always first consider other sleep solutions that involve less crying. This is especially true if your child does not have extreme fussiness/colic.

One way to think about different sleep solutions and help you choose one is to organize them into three groups:

1. "No-cry" sleep solutions
   Teach self-soothing
      Many hands, father care
      Drowsy but awake, soothing
      Many naps
   Sleep log
   Bedtime routines
   Motionless sleep
   Sound machine, room-darkening curtains
   Positive routines plus faded bedtime with response cost

Scheduled awakening
Control the wake-up time
Relaxation training
Stimulus control
2. "Maybe-cry" sleep solutions
Fade procedure
Nap drill
Parent-set bedtimes, regular bedtimes, earlier bedtimes
Swings
Crib tent
Sleep Rules and silent return to sleep
Pass system
Day correction of bedtime problems
3. "Let-cry" sleep solutions
Extinction: with or without cap, with or without parent
   presence
Graduated extinction
Check and console

Parents have told me that the sleep solution that needs to be emphasized is many naps or brief intervals of wakefulness because it is not intuitively obvious that babies, who sleep so much, need to return to sleep within one to two hours after waking up.

MAJOR POINT
Babies need to sleep within one to two hours after waking up.

For some parents, the major decision is whether to ever let their child cry. Some parents are strong believers in only one approach to soothing to sleep. They believe there should never be any crying and that by always holding their baby, frequently nursing their baby, and sleeping with their baby, they can prevent extreme fussiness/colic from occurring and prevent sleep problems. They characterize their approach as "gently to sleep" or "attachment parenting," a gentle, warm, child-centered style that enhances a sense of security because the baby is taught that the mother is always there. They are proud to "wear their baby" and proclaim themselves "twenty-four-hour parents." They characterize other approaches as "cry it out" or "detached parenting," a cold, rigid, parent-centered style that creates a sense of abandonment because the baby is taught that the mother is unresponsive. These parents say that when the baby stops crying and sleeps, he has "given up" trying to communicate with his mother and will grow up with feelings of insecurity. This stark contrast in parenting styles is supposed to produce differences in babies and differences in the bonding between the child and her parents.

However, there are some major problems with this way of thinking. First, there is no evidence that one style or another produces a specific outcome. Second, babies themselves contribute a lot to what will easily work or not work. Third, it's not just about the bond between babies and mothers; fathers, siblings, and real-life family issues help shape your ability to soothe, comfort, and put your baby to sleep. Fourth, there are methods in between always attending to night crying and never attending to night crying, such as those listed under "maybe-cry" above. "Attachment parenting" may or may not be your decision, but it may work well for babies who have common fussiness and develop an easy temperament. For these babies, everything you read in popular books about soothing and sleeping will likely work. Perhaps, for the majority of parents, the path to healthy sleep does not involve any crying. There is no reason to be judgmental and criticize other parents who are not so fortunate.

A minority of families become distressed or overwhelmed with the arrival of their baby because they lack sufficient resources to soothe the baby or the baby has extreme fussiness/colic, with the result being that the baby develops into an overtired 4-month-old with a difficult temperament. These parents may have started out with the crib and decided later to use the family bed for soothing and sleeping, and were still frustrated when, after 4 months, the baby still did not sleep well. Flexibility and sensitivity to your baby is important in choosing a sleep solution that fits your family.

Another important factor in choosing a sleep solution is sensitivity to your own personality and makeup. As mentioned previously, some parents feel more stressed, and for them graduated extinction is more acceptable than extinction. Some mothers have depressive symptoms and might find extinction too stressful, or they have anxiety symptoms that appear to be associated with infant colic (discussed below).

Also, one study used a parenting scale to measure parental discipline style and discovered that certain maternal factors were associated with success in using extinction. The two main factors studied were laxness (the extent to which parents notice but do not discipline misbehavior), and verbosity (the extent to which parents respond to misbehavior with coaxing, begging, or lengthy explanations—not to be confused with appropriate parental reasoning, explanations, and conversations that are associated with greater compliance in toddlers and preschoolers).

For mothers who were less distressed with their roles as parents and "who made fewer lax and verbose disciplinary mistakes," there were better outcomes with extinction. These mothers were more compliant with the treatment protocol; that is, they more consistently followed the plan. So the recommendation or choice to use extinction might also be influenced by maternal discipline style. In this study, there were no maternal characteristics associated with graduated extinction. Graduated extinction, though, was easier to implement. As stated before, other research has shown that graduated extinction is more acceptable when parents report more stress in their marriage. Often, families start with graduated extinction and see some improvement in their child's sleeping, demeanor, and behavior and then shift to extinction. Both methods improve bedtime and nighttime sleep problems.

Another study followed a group of young women prior to, during, and after pregnancy. About 10 percent of the babies born had extreme fussiness/colic. Mothers who had anxiety before, during, or after the pregnancy were more likely to have a baby with extreme fussiness/colic. In this study, unlike others, there was no association between maternal depression and extreme fussiness/colic.

This study associating maternal anxiety before the pregnancy and extreme fussiness/colic and the previous study regarding discipline style and ability to use extinction highlights the interplay between maternal issues and baby issues. Sometimes this combination of maternal issues and baby issues is expressed as a fear of ever letting your baby cry.

WHY CAN'T I LET MY BABY CRY?

1. *Unpleasant childhood memories.* These may surface and remind you of feelings of loneliness or being unwanted.

2. *Working parent's guilt.* You may feel guilty about being away from your child so much.

3. *We already tried and it didn't work.* Maybe your child was too young then; maybe you taught her, by your behavior, that if she cried for more than a certain amount of time you would go to her; maybe you unknowingly provided intermittent reinforcement by going to her at some times but not at others.

4. *I enjoy my baby's company too much at night.* This may be because you're not a good sleeper yourself.

5. *If I don't nurse my baby at night, she might lose weight.* This is usually not true.

6. *We're under a lot of stress.* In *My Child Won't Sleep*, Jo Douglas and Naomi Richman wrote: "If you are feeling stressed,

your child may respond by not sleeping so well. If the stress is related to difficulties between you as parents, you may think that your young child will not notice, but the chances are that he will. His way of waking at night and coming into your bed can be a way of preventing you from talking to each other and sorting out your problems, and his presence can act as a useful contraceptive." Although this quote applies to older children, it's possible that maintaining the baby's night waking or having the baby sleep with you when he or she is younger also serves the purpose of avoiding marital problems.

7. *I feel that I am a bad parent if my baby cries.* You are not a bad parent if you are helping your baby learn healthy sleep habits.

What does it mean to be a "good parent"? Parents feed and protect their young and provide comfort and guidance. When your baby cries, you go to her. On the surface, it certainly seems reasonable to say that the cry of your baby communicates messages: "feed me," "change me," "pick me up," "hold me," "hug me," or "rock me." The question is, why is it that when a parent makes an immediate and complete response to these messages, some babies still cry? Alternatively, if crying is a form of necessary communication, why is it that many parents will deliver complete, loving, and sensitive care even when their babies do not cry? Perhaps crying as a signal system is not perfect: some babies cry even when they don't need to cry, because their needs are being cared for, and other babies don't cry but still receive the care they need. Crying may be a fundamental part of what it means to be a baby: birds fly, babies cry.

Some baby animals make sounds that always cause the mother to move closer to the baby animal; these have been called "proximity-promoting calls." The obvious benefit for the baby animal is protection, nurturing, and not getting separated from the group. In infants, it is possible that crying originated as a similar signal that is no longer tightly linked to infant survival, but still occurs as a behavioral remnant of some distant past. For example, babies might have originally had gestations of more than nine months before our ancestors assumed an upright posture; now babies' brains at birth may be a few months biologically immature. The result is that during the first few months, some aspects of brain development may not be well attuned to the outside world, and this misalignment expresses itself as crying.

Another important fact is that the meaning of crying changes with age. Your baby may cry because she is hungry and needs food to survive. But during the first few months, your baby may also cry, smile, or suck when asleep. Your toddler may cry because she wants a second helping of dessert after dinner. Your child may cry when afraid. Your teenager may cry when feeling hopeless. You may cry from happiness at a wedding. Not all crying signifies pain. Unfortunately, when parents talk about crying babies, the assumption is that all crying equals pain. This leads to the sometimes hidden thought, "If my baby cries, I am a bad parent."

Thinking about how mothers relate to their babies during these early times and how they forge close relationships led to two popular concepts: infant bonding and attachment theory. Both focused almost exclusively on mothers and both claimed that future events would be strongly influenced by early experiences.

Infant bonding theories promoted the importance of early physical contact between baby and mother as a mechanism to a better adjustment later in life. The good news was that this concept caused the delivery of babies to become more comfortable, taking place in surroundings more like a hotel room than the cold, impersonal environment of a traditional delivery room. The bad news was that mothers who missed this experience because of complications around the delivery, and mothers who adopted older children, felt deprived and worried about their future relationship with their children. You see, infant bonding was thought to take place only during a critical period, very much like the imprinting of baby geese, who will follow any large, moving object they see at a specific time in their development. The fact is that there is no scientific evidence that a similar critical period exists for human babies, and there is no evidence that lack of "bonding" at a specific time right at birth affects subsequent behavior in either infant or mother.

Attachment theory not only considered the interaction between the mother and the child but claimed that if attachment didn't develop well, the infant would grow into an adult who had difficulty in peer relationships, romantic relationships, or parenthood. The good news was that mothers were encouraged to be affectionate, tactile, and warm without fear of spoiling their child. The bad news was that attention to children twenty-four hours a day was thought to be good. Today's "helicopter parents" are one result.

Popular distortions of attachment theory claimed that a "twenty-four-hour parent"—meaning one who attends to every cry day and night—would produce a more securely attached child than would a "selfish" parent who ignores a cry at night so she can get some sleep. Accumulated scientific data do not support these claims. In fact, published research on children between 7 and 27 months of age has shown that when parents are instructed not to attend to their children's protest crying (extinction), *measurements of infant security significantly improve and all the mothers become less anxious over time.* A similar study in sleep-disturbed infants also showed no evidence of detrimental effects on security. It's a simple but true statement that when the entire family gets more sleep, everyone feels better, even if the cries of one member of the family have to be ignored for a while to get there.

In discussing the myth of popular attachment theory, the famous child psychologist Michael Lewis emphasizes how the development of social skills and peer relation skills are encouraged and protected both by family members other than the mother and by people outside the family. Further, in his aptly titled book *Altering Fate: Why the Past Does Not Predict the Future,* he explains how this development depends more on current, ongoing relationships than on past experiences.

Extremely violent or catastrophic events aside, for ordinary families the power of past events has been extremely exaggerated, and the singular influence ascribed to the mother is unjustified. Strong proponents of the importance of early events have created in the minds of many mothers a *false* conclusion: "I am a bad mother if my child cries, because crying may cause permanent emotional damage."

The sad fact is that older theorists were unaware of the benefits of healthy sleep and how we are fundamentally different in sleep and wake modes. Child psychologists, child psychiatrists, and pediatricians did not know the benefits of healthy sleep until recently. Unfortunately, even today there are too many professionals who lack training regarding children's sleep.

The improvement in educating child health care professionals has been slow; a 2013 national survey of pediatric residency programs showed that half of all programs had only two hours of instruction on sleep and sleep disorders during their three years of training; the average number of hours was 4.4, but 23 percent of the programs provided no sleep education. In 1994, the mean number of hours was 4.8, and 46 percent of programs offered no education to pediatricians. So in nineteen years, the percent of pediatric residency programs that include instruction on sleep issues increased from 54 percent to 77 percent, but the average number of hours remained about the same, only about four to five hours. This partially explains why there is so much misunderstanding about the prevention and treatment of sleep issues in children and why, because they have not received much or any formal education in this area, pediatricians in practice so often incorrectly advise parents that their child is likely to "outgrow" the sleep problem.

When your baby was younger, she slept when she needed to. She controlled your relationship with her, in the sense that you met her needs whether you wanted to or not. You didn't let her go hungry simply because you didn't feel like feeding her just then. You didn't let her stay wet because you didn't feel like changing her. Her needs determined your behavior.

But later on, a shift should occur so that *you* become in charge.

For example, when your child is older, you may decide not to give her junk food simply because she asks for it. You will not risk her physical safety by letting her climb too high on a tree simply because she wants to. And you will not let her stay up late at night to play when she needs to sleep. What, then, are we to do when the child does not cooperate, crying because she does not *want* to go to sleep even though she *needs* to sleep?

"Let Them Cry": A Division of Popular Opinions

There is a long-standing disagreement among those who write for popular magazines or now online about what happens when children cry after being left alone at night to sleep. In September 1984, *McCall's* said: "Letting a baby 'cry it out' will not teach him the basic trust or confidence he needs to feel secure in his new world." *Parents* magazine, in November 1983, said: "It may give him the feeling that there's nobody out there who cares. The child may become a passive, ineffective person, or he may become angry or hostile."

However, the editor in chief of *Parents* wrote in the October 1985 issue, after the birth of her third child: "The trick was that after eight years of parenthood, my husband and I have discovered . . . [that] the first sound does not mean that the baby needs to be picked up immediately." Don't wait eight years to learn what she discovered a long time ago!

"Let Them Cry": An Agreement of Expert Opinions

While the popular press and the Internet may give all types of conflicting evidence from a variety of sources, expert opinion is solidly together. In fact, all evidence from an array of child health specialists concludes that ignoring "protest" crying at bedtime will not cause permanent emotional or psychological problems. In plain fact, the contrary is true. For example, while Dr. D. W. Winnicott, a British pediatrician and child psychiatrist, stressed the importance of mothers' attentive holding of their child, he also emphasized that the *capacity to be alone* is one of the most important signs of maturity in emotional development. In his view, parents can facilitate the development of the child's ability to soothe herself when left alone. Please don't confuse this with abandonment or, on the other hand, use this notion as an excuse for negligence.

Margaret S. Mahler, a prominent child psychoanalyst, identified the beginning of the separation-individuation process whereby the infant begins to differentiate from the mother at 4 to 5 months of age. This is the age when children naturally begin to develop some independence.

Dr. Alexander Thomas and Dr. Stella Chess, two American child psychiatrists, followed more than a hundred children from infancy through young adulthood. One item they examined was the regularity or irregularity of sleep and how parents responded. They wrote: "Removal of symptoms by a successful parent guidance procedure has had positive consequences for the child's functioning and has not resulted in the appearance of overt anxiety or new substitute symptoms. . . . The basic emphasis [of the] treatment technique is a change in the parents' behavior." So please don't fear when your child cries in protest at night, because he is being allowed to "practice" falling asleep, that this crying will cause emotional or psychological problems later. By itself, it will not.

Let me be very clear about this. During the periods of normally occurring day and night sleep times, emotional problems do *not* develop if parents ignore protest crying.

Drs. Thomas and Chess were sensitive to irregular sleep patterns in the infants in their study. Many of those infants also had frequent and prolonged bouts of loud crying. When I asked Dr. Thomas what advice he had given to the parents of those crying babies who did not sleep at night, he responded, "Close the door and walk away." Did this create or produce any problems? His answer: "No. None at all."

Always going to your crying child at night interferes with this natural learning and growth. Such behavior produces sleep fragmentation, destroys sleep continuity, and creates insomnia in your child.

One study examined infant crying at 1 year of age. It compared children over 6 months of age whose parents indiscriminately responded to every cry, day or night, to those children whose parents were trained to respond promptly to every intense, stressed, or demanding cry but to delay their response to quiet vocalizations or weak cries. The children in the first group, whose parents indiscriminately responded, cried much more than children in the second group. This study suggests that crying for attention can be learned or taught by at least 6 months of age. I suspect that this learning can occur even earlier, so I encourage parents to try to be discriminating in their responses to their baby's cries at night as early as possible. This is easier said than done for first-time mothers but much easier for second-time mothers.

Mothers who in general do not feel loving or empathetic toward their children, who are insensitive or emotionally unavailable to them, and who have a lack of warmth or affection are more likely to be referred to psychologists or psychiatrists. Consequently, these specialists sometimes take the attitude that *all* parents should be encouraged to *never* let their child cry, for fear of encouraging a cold parent-child relationship. Based on their observations of a small group of clinically referred families, they make this recommendation to all families. As a general-practice pediatrician, however, I don't share this view, because I see that the vast majority of parents are loving and sensitive to their child's needs. These parents should not fear letting their child cry at night to learn to sleep. Fading (see page 192) is an alternative method and is effective even for mothers receiving psychiatric care.

DOES LETTING MY CHILD CRY TO HELP HER SLEEP BETTER
ACTUALLY HARM HER INSTEAD?

Some parents worry, *"I am afraid that letting my baby cry will cause her permanent emotional harm."* There is no evidence that protest crying while your child is learning how to sleep better will cause any kind of emotional problems later in life. However, because many parents have this fear, I welcome the opportunity to directly address it.

The short answer is no—there is absolutely no scientific evidence to indicate harmful effects of crying to help a child sleep. However, some parents understandably have difficulty allowing their child to cry. For those parents, the following information should set your mind at ease on this point. If you are already secure in the knowledge that you can safely let your child cry in order to teach self-soothing skills, then you can skip this section.

One of the world's foremost researchers in sleep, William C. Dement, taught me at Stanford University Medical School in 1967 that we exist in three distinctly different biological domains: awake, REM sleep, and non-REM sleep. Although all three domains interact with one another, there are specific problems that can occur within each domain.

According to Dr. Dement, traditional medical science historically focused on only the first domain: wakefulness. His major point was that we are fundamentally different when we are asleep than when we are awake. The body's clock knows when we should be asleep and adjusts our brain, our temperature, and our hormone levels to the sleep mode. In sleep mode, we do not respond, think, or feel as we do when awake. If you do not believe this, ask any mother of a 6-week-old infant how she is when she is up at night soothing her baby!

There has been much misunderstanding about "insecurity" and "crying to sleep" because of a failure to make the distinction between (1) *the importance of sleeping well when we are in a biologi-*

cal sleep mode and (2) *the importance of security of attachment when we are in a biological awake mode.* This failure is understandable, because most child psychologists, child psychiatrists, and pediatricians have not had the opportunity to do research or to receive training regarding the benefits of healthy sleep. They do not fully understand or appreciate the degree to which the sleeping brain is different from the awake brain. As previously mentioned, even today very little teaching regarding sleep (only about four to five hours) takes place during the standard three-year pediatric residency program. Sad to say, "expert" advice in popular magazines, books, and blogs often reflects this lack of knowledge.

Because there is a basic difference between the sleeping brain and the awake brain, different types of problems can develop. When the brain enters the biologic domain of sleep, problems such as night terrors might appear. Night terrors and other sleep problems simply do not occur when the brain shifts to the awake domain.

Similarly, we are fundamentally different when we are awake. When our children are awake, we worry about problems such as temper tantrums, fighting, not sharing, or not eating well. Also, we sometimes wonder if we are making the appropriate emotional connection. Are our children getting enough love? Are they happy? Are they securely attached, or do they feel insecure? How we interact with our children while we feed them, bathe them, dress them, and play with them is very important. However, insecurity of attachment as a concept makes no sense when the brain shifts to the sleep domain. When your child's brain is in the sleep mode, he needs sleep and not more social interaction with parents. As stated before, during the periods of normally occurring day and night sleep times, emotional problems do *not* develop if parents ignore protest crying.

Still, you might wonder about what goes on at the borderland between awake and asleep. Does crying harm your child when he is left alone to cross that border and fall asleep?

Dr. William Sears, a champion of attachment parenting, writes in the revised edition of *Nighttime Parenting:*

Attachment parenting builds family harmony but detachment parenting leads to disharmony. . . . [*Detachment parenting*] preach[es]: "Let the baby cry it out." . . . Children are too valuable and their needs too important to be made victims of cheap, shallow advice. . . . Avoid non-supportive and negative advice such as "Let your baby cry it out." . . . These advisors give you the subtle message that your baby is fussing because of something you're doing or not doing. . . . This leads to a vicious cycle . . . result[ing] in *escape mothering*, seeking alternative fulfillment such as a career or other activity outside the home. . . . Researchers found that the harmony between a mother and her suckling infant had an organizing effect on the baby's sleep pattern. [*Note:* This is true—in a study on rats! For more examples of Dr. Sears's selective and misleading use of data, see below.] . . . If, in a difficult situation, you've tried all the natural methods of nighttime parenting, but the family is nevertheless falling apart . . . use of a sleeping medication seems appropriate. . . . In my medical experience, the prescription drug chloral hydrate (Noctec) is the most safe and effective sleep-inducing medication for infants and children. (Emphasis added.)

Noctec is used as a procedural sedative primarily in hospitals for MRI, EEG, cochlear implant, dental procedures, and so forth. It has never been proven to be safe or effective as a sleep aid for children, as described by Dr. Sears.

There you have it. In Dr. Sears's opinion, parents should embrace attachment parenting and all the "natural" methods because research on rats explains how to mother your baby! Let's assume you followed his prescriptions. You ignored those who preach cheap, shallow advice, and you did not practice "detachment parenting" or "escape mothering" by pursuing a career or activity outside the home. But for some reason, your child is still not sleeping well. So what do you do, according to Dr. Sears? You drug your baby to make him sleep!

Well, according to Dr. Weissbluth, drugs are not the answer to this problem!

Unfortunately, unlike me, Dr. Sears has never had the opportunity to do research on sleeping in children, and his fear of "crying it out" (extinction) as a method to help children sleep better appears to blind him to the real harm children suffer when they do not sleep well. It is dangerous to advocate drugs, and it is dangerous to ignore the consequences of not sleeping well.

On his website there is a list of publications that Dr. Sears falsely claims support his position. Actually, *none* of the published research he cites is on the subject of using extinction to help a child sleep better. Instead, his list of publications describes many irrelevant subjects, including studies on rats and nonhuman primates and two discussions on childhood maltreatment.

As an example of how grossly irrelevant and misleading Dr. Sears's list of publications is, he cites Dr. Bruce Perry's "Incubated in Terror: Neurodevelopmental Factors in the Cycle of Violence." Referring to this work, Dr. Sears writes on his website, "He [Dr. Perry] found when chronic stress over-stimulates an infant's brain stem . . . [the] child will display increased aggression, impulsivity, and violence." But wait! What is the "chronic stress" that Dr. Perry studied? Is it some stress that babies undergo while learning to sleep better through extinction? No! The subject of Dr. Perry's research on children is the long-term effects of trauma/neglect such as the Columbine school shootings, the September 11 terrorist attacks, being raised in closets or cages, and family violence. Dr. Perry is not writing about "crying it out" to help infants sleep. Because Dr. Sears's list of citations is widely circulated, it bears restatement: *not a single item in his presentation deals with the question of whether using extinction to help a child sleep better harms the child.* For more information on how dramatically Dr. Sears mis-

uses published studies, see http://mainstreamparenting.wordpress
.com/2008/06/25/of-sources-and-straw-houses-the-annotated-dr-sears
-handout-on-cio.

The assessment that extinction or graduated extinction hurts the
child or damages the relationship between the child and parent is
false. It is irresponsible for a professional such as Dr. Sears to claim
that studies performed only on animals and severely abused or neglected children constitute evidence in support of his position that
"crying it out" in children to help them sleep better is harmful.
Dr. Sears is not a researcher, but among researchers, wildly inappropriate citations or selectively including only those citations that
support your point of view is called intellectual dishonesty.

Dr. Sears's pseudoscientific approach makes it more difficult for
mothers to get a handle on their child's sleeping, because he creates
unwarranted fears that extinction will cause harm. Mothers usually
become sleep deprived after the baby is born, and this alone may
cause significant mental stress. There is a complex interplay between a mother's anxiety, mood, and child sleep issues, and
Dr. Sears's opinions interfere with finding solutions.

Contrary to Dr. Sears's irresponsible opinions, scientific research
has been published in peer-reviewed journals showing that extinction to help an infant or child sleep better does not cause harm. In
fact, the opposite is true: after extinction, there are improvements in
the mother, the child, and the bond between them.

Here are several studies (see also page 181):

Journal of Abnormal and Social Psychology (1959): "No unfortunate side- or after-effects of this treatment were observed. At three and three-quarters years of age, the child
appears to be a friendly, expressive, outgoing child."

Journal of Developmental and Behavioral Pediatrics (1991):
"Extinction is an effective, reasonably rapid, and durable
treatment for infant sleep disturbance [three citations] . . .
mothers became less anxious as the study proceeded. . . .

[The data show that extinction] is consistent with previous reports on improvements in parental self-esteem, depression, marital satisfaction, and sense of control following extinction-based treatments of sleep disturbances [cites two additional supporting studies]. Some have argued, sometimes forcefully, against the use of extinction procedures with infants, on the grounds that such procedures will damage the infant-caregiver (mother) bond and impair the infant's sense of security. A measure of infant security was explicitly included in this study to test this hypothesis, and again, the results are clear. Infant security improved significantly over the course of the study . . . we can reject the hypothesis that exposure to extinction . . . will impair security."

Journal of Pediatric Psychology (1992): "Measured and compared the behavior characteristics and security scores of infants (6–24 months) treated with extinction for sleep disturbances . . . There was no evidence of detrimental effects on the treated infants whose security, emotionality/tension, and likeability scores improved."

Journal of the American Academy of Child and Adolescent Psychiatry (1994): Sleep training improves daytime mother-infant interactions.

Journal of Paediatrics and Child Health (1998): "Cold turkey [extinction and other methods improved] problematic childhood sleep behavior [and] is associated with significant improvement in maternal mood. It is likely significant numbers of mothers diagnosed as having postnatal depression are suffering the effects of chronic sleep deprivation."

Journal of Abnormal Child Psychology (1999): "Both [extinction and graduated extinction] treatments improved bedtime and nighttime sleep problems and only positive side effects were associated with both treatments. Graduated extinction was easier to implement."

Sleep (2006): "Adverse secondary effects [for behavioral treatment of bedtime problems and night waking in infants and young children] as the result of participating were not identified in any of the studies. On the contrary, infants who participated in sleep interventions were found to be more secure, predictable, less irritable, and to cry and fuss less following treatment. . . . It is important to indicate that sleep related behavioral intervention also led to improvement in the well-being of the parents beyond the specific benefits in sleep patterns in the children. . . . The results were remarkably consistent across studies. Following intervention for their child's sleep disturbance, parents exhibited rapid and dramatic improvements in their overall mental health status, reporting fewer symptoms of depression . . . an increased sense of parenting efficiency, enhanced marital satisfaction, and reduced parenting stress."

Sleep (2006): "A total of 13 studies [of behavioral management of sleep problems] have assessed a number of secondary treatment outcomes related to daytime functioning in the child (including behavior, mood, self-esteem, parent-child interactions). The majority of these studies reported positive effects on daytime functioning; no adverse secondary effects were identified in any of these studies. Parental (largely maternal) well-being (including mood, overall mental health status, parenting stress, marital satisfaction) has been included as an outcome measure in 12 studies: results have been consistent in demonstrating improvements in perceived parenting efficacy, marital satisfaction, parenting stress, and maternal mood."

Journal of Child Psychology and Psychiatry (2008): "Maternal separation anxiety as a regulator of infants' sleep . . . [T]he current research documented an interplay between maternal separation anxiety and aspects of the child's sleep-wake transitions."

Early Child Development (2012): For 6-month-old infants with sleep problems, on both the first and third days of a sleep training program, they showed no increase in cortisol levels from before to after "crying it out" (extinction). Also, from the baseline (pre-sleep-training) on the first day to post-sleep-training on the third day there was no increase in cortisol levels. In fact, although not statistically significant, the post-intervention cortisol level after "crying it out" on the third day was lower than the baseline pre-intervention level on the first day. This observation is so important it bears restatement. Cortisol levels after three days of "crying it out" on average showed *no increase* compared to before the sleep training program began. Further, the cortisol level on the fourth day was less than the third day (personal communication). Also, Dr. Wendy Middlemiss wrote, "All infants exhibited behavioral distress on the first day. . . . On the first day of the sleep training program, all infants engaged in 2 or more bouts of crying [one bout of crying was defined as sustained distress for five to ten minutes or more]. In contrast, by the third day of the program, all infants settled to sleep independently without a bout of distress . . . also, the fussing [shorter than one bout of crying] was less intense as well as shorter than the bouts of distress on the first day. . . . Overall, outward displays of internal stress were extinguished by sleep training." Additionally, by the third day, the mothers' cortisol levels were significantly lower, presumably because their infants were crying less or sleeping better or both.

Pediatrics (2012): Behavioral sleep techniques have no harmful effect on measures of children's emotions, behaviors, psychosocial functioning, child-parent closeness, or attachment five years later.

Developmental Psychology (2012): "It is important for babies to learn how to fall asleep on their own . . . learning how to self-soothe is critical for regular sleep."

My observations and sound scientific data show that if children are well rested during the day, and if the bedtime is early enough to prevent a second wind, and if parents do not reinforce the crying by going in to comfort the child, then crying occurring with extinction lasts only a few days, after which the entire family enjoys the physical and psychological benefits of more sleep. My research shows that with extinction in children younger than 4 months, the average amount of crying is as follows:

Night 1:   Crying lasts 30–45 minutes
Night 2:   Crying lasts 10–30 minutes
Night 3:   Crying lasts 0–10 minutes
Night 4:   No crying

In children 4 months of age and older, the usual pattern is:

Night 1:   Crying lasts 45–55 minutes
Night 2:   A little more or a little less crying than night 1
Night 3:   Crying lasts 20–40 minutes
Night 4 or 5:   No crying

If the bedtime is too late or naps are not going well, the process might take longer or not work.

There are a few possible explanations for why there is so much misunderstanding and controversy regarding the subject of children, parents, and sleep. As mentioned previously, pediatricians between 1994 and 2013 spent only about four hours of their three-year training studying sleep, so they have at best only a cursory understanding of the benefits for the child and parents of sleeping well (Chapter 2). Also, as will be discussed later, there is a trade-off in attachment parenting between less fussing/crying when younger and more night waking (signaling) when older, so it is not correct to state that one method of parenting is better than another. Finally, there may be more anxiety about parenting today than in previous generations. If true, this heightened anxiety creates not just fear but uncertainty, with parents worrying, "How do I start helping my child sleep better?"

I WANT TO START A SLEEP SOLUTION, BUT I AM NOT SURE HOW TO DO IT

There is not a one-size-fits-all approach to implementing a sleep solution. Here are several factors to help you think about your particular situation.

Family

When a bedtime is way too late because of one or both parents' work schedule, sometimes a sleep solution depends on having someone other than the parent put the child to sleep earlier or having a parent come home earlier. For some families, neither option may be possible. In others, a parent might be able to come home a little earlier, but still not early enough for an improved bedtime. Even so, small improvements are better than none. Do what you can during the week, and then shift your focus to paying back the sleep debt on weekends, with good-quality naps and super-early bedtimes.

Sometimes a sleep solution should begin on a Saturday when both parents are available to support each other or care for other children. Parents should not start a sleep solution unless they are in complete agreement and can both commit to four to seven days. Teamwork and communication are the bedrock that will support your sleep solution success. As mentioned previously, humans are not robots and cannot realistically expect to achieve perfection. Nevertheless, during the first few days of implementing a new sleep plan, try hard to be 100 percent consistent. If you are inconsistent or cave after one or two days, you'll pay. You will have taught your child that crying is how to get more parental attention. If this happens, don't beat yourself up; try again a few days or weeks later. Often, after that time, families are more determined than ever to persevere, and this new resolve allows them to successfully execute the plan of action. I think this is worth restating, because some parents reading this are surely struggling with their own severe sleep deprivation and the guilt of previous failure to help their child sleep better. It's all right to take breaks when sleep solutions are not working, you feel overwhelmed, or you cannot take any more crying. Waving the white flag is fine when you get discouraged. You can retreat to swing sleep or naps in the stroller or car to regroup and get everyone better rested. Later, try again. Success often occurs on the second try.

It is smart, not selfish, for the mother to take breaks without guilt to recharge her battery, because she is the power source of most of the soothing effort.

Yet success does not rest on the mother alone. It often depends on whether the father remains calm, is willing to help solve the problem, and actively participates in the solution (see Chapter 3). If the father is not willing or able, then the mother might have to wait until he is away from home for an extended period, on a business trip or family visit, to fix a sleep problem. Alternatively, sometimes it's the father who sends the wife to a hotel for the first night of the solution because she is too sleep deprived to tolerate any crying. Sometimes, though, a family feels stuck and has trouble making a start. If that describes your situation, try starting with a baby step.

Start with Small Steps and Simple Solutions
Sometimes a family is reluctant to begin a sleep solution because the mother is severely sleep deprived and feels overwhelmed. Although she intellectually understands what to do, she is unable to execute because she is emotionally strung out. She is fearful that there will be more stress from her baby's crying, and she cannot handle any more stress. She is at her limit. Or she is in a sleep-deprived fog and cannot really see or believe in any viable sleep solution. In either case, try to get the father or others to take over; convince Mom to take a break. Fathers are usually less sleep deprived than mothers, so dads need to step up in this situation and create a plan, if possi-

ble. Some dads need extra motivation, and being optimistic that he can succeed will go a long way toward giving him the confidence to try. Realistically, however, all dads are not always available or willing.

If the mother is doing the heavy lifting by herself, try small, simple, and acceptable steps first and later try to reach optimal sleep for the child. The simpler the solution, the more likely you will remember what to do and do it consistently. For example, a small step that is simple to remember might be a slightly earlier bedtime. Another example might be letting someone else put your baby down drowsy but awake just once a day or once a week. The benefit is that when you see how improvement in your child's sleep causes improvement in his mood and performance, you will be emboldened to try more complex solutions and fine-tuning to improve sleep even though he might protest. Seeing is believing. Of course, a possible outcome is that no improvement might occur because the change in the bedtime is too small to be beneficial. But go ahead anyway and give it a try. What do you have to lose?

An optimal sleep plan for your child might be complex in order to accommodate many variables for your particular family, but it is not always practical to tackle the whole problem at once, and it may not be clear whether to go slowly or quickly.

Gradual Versus Abrupt Changes

There is no hard-and-fast rule as to whether a sleep solution change should be implemented gradually (a check-and-console strategy or graduated extinction) or abruptly (extinction or extinction with a cap). For some parents, gradual changes appear gentler and abrupt changes appear harsher. But gradual changes might take longer to see results. Often a family wishes to move gradually, but after seeing some improvement, they change course and make more dramatic changes. For example, they move quickly from graduated extinction to extinction.

Parents who favor a more gradual approach (check-and-console or graduated extinction) over an abrupt approach (extinction) often complain of frequent "relapses." The general reason a gradual approach tends to be less successful in the long run is that it takes longer and there are always natural disruptions of sleep, such as illnesses or vacations. The subsequent reestablishment of healthy sleep routines using a gradual approach becomes very stressful to the parents. Several days of a gradual approach often wear down parents, so they give up and revert to their old inconsistencies. Parents who have successfully used extinction know that they might have one, and only one, nasty reentry night of crying after they return home from several days on vacation or from a visit to a relative's house.

The truth is that some parents swing back and forth between firmness and permissiveness so often that they cannot make any cure stick. They confuse their wishful thinking with the child's actual behavior. This is why a sleep log can be an important tool to help document what you are really doing and how your child is really responding. After all, short-term "successes" might only reflect brief periods when your child crashes at night from chronic exhaustion. Or the actual improvement in sleep habits may be so marginal that the normal disruptions of vacations, trips, illnesses, or other irregularities constantly buffet the still-tired child and cause repeated "relapses" in which he wakes often during the night or fights going to sleep.

In contrast, parents who successfully carry out an abrupt retraining program—the cold-turkey approach—to improve sleep habits see immediate and dramatic improvement without any lasting ill effects. These children have fewer relapses and recover faster and more completely from natural disruptions of sleep routines. Seeing a cure really "stick" for a while gives you the confidence to keep tighter control over sleep patterns and to repeat the process again if needed.

Sometimes it appears more practical to gradually make a change in a daily sleep schedule, such as when there is a natural nap transition from two naps to one nap and the single midmorning nap is slowly pushed, over the course of a few weeks, toward midday. If you tried to do this abruptly, your child might get a second wind and take no nap! Other times it appears more practical to abruptly make a change, such as when there is a short nap around 6:00 p.m. and a way-too-late bedtime; in fact, this so-called nap should really be the bedtime. But here also, a family might fear that it is too much of a "shock to his system" to abruptly move the bedtime much earlier. Or perhaps they have difficulty themselves with such an early bedtime and want time to gradually make the adjustment. Here is a guideline: When you are keeping your child up later (for example, trying for a single midday nap by delaying the midmorning nap), do it gradually. When you want your child to have an earlier bedtime, if you wish, do it abruptly. But many families are reluctant to move the bedtime earlier.

Fear of an Early Bedtime

Parents often fear that an earlier bedtime will automatically produce an earlier wake-up time that is inconvenient for them. This usually does not occur because an earlier bedtime produces a better-sleeping child who is more able to self-soothe, even in the very early morning hours. This is why sleep begets sleep. Also, a bedtime that is too late might occur because parents coming home late from work want to play with their child and think that the playtime is more important than sleep.

But an earlier bedtime directly benefits your child. And there are indirect benefits for the family as well: the stay-at-home mother doesn't have to deal with a "witching hour" in the late afternoon, and no "witching hour" means the father comes home from work to a calm, well-rested mother; both parents have relaxed private time in the evenings and overnight, which strengthens the marriage; the child is raised by well-rested parents.

How early is early? To repay a sleep debt as part of a sleep solution, a temporary super-early bedtime of 5:30 p.m. (under age 3) or

6:30 p.m. (for older children) might be needed for one or only a few nights. But if this super-early bedtime is kept in place too long, it may backfire and cause the now well-rested child to have a long latency to sleep or create a wake-up time that is way too early. So after a few days, when he is sleeping better, gradually move the bedtime back a little. Through trial and error, find that sweet spot for the new later bedtime hour that is not as late as the original too-late bedtime hour.

A 5:30 p.m. bedtime might also be used for only one night after a natural sleep disruption caused by an illness or family holiday. I call this a "reset." Put your child to bed super early and ignore protest crying. One, but only one, night of protest might be the price you pay for a lovely family holiday. But this single super-early bedtime might be employed several times a year because of frequent grandparent visits or illnesses. Be firm.

So the bedtime is not a fixed clock time but is moved earlier when needed, then readjusted later again to keep your child well rested, which is the overall goal.

Competing Goals

One important goal is to synchronize soothing with the onset of the rising biological wave of sleepiness at nap times and bedtimes. So after your child reaches about 4 months of age, the advice is to keep him up until the anticipated time this wave is expected to occur, even if he is sleepy earlier. Keep him up to catch the wave!

Another important goal is to avoid a second wind by not keeping him up when he is short on sleep, because if he gets extremely short on sleep it will be harder for him to fall asleep and stay asleep. Put him down early before he gets keyed up!

These two goals may be in conflict, especially when your child is short on sleep. So to achieve the first goal, adopt a gradual approach and keep him up a little later each day or so to get closer to his natural sleep time. To do that, you might have to tolerate a little second wind and deal with it by distraction, entertainment, amusement, and longer soothing to sleep. Temporarily, the bedtime might be super early (5:30 p.m.) while you search for his best nap time and bedtime. Keeping track with a sleep log may help you discover his best sleep times by seeing the forest and not the trees. The big picture is most important, but when you are sleep deprived, it may be hard to see.

Details and the Whole Picture

We often get caught up in the day-to-day details of our children's sleep and sometimes have to take a step back and look at the whole picture. For example, a parent might say, "Help! My son gets up too early, around 5:00 a.m." It is important to know how often this too-early wake-up time occurs. If the 5:00 a.m. wake-up time occurs 10–20 percent of the time, there may be circumstances in the family that render this too-early wake-up unavoidable. For instance, occasional late scheduled sports for an older sibling might cause the bedtime for the baby to be too late, which will cause him occasionally to awaken too early in the morning. Perhaps the family will be able to hire a babysitter or have a relative or neighbor watch the baby when the older sibling has a late sports event. Or maybe they will have to accept this as an untreatable minor sleep problem and learn to live with it. On the other hand, if the 5:00 a.m. wake-up time occurs 80–90 percent of the time, the baby will eventually exhibit major adverse effects from cumulative sleepiness, and this should be viewed as definitely change-worthy.

Don't fret about naps or night sleep on a day-to-day or night-to-night basis. It will drive you crazy. That is missing the forest for the trees. When starting a sleep solution, be patient with your plan, and remember that it may take several days or several weeks before you see the benefits. Try something for at least several days before you conclude it is or it is not helpful. If you do not see improvement, step back and look at all the elements of healthy sleep (Chapter 1), because focusing on only one sleep issue might have distracted you from noticing that other aspects of your child's sleep also need improvement. Improvement may be sequential (first night sleep, then the midmorning nap, and then the midday nap), not simultaneous. It may take weeks for naps to improve after night sleep has improved.

Relatives and Friends

There are individual variations in sleep patterns at any given age, even though there are general patterns that apply for every age. There is enormous variation among families regarding teamwork, number of rooms, the presence or absence of colic, and so forth. *Don't compare your child to other children;* just focus on your own child. For example, your child's naps might be shorter than your sister's child's naps, so your child should be going to bed a little earlier. What works for your relatives and friends may not work for you. Often a mother in my practice, who was successful in helping her child sleep well, might complain to me that her advice to a relative or friend went unheeded and wonder why their child's sleep deprivation was ongoing. Knowing that her husband had cooperated, I would ask whether the husband of her relative or friend was as supportive as her own husband, and the usual answer was no.

Regular sleep schedules in general help anchor healthy sleep. But *don't be a slave to a sleep schedule.* Exceptions to your sleep plan, such as skipping naps or staying up late for holidays or special occasions, are fine once or twice a month, but not much more often. Well-rested children tolerate these events and recover quickly. Early bedtimes or naps at home are *socially limiting.* But it is *liberating* to be out with a well-rested child who never fusses, and it is liberating for a couple to have relaxed private time in the evening when their child easily falls asleep early at night.

When starting a sleep solution, *be discreet* in confiding details of your plan to other people. You are in a vulnerable state because of your own sleep deprivation and therefore do not want to invite critical comments from relatives or friends who may not be supportive. Talk to your pediatrician, especially if your child has eczema or chronic snoring or mouth breathing during sleep before embarking on any sleep-solution plan.

The Sleep Wheel: Sleep as a Twenty-Four-Hour Cycle

Imagine an upright wheel slowly rotating to make a complete revolution every twenty-four hours. It looks like a Ferris wheel, but I call it a Sleep Wheel. The Sleep Wheel illustrates how your child's sleep is not made up of independent, isolated parts but instead is composed of different but related parts.

The Sleep Wheel is driven by a giant engine, perhaps the largest motor you can imagine: the rotation of the Earth on its axis. As the Earth rotates, it creates alternating periods of light and darkness. You have no control over the speed of the Sleep Wheel. It turns round and round no matter what you do as a parent.

However, as a parent, you can build the spokes that radiate from the center to the rim and create the structural integrity of the wheel. The four spokes of the Sleep Wheel support the rim:

1. Start early
2. Many hands (get Dad and others on board)
3. Put your child down while drowsy but awake
4. Many naps (no cumulative sleepiness, no second wind)

These spokes support the structure because they allow your baby to begin to learn self-soothing. If the spokes are strong, your child will have a smooth ride as the wheel turns round. If the spokes are weak, the rim will wobble in the wind. If some spokes are missing or there are no spokes at all, the rim will bend or collapse altogether.

Attached to the rim of a Ferris wheel are passenger cars, but attached to the Sleep Wheel are the six different parts of your child's twenty-four-hour sleep/wake cycle. Let's follow the Sleep Wheel through one complete revolution, beginning with the evening bedtime.

1. At 6 weeks of age (all ages are counted from the due date), an *early bedtime* develops. The failure to establish an early bed-time will result in a second wind that causes bedtime battles, difficulty in falling asleep, and difficulty staying asleep, such as night awakenings (fragmented night sleep) or waking up too early in the morning. If day sleep is deficient, a second wind will develop in the late afternoon or evening and make it dif-ficult to easily fall asleep unattended (drowsy but awake) or stay asleep (consolidated sleep). You then might see bedtime battles and fragmented sleep (signaling).

2. *Consolidated night sleep* develops before or between 6 and 9 months of age, when babies no longer need to be fed at night. Feed your baby at night when hungry but do not re-spond to every sound. Responding to your baby at night for soothing when he is not hungry will create a night crying habit around or after 4–6 months of age. At that point, soothing becomes more socially stimulating. Fragmented night sleep is as harmful as brief night sleep and might cause your baby to wake up too early in the morning.

3. *Wake-up time* is not too early. If you go to your baby too early to start the day, she will not be able to nap well later because she starts the day too tired. Many young babies start the day between 5:30–6:30 a.m.

4. The *midmorning nap* is regular but initially brief and develops around 3–4 months of age. This nap should start around 9:00 a.m. If it starts much earlier than that because your child woke up tired (whether because the bedtime was too late, there was fragmented night sleep, or too early a wake-up time in the morning), then the rest of the day's sleep will be thrown off schedule. On the other hand, if the nap starts too late, a second wind will make self-soothing for the midmorning nap

difficult or impossible, or it may cause the nap to be way too brief. This nap may naturally become longer until 6 months of age, after which it will become shorter.

5. The *midday nap* is regular but initially brief and develops shortly after the midmorning nap. This nap starts around 12:00–2:00 p.m. If it starts too early because your child wakes up too tired from his midmorning nap (whether because the bedtime was too late, there was fragmented night sleep, too early a wake-up time in the morning, or a midmorning nap that took place too early or too late), then the rest of the day's sleep will be thrown off schedule. On the other hand, if the nap starts too late, a second wind will make self-soothing difficult or impossible for the midday nap, or the midday nap might be too brief. This nap may naturally become longer until 6 months of age, after which it will become shorter.

6. *Late afternoon nap(s)* tend(s) to be irregular and brief. They usually disappear by 9 months of age.

Good naps prevent a second wind in the evening and make it easier for your child to self-soothe for bedtime.

Whether you have a newborn or an older child of any age, your first task as a parent is to build the spokes of the Sleep Wheel. Then you start to assemble the six different parts of your child's twenty-four-hour sleep/wake cycle based on your child's age. There are two common pitfalls: one is that a parent is focused on one or more of the six parts but has not yet constructed the spokes, and the other is that a parent is focused on only one (or two or three) of the six parts and ignores the others.

Each of the six parts affects the other five. If one is not developed at the appropriate age, the entire Sleep Wheel becomes unbalanced.

My Child Is Different; I Don't Believe You

Q: *All children are different, and your suggestions to fix sleep problems will not work for my child.*

A: Some success occurs in *all* children when parents keep their children well rested during the day, establish a reasonably early bedtime that prevents a second wind, and consistently do not reinforce crying at night. All of these elements are necessary.

Q: *I think that you cherry-picked or faked the success stories in your book.*

A: Read at random a few of the more than 1,400 five-star parent reviews of the prior edition of this book online to see how quickly children can be helped to sleep better. Success is more elusive when the bedtime is too late, when the child does not sleep well during the day, and when there is too much parental attention during the night.

Q: *All children are different, and my child does not need to sleep when you suggest.*

A: The fundamental fact is that you can't fight circadian rhythms, and if you try to do so, it is your child who will pay the price. This is true for *all* children.

Q: *I think you are wrong that early bedtimes are such a big deal.*

A: During my forty years of general pediatric practice, I cared for many children from their first day to age 18–22. During a routine office visit, I might discuss a minor sleep issue such as a newly observed slightly longer time required for the child to fall asleep. In such a case, I would ask how the child appears between 4:00 and 5:00 p.m., and the mother might report, "She's fine. She's always sweet and charming, active and playful." Nevertheless, I would often suggest a slightly earlier bedtime for one to three nights as a trial. Usually, three days later the child would be falling asleep faster, the total night-sleep duration would be slightly longer, and the mother's report would be, to her surprise, that her child was now even sweeter, calmer, more alert, and more patient between 4:00 and 5:00 p.m. than before. Skepticism about this scenario is a normal response.

When I would ask the mother if she'd ever thought her daughter would actually become sweeter with a slightly earlier bedtime, the answer would almost invariably come back as no. Still, the mother might protest that the earlier bedtime is inconvenient. My reply to this objection was to remind the mother that her child did in fact fall asleep at the earlier bedtime, with good results, which proves that her child needed the earlier bedtime and that the previous bedtime was too late. In this common scenario, the shift to an earlier bedtime might be as little as ten to twenty minutes! The fact that small changes like this may have profound consequences is discussed in Chapter 1. Obviously, this slightly earlier bedtime will not help for major sleep problems caused by a bedtime that is way too late.

Q: *I think you are wrong that sleep is more important than classes.*
A: It is common for first-time parents to be anxious because of their inexperience. There is an enormous parenting-education industry trying to sell their goods and services to parents, and the industry deliberately preys on parents' worries and insecurities. The industry succeeds by implied fake promises: "Your child will be better (smarter, brighter, stronger, more successful) if you buy this product or take this class." Please stop eating the baloney sandwiches that they are trying to feed you.

Parents need to understand that much of what is being promoted to them is not based on any scientific evidence of benefit to their child. There is a long history of once popular but now thoroughly discredited parenting enterprises: "patterning" as a treatment for children with developmental delays was sold by the Institutes for the Achievement of Human Potential (1955);

therapy for autism, based on the false premise that autism is caused by "refrigerator mothers," was promoted by the Orthogenic School at the University of Chicago (1967); the now-debunked "Mozart Effect" to raise your child's IQ (1997) was sold by CD purveyors; Baby Einstein DVD videos, advertised as educational for babies and sold by Disney, were recalled (2009); and probiotics, a $24 billion industry, were shown to not soothe babies' colic (2013). Yet even today, innumerable "educational" toys, videos, games, and computer-based activities are being marketed to naive parents who only want the best for their children.

A contributing factor in today's rush to "improve my child" is that parents' challenges have increased in modern times. There are more mothers in the workforce and away from their children (contributing to so-called working mother's guilt); the global economy means that there are more people competing for fewer good jobs; parents want more educational activities for their children because there is more information available and more facts to be learned. And it is harder for parents to pay close attention to their children and harder for children to pay close attention to their parents and other children because of screen-based distractions. All these factors tend to inhibit early bedtimes or displace naps.

Simply ask yourself: what is the power of a nap that can turn a raving, ranting, and out-of-control toddler into a sweet and charming human being?

I know that I am ruffling some feathers to suggest that sleep may sometimes be more important than a scheduled activity. If you are skeptical that sleep is more important than another lesson, class, or sports activity, talk to a disinterested party such as your pediatrician, a child psychologist or child psychiatrist, or a specialist in early child development. Of course, you might get a different opinion from someone who will personally benefit, such as a coach, tutor, or preschool operator/owner. Even a mother who is using a drop-off class as a babysitter so she has more self-maintenance time might highly praise a class in order to feel better about not spending time with her child. So be careful whom you listen to and consider what is behind their recommendations. Again and again in this book, I show you what stands behind my recommendations: deep experience and solid scientific research.

My position is that sleep is of vital importance and well-rested children soak up knowledge like a dry sponge. Colors are more vivid, sounds are more interesting, smells and tastes are more exciting. Life and being with others is more enjoyable. Sleepy children experience a drabber, duller world, as through a glass darkly. Remember how it is for you when you get foggy or nod off at a class, concert, meeting, or party. Think of all that you have missed in your life because you were too sleepy or sleep deprived. Is that how you want your child to grow up?

Of course, in real life it's often a matter of degree. We don't go through our days alternating between being fully alert and calm and being groggy and crabby. Most of us live in a gray zone somewhere in the middle of these extremes, occasionally moving more in one direction and then in the other. It's no different with your child, and part of your job as parent is to decide when it is more important to schedule an activity for your child and when you should focus on letting your child get the sleep she needs. My observation is that when parents routinely keep their child well rested, then that child is more able to deal with occasional sleep disruptions such as classes or family outings.

But it is absurd to think that your child will get much benefit from some activity when he has a strong biological need for sleep.

Because marital disharmony or mental health problems in parents may express themselves in choices involving their children, such as classes versus extra sleep, and since these conflicts interfere with rapid success in correcting a sleep problem, these and similar challenges should be explicitly dealt with first, if at all possible.

REMEMBER
Different children require different approaches.

An easy, regular, common fussy baby may respond quickly to sleep-training strategies at around 6 weeks. A more irregular, extremely fussy/colicky child may respond well when 3 to 4 months of age.

Summary and Action Plan for Exhausted Parents

Young children and infants cannot tell us how they feel, so parents need to be watchful. Is your child active, alert, vital, and wide awake, or is he fighting sleep and woozy?

MAJOR POINT
Junk food is bad for the body. Junk sleep is bad for the brain.

Obviously, sleeping is not an automatically regulated process like the control of body temperature. Sleeping is more like feeding. We do not expect children to grow well if all they eat is junk food. Children need a well-balanced diet in order to grow. If the food that is provided is insufficient or unbalanced, this unhealthy diet will interfere with the child's growth and development. The same is true for unhealthy sleep patterns.

REAL LIFE
If your child has a sleep problem that requires multiple changes, but you are only able to make some of the changes, go ahead and do the best you can.

Be consistent. Anytime you make a change, allow at least four to five days before making another change to see whether you have helped your child. Be patient.

1. Keep a sleep log as described on page 216.
2. Identify the main sleep problem; review the chapter that fits your child's age.
3. Identify the elements of sleep that need improvement or correction for your child's sleep problem:
   Self-soothing (see Chapter 3)
   Sleep duration: night sleep and day sleep
   Naps
   Sleep consolidation
   Sleep schedule
   Sleep regularity
4. Determine what you can and cannot do ("let cry," "maybe cry," "no cry" sleep solutions). Are there parent issues that need to be addressed (see Chapter 3)?

IMPORTANT POINTS

Sleeping well is a 24/7 process. It's not just about how we get our children to go to bed at night without crying. Solving sleep problems may be a very tough prescription and demands a consistent approach. There may be increased crying in the beginning, but the payoff is that crying around sleep will be eliminated altogether in the end. Children benefit by becoming healthy sleepers and self-soothers who welcome each day with the resources of the well rested. Parents benefit by sleeping better themselves, which makes them better parents and partners.

How to Live with Your Choice

If you alone are doing the heavy lifting, keep it simple. There may be many variables and specific features about your family that you wish to change, but you are likely to be sleep deprived yourself, so a single change in routine might be all that you can handle for now. For example, moving the bedtime earlier is usually a powerful part of any sleep solution, so start with that. Complex solutions and fine-tuning might be left to a later time, when you get some help or you are less sleep deprived.

If you have help and the ability to make a full-court press, work on all the age-appropriate sleep elements simultaneously.

Collect data. However, diary data are too detailed to be useful; instead, make a sleep log so you can see the forest for the trees. Look at the big picture to see if there is a pattern that explains why there are good sleep times and not-good sleep times.

Fathers are usually less sleep deprived than mothers, so try to get the father to create a plan. Many fathers want to cooperate with helping their child sleep, but only in the sense that they will do what their wife tells them to do. They expect her to be the leader in all things related to child rearing and view themselves as the helpful follower. This does not work for finding and successfully executing a sleep solution when the mother is very sleep deprived. Assign Dad the responsibility of reading about sleep, collecting and analyzing data, and, with feedback from Mom if practicable, creating and executing a plan. Make it his job! Even if Mom isn't crazy about the plan, she should stand down for a few days to give it a chance . . . and to give herself time to recover energy, equilibrium, and insight. Remember: allow a few days to go by before tweaking or abandoning the plan. Once you see some improvement, be patient; it may take several days or a few weeks to see the full benefit of your plan.

If you feel overwhelmed, take a break from your plan to give yourself time to regroup, and consider restarting it later. Success often occurs on the second try.

Don't compare children. There is individual variation in sleep patterns at any given age. Don't compare results. There is enormous variation among families regarding teamwork, number of bedrooms, the presence or absence of colic, and parent issues.

Exceptions to your sleep plan such as skipping naps or staying up late for holidays or special occasions are fine once or twice a month, but not much more often. Well-rested children tolerate these events and recover quickly.

Talk to your pediatrician if your child has eczema or chronic snoring or mouth breathing during sleep.

PART II

Establishing Healthy Sleep Habits from Infancy to Adolescence

CHAPTER 5

Healthy Sleep Habits in the First Month

A main goal at this age is to encourage the development of self-soothing skills.

Every newborn baby is unique. And the closer we look, the more differences we see. Some of these differences reflect genetic or inborn traits. Recent sleep research has focused on genes that control our biological clocks. For mothers of fraternal twins, the finding that sleep periods occur at different clock times will not be surprising. There are other differences present at birth that are not inherited but are caused by whether the baby was born at 37 or 42 weeks of gestation, or whether the mother smoked or drank large amounts of alcohol during her pregnancy. One area of research, based on animal studies, is how the mother's biological rhythms may help set or influence the rhythms of the fetus and the newborn baby: based on the regularity or irregularity of the mother's sleep/wake patterns, activity/rest patterns, or eating patterns, there may be a kind of prenatal programming affecting the baby's own rhythms.

All of these differences—in smiling, sucking, sleeping, physical activity, and so on—combine to make a baby an individual. This chapter will describe the individual sleeping patterns in babies and how these patterns change as babies grow. Despite individual differences, there is some advice that applies to all babies:

Think and plan *how* you want to soothe your baby but, more important, *when* you soothe your baby.

- Babies quickly become overtired after only one or two hours of wakefulness, and some cannot comfortably stay up for even one hour! During the day, note the time when your baby wakes up and try to help her nap by soothing within the next one or two hours, before she becomes overtired. Try to keep the intervals of wakefulness brief.
- Babies less than 6 weeks old may fall asleep very late at night, and each bout of sleep may not be very long during the day or night. Try to soothe your baby to sleep during the day before she becomes overtired. Always respond to your baby when you think your baby is hungry or in distress. Avoid the overtired state by keeping the intervals of wakefulness brief.
- Eighty percent of babies more than 6 weeks old become more settled at night, sleep a little longer at night, and begin to become drowsy for night sleep at an earlier hour. If your baby shows signs of drowsiness earlier, try to soothe her to sleep at an earlier hour.
- Twenty percent of babies more than 6 weeks old do not appear to become more settled at night, do not appear to sleep longer at night, and do not become drowsy at an earlier hour. Nevertheless, try to soothe your baby to sleep at an earlier hour even if she does not show signs of drowsiness earlier. Spend extra time soothing: prolonged swinging, long luxurious baths, and never-ending car rides. Fathers should put forth extra effort to help out.

Newborn: The First Week

Night sleep: No established rhythms
Day sleep: No established rhythms
Bedtimes: No established rhythms

Begin to teach self-soothing and bedtime routines (see Chapter 3)
and feed only when your baby is hungry at night.

After your baby is born, you will experience the joy of becoming a parent along with the exhaustion that follows labor and delivery and perhaps the groggy aftereffects of anesthesia or pain medication. During the first few days, you don't have to worry about when to feed your baby and put him to sleep because in hospitals without total rooming-in, a feed/sleep schedule is imposed on baby care activities. The feed/sleep schedule is determined by general guidelines to prevent low blood sugar, changes of nursing shifts, visiting hours, and the need to measure vital signs. You will receive instructions regarding when to feed your baby when you are discharged but not when or how to put your baby to sleep. Feelings of uncertainty or anxiety regarding feeding and sleeping may surface as you prepare to go home. This is normal, because the first-time parent is a rookie. Even the second-time parent is worried about how to manage more than one child. Only the third-time parent is a true veteran!

Your baby has no circadian rhythms or internal biological clocks
yet, so you can't set your baby to clock time.

For most full-term babies, as soon as the parents arrive home, they will need to disregard the clock and feed their baby whenever she seems hungry, change her when she wets, and let her sleep when she needs to sleep. Full-term babies sleep a lot during the first several days; pre-term babies sleep even more, while post-term babies sleep less. For a few days, full-term babies eat very little and often lose weight. This is all very natural and should not alarm you. If your baby sleeps a lot, don't confuse sweetness with weakness.

Turn off your phone when nursing, when napping, and when with
your husband. After a few weeks, if you are nursing, consider a
once-a-day relief bottle (formula or expressed breast milk).

Presumably this calm, quiet period during the first days is syn-chronized with the few days it takes for the mother's breast milk to come in. Babies sleep a lot, fifteen to eighteen hours a day, but usu-ally in short stretches of two to four hours. These sleep periods do not follow a pattern related to day and night, so get your own rest whenever you are able.

Q: *I heard that I am supposed to put my baby to sleep when drowsy but awake. But every time I feed her, she quickly falls asleep. Am I supposed to wake her up and then put her down to sleep?*

A: Newborns usually fall asleep during a feeding, and it does not make sense to wake them simply in order to put them back to sleep. It goes against Mother Nature! But older babies, when they really slow down or finish sucking, may be almost but not quite asleep. When the breast or bottle is removed, older babies momentarily look around in a dazed fashion, just to check out that everything is okay, and then go into a deep, comfortable snooze.

Why, then, have you heard that you should not let your child fall asleep during soothing or feeding? The theory is that your child needs to learn self-soothing skills, and that she will not learn these skills if she comes to associate soothing or feeding with sleep. Con-sider two scenarios. In the first scenario, you keep the intervals of wakefulness brief, less than one to two hours, and you watch for signs of drowsiness (see Chapter 3). At the drowsy time, you soothe and feed your baby. She now may be drowsier and entering the sleep zone, but she is not completely asleep at the end of the soothing and feeding. That is when you put her down. Now she is able to self-soothe herself to deep slumber. This is easy because she was not overtired, and 80 percent of babies (those who display common fussiness/crying) can handle this well. But this scenario does not require you to awaken your baby if she occasionally falls asleep dur-ing a feeding. There may be a lot of non-nutritive sucking after a feeding, so if your baby often falls into a deep sleep at the breast, slightly shorten the duration of the feeding plus sucking in order to be able to put her in her crib drowsy but awake. As long as weight gain is fine, there is no harm in trying this.

In the second scenario, you allow your child to stay up too long and she becomes overtired. She has passed through the drowsy zone and is entering the fatigue zone. Now, when you soothe and feed your baby, you discover that she will not be easily placed in her crib or stay asleep unless she is already in a deep sleep at the end of the soothing and feeding. Soothing herself to sleep is difficult because she develops a second wind or she belongs to the 20 percent of babies (those afflicted with extreme fussiness/colic) who are often this way during the first few months. The problem is not your failure to "put her to sleep when drowsy but awake"; rather, the problem is allowing your baby to become overtired or being unlucky and having an extremely fussy/colicky baby.

WARNING!
The first week of life is like a honeymoon. Newborns "sleep like a baby" except when your baby is born post-term.
For all babies: **It will become more and more difficult to soothe and put to sleep your baby in the evening hours at 6 weeks of age, counting from the due date.**
For 80 percent of babies: **They will settle down at night after 6 weeks.**
For 20 percent of babies: **It will become more and more difficult to soothe and put to sleep your baby all the time starting at several days of age, counting from the due date. All these babies settle down at night around 3 to 4 months of age, some even at 2 months.**

When your baby becomes more and more difficult to soothe and put to sleep, he appears to be completely out of your control, and your life will not be easy. Sleep training is described in detail in

Chapter 3 and does not mean simply letting your baby cry. Sleep training involves:

Teaching self-soothing
  Start early
  Many hands (enlist Dad and others)
  Put your baby down drowsy but awake
Many naps, with brief intervals of wakefulness
Bedtime routines

Weeks 2 to 4: More Fussiness

Night sleep: No established rhythms
Day sleep: No established rhythms
Bedtimes: No established rhythms

All babies are a little hard to "read" during the first few weeks. Most activities such as feeding, changing diapers, and soothing to sleep occur at irregular times. Do not expect your baby to adhere to a schedule because the baby's needs for food, cuddling, and sleeping are going to occur erratically and unpredictably. When your baby needs to be fed, feed him; when he needs to have his diaper changed, change him; and when he needs to sleep, allow him to sleep.

What do I mean by "allow him to sleep"? Try to provide a calm, quiet place for your baby if he sleeps better this way. Many babies are very portable at this age and seem to sleep well anywhere. You're lucky if your baby is like this, and you're even luckier if he is one of the few who have long night-sleep periods. During weeks 2 to 4, most newborns don't sleep for long periods at night.

Studies have shown that for babies a few weeks old, the longest single sleep period may be only three to four hours, and it can occur at any time during the day or night. (This is known as day/night confusion, though the term is a bit misleading. It's not that your baby gets day and night mixed up; instead, your baby has not yet developed her internal timekeeping mechanisms that distinguish night from day.) Extremely fussy/colicky babies may not even have a single sleep period that is this long; premature babies may have longer sleep periods.

Parenting strategies such as changes in the amount of light or noise don't appear to greatly influence babies' sleep patterns at this stage. In fact, specific styles or methods of burping, changing, or feeding do not seem to really affect the baby at all. Try not to think of doing things *to* or *for* the baby. Instead, take time to enjoy doing things *with* your baby. Do the things that give you both pleasure: holding, cuddling, talking, singing, listening to music, walking, and bathing. This active love is sufficient stimulation for now; you don't have to worry about buying the right toy to stimulate your baby. Here are some concrete steps you can take to make it easier for everyone:

1. Take naps during the day when your baby is sleeping.
2. Turn off all phones in the house when your baby is sleeping.
3. Go out, without your baby, for breaks: a walk, a coffee date, or a movie.
4. Plan or arrange for a few hours of private time to take care of yourself.
5. Do whatever comes naturally to soothe your baby; don't worry about spoiling her or creating bad habits. But do try to ignore the very quiet vocalizations that normally occur during sleep and which do not indicate hunger or distress.
6. Use swings, pacifiers, or anything else that safely provides rhythmic, rocking motions or engages the sucking reflex.

If you find that your baby sleeps well everywhere and whenever she is tired, enjoy your freedom while you can. A time will come when you will be less able to visit friends, shop, or go to exercise classes, because your baby will need a more consistent soothing-to-sleep routine and a less stimulating sleep environment.

Q: *Why are breast-fed babies fed more often at night than formula-fed babies?*

A: It may be that breast milk takes less time to digest, so the breast-fed baby is hungrier sooner. It may be that the mother who has chosen to breast-feed is more sensitive or attuned to her baby and responds more frequently to the baby's sounds: both hungry sounds and sleep sounds. Maybe the breast-feeding mother is more committed to soothing or nurturing her baby, using her breasts as a pacifier even when her baby is just fussy and not hungry. Perhaps the breast-feeding mother responds more often because her breasts feel uncomfortably full. Or the mother who is breast-feeding is unsure whether her baby has gotten enough, because, unlike the formula-fed baby, she cannot see how much her baby has taken. Both breast milk and formula have the same number of calories per ounce even though formula appears to be thicker.

Q: *I've heard that my newborn should not sleep in the bassinet in my room because it will spoil him.*

A: Nonsense. For feeding or nursing, it makes it easier for both of you if your newborn is close. When your baby is older, say 3 or 4 months, both of you may sleep better if he is not in your room. Anyway, by then the number of night feedings is usually fewer.

Brief awakenings or complete arousals at night occur normally, at all ages, as discussed in Chapter 1. Quiet or brief vocalizations may accompany these arousals. In young infants, especially under 4 months of age, babies are fed at night and some of these arousals might be misinterpreted as hunger. At any age, if parents attend to these normal arousals too frequently or provide too much intervention, the child may develop a night-crying or night-feeding habit. This becomes a sleep problem called signaling, and because it fragments both the child's and parent's sleep, the result is a sleep-deprived family. Signaling describes children who have difficulty or are unable or unwilling to return to sleep unassisted. Over time, the number of times the child awakens and signals tends to increase and the duration of wakefulness of each event also increases.

Q: *When will my child sleep through the night?*

A: After 6 weeks, infants tend to go to sleep earlier, around 6:00 to 8:00 p.m., and most need to be fed before they wake up to start the day. The need for night feedings disappears slowly over the next several months. After a few months, most babies do not need to be fed more than twice at night: in the middle of the night and early in the morning. Except for breast-fed babies in a family bed, more than two night feedings after a few months will begin to create a night-waking habit. After 9 months, these night feedings are not needed. Sleeping through the night is discussed in detail in Chapters 7 and 8.

A change occurs in all babies during these first few weeks, and you should prepare for it. When your baby is about to fall asleep or is just about to wake up, a sudden single jerk or massive twitch of his entire body may occur. As the drowsy baby drifts into a deeper sleep, the eyes sometimes appear to roll upward. This is normal behavior during sleep/wake transitions. Also, all babies become somewhat more alert, wakeful, and aroused as the brain develops. You may notice restless movements, such as shuddering, quivering, tremulousness, shaking or jerking, twisting or turning, and hiccoughs. There may be moments when your sweet little baby appears impatient, distressed, or agitated for no identifiable reason. This is all normal newborn behavior. These behaviors will soon disappear as the brain develops more inhibitory control, especially after 6 weeks of age.

During these spells of unexplainable restlessness or fussiness, your baby may swallow air and become gassy. Often he appears to be in pain. Sometimes he cries and you can't figure out why. The crying baby may be hungry or just fussy. This is confusing and frustrating to all parents.

All in all, at this point you may not have the baby you dreamed of having. She fusses or cries too much, sleeps too little, and spits up on you whenever you forget to cover your shoulder with a towel. This is known as reality, and the sooner parents learn to accept the baby they have, rather than stressing about some hypothetical perfect dream baby, the better everyone will be.

Fussiness and Crying

Baby-Driven Path, the Role of the Baby

COMMON FUSSINESS /CRYING

Fussiness
Fussiness is an unsettled or agitated state that often precedes crying if not attended to by parents with soothing efforts. A fussy child appears to be in mild distress or mildly uncomfortable. But not all fussiness in children is created equal. How do you judge the degree of your child's fussiness? Measurements of fussiness are used by researchers and pediatricians to *arbitrarily* divide infants into groups with names like "common fussiness" or "extreme fussiness." But these measurements don't paint a complete picture, just as the measure of your weight in pounds does not say everything about your total health picture. That's why I advise parents not to worry about measurements and labels. Instead, keep in mind that your child will have a little, a medium amount, or a lot of unexplained fussiness and crying that is likely to first increase, then decrease after 6 weeks (counting from the due date), and then disappear more or less completely around 2–4 months of age.

But at 2 to 4 weeks, as fussiness and crying increase with attendant swallowed air (gassiness), you cannot predict how much fussiness and crying there will be in the future, so it is worthwhile to read this entire section to prepare yourself for possible challenges ahead.

Eighty percent of babies have common fussiness, and the parents of these babies are fortunate. These babies do not require a lot of parental soothing. They tend to be naturally self-soothing, mild, and calm; they fall asleep easily and sleep for long periods.

Breast-feeding these babies is relatively easy because the mothers tend to be better rested and the babies tend to be more regular in their habits. Feedings may be relatively short and infrequent because nursing is mainly for satisfying thirst and hunger. When these babies are fussy, methods of soothing other than breast-feeding often work. In fact, the popularity of many techniques or strategies for soothing babies is due to the fact that for these babies—the majority of babies—most everything for soothing works well!

Bottle-feeding these babies either formula or expressed breast milk with or without breast-feeding is a family decision that is usually easily made. Some considerations are to allow the father or other children the pleasure of feeding the baby, thus enabling the mother to get some needed extra sleep at night or to return to work by continuing to pump her breasts at work, or to make it easier for the parents to arrange an evening for an old-fashioned date.

Before your baby is born, you might decide that you want to sleep with your baby (see SIDS, Chapter 1) or that you want to use a crib or bassinet. For 80 percent of all babies, those with common fussiness, it doesn't matter which you choose; these babies are fairly adaptable and self-soothing. You might sleep with your baby both during naps and at night, or only at night. Or you might lie down with your baby when she first falls asleep, put her down in her crib, and then, at the first night feeding, bring her into bed with you. Or you might have a co-sleeper attached to your bed and use it for part or all of the night. You can easily put your baby to sleep within one to two hours of wakefulness, because drowsy cues are usually obvious in these babies. Any soothing-to-sleep method is likely to work, and the baby and parents usually sleep well. Parents are at a low risk for feeling distressed, and I think maternal depression is not very likely. Some of these common fussy babies, however, will occasionally behave like the extremely fussy baby, and your plans might have to be altered. Only about 5 percent of these babies seem to develop into overtired 4-month-olds.

During the first 4 weeks after birth, your baby really is "sleeping like a baby." Elliot, my first son, described his own first son as having a look on his face like "I didn't do it," or seeming almost intoxicated, during this time because he slept so much. Placing your baby in the crib is usually a piece of cake. During weeks 4 through 8, your baby will become more wakeful and alert and have more evening fussiness. Elliot said that his son now had a more quizzical look, like "Who are you?" and "Give me back my pacifier!"

Helping babies with common fussiness to sleep well using graduated extinction, extinction with a cap, or extinction may start early, even before 2 months of age, as described in Chapter 3 (for soothing and crying) and in Chapter 4 (for extinction).

Crying: All Babies Cry Some of the Time

Crying in infants was first intensively studied in 1945 by a group of dedicated researchers at the Mayo Clinic led by Dr. C. Anderson Aldrich. In their first study, they observed seventy-two newborn babies in a nursery. The researchers worked in shifts so that each baby was observed twenty-four hours a day. They recorded the onset of crying and how long it lasted. They tried to attribute a cause to the crying—wet or soiled diapers, hunger, cramped positions, chilling, and the like—if one was apparent. They found that most of the newborns cried between one and eleven minutes per hour for the duration of their stay in the nursery. The average daily total duration of crying was about *two hours* for these seventy-two babies. *All* of the infants cried for some time *every* day.

Continuous observations were also made for fifty of the original seventy-two babies staying in the nursery for eight days—the recommended stay at that time. Remember, these babies were being observed every minute during those eight days. Researchers found that the minimum amount of crying per day in this group was 48 minutes and the maximum amount was 243 minutes. *All* of the infants cried some of the time—at least forty-eight minutes per day. The average duration of crying was, as before, about *two hours* per day.

Some Crying Can't Be Attributed to an Obvious Cause

The researchers attempted to classify the causes of crying: hunger, vomiting, wet or soiled diapers, and unknown reasons. For example, if the baby was crying and sucking around feeding time, and was calmed by feeding, then the crying was attributed to hunger. They found that hunger appeared to cause 36 percent of all time spent crying. Wet diapers caused about 21 percent of crying time, and soiled diapers about 8 percent. Specifically interesting was that 35 percent of all time spent crying was due to "unknown reasons." The researchers were surprised that such a large part of crying— over one-third—could not be explained by any obvious causes.

Then they examined the number of separate crying spells. Each spell was counted once, regardless of its duration. They found that the number of crying spells for "unknown reasons" was greater than any other cause, including hunger. Their conclusion: crying spells caused by hunger were slightly longer in duration, though less frequent, than those caused by "unknown reasons."

Thus, the findings of the Mayo study were that all babies cry during the newborn period and that much of this crying cannot be attributed to any obvious cause. The authors made some guesses about non-obvious causes: bright lights, peristaltic movements or contractions in the gut, loud noises, and loss of equilibrium. They added, almost as an afterthought, that perhaps the infants' crying expressed a need for fondling or rhythmic motion.

The authors continued the study at home on forty-two infants, using a detailed diary filled in by the mothers. These data covered about twenty-one days at home, after a nine- or ten-day stay in the nursery. The babies averaged four crying spells a day. *All* babies had some crying spells. Fifty-five percent of these spells were attributed to hunger. Crying associated with vomiting, stooling, urination, overheating, bathing, chilling, lights, or noises (the mothers making these attributions) were individually less common than crying for unknown reasons. Again, *crying for unknown reasons (20 percent) seemed to be second only to hunger (25 percent) as a cause of crying.*

Two to Three Hours of Crying Per Day Is Average

The well-known Cambridge pediatrician T. Berry Brazelton performed an important study on crying in 1962, utilizing diaries completed by parents to study crying in eighty infants. Fussy crying spells unrelated to hunger or to wet or soiled diapers occurred in virtually *all* the babies. Only twelve of the eighty fussed less than one and a half hours per day. About half cried for about two hours per day. This increased to an average of about three hours per day at age 6 weeks. Thereafter the amount of crying declined to about one hour per day by age 12 weeks.

Many Babies Have Evening Crying Spells

Dr. Brazelton also found that crying spells became much more focused or concentrated in the evening by the time the infants were about 6 weeks of age, when the crying peaked. By this time, very little crying occurred during the day. The spells of crying in the evening occurred around the same time every evening and began suddenly. The reason for this rapid shift in behavior from a calm/quiet state to a crying state is not known. This was also observed in an unpublished study by Dr. James A. Kleeman and Dr. John C. Cobb, in which out of seventy-eight mothers questioned about their infants, sixty-eight reported "fussy periods," fifty of whom said that the periods occurred in the later afternoon or evening, with the fussiest hours coming between 7:00 p.m. and 9:00 p.m.

Crying Decreases at About 3 Months

Dr. Brazelton found that, on average, crying decreased to about one hour per day by age 12 weeks. Another Harvard study verified

Dr. Brazelton's observations using tape recordings of infants crying in their homes. This study observed the same time course: an increase in crying at about 6 weeks, and a decrease by about 12 weeks. Although the amount of daily crying was less than that observed by Dr. Brazelton, this may be because only ten infants were studied. This means that the natural history of unexplained crying runs the same time course as that of colicky behavior. In both cases, babies calmed down at about 3 months of age.

You can see that, in at least five important particulars, what has been called "colic" is just an extreme form of normal crying. Colic may just be a lot of normal fussing/crying. In fact, even Dr. Brazelton suggested that those infants in his study who cried more than the others were indistinguishable from infants with colic. I think this is a very plausible suggestion. There is not a great gulf between normal crying and colic. The idea that colic is an all-or-nothing event (like pregnancy) is probably wrong. Colicky babies cry like other babies, only more so. Or, if you prefer, most babies cry like colicky babies, only less so.

This is not to diminish the distress caused to parents because of their inability to deal with this crying. That difficulty cannot be overstated. Government data have shown that infant homicides increase after the second week and peak at the eighth week, and the researchers concluded that the "peak in risk in week eight might reflect the peak in the daily duration of crying among normal infants between weeks six and eight."

There are no clear cutoff points in measurements of irritability, fussing, or crying, whether by direct observation in hospital nurseries, voice-activated tape recordings in homes, or parent diaries. Thus, extreme fussiness/colic appears to represent an extreme amount of normally occurring, unexplained fussing/crying that is present in all healthy babies.

Because the spells of fussing or crying are universal, differing only in degree among infants; because the occurrence of spells peaks at 46 weeks after conception and seems to be independent of parenting practices; and because the behaviors exhibit behavioral state specificity (the babies are awake when the crying begins and fall asleep when the crying ends) and a day-night rhythm, it is reasonable to conclude that these behaviors reflect normal biological processes. One example is the normal biological process involving the development of sleep/wake control mechanisms: In all babies, the consolidation of night sleep develops during the second month (after the peak of crying occurs), and the periodic alternation of wake and sleep states during the day is well developed by 3 to 4 months of age (when colic ends).

Because *all* babies fuss and cry, some a little and some a lot, it's best to think of colic as something a baby *does*, not something a baby *has*. It's a stage of life, not a medical problem.

EXTREME FUSSINESS/COLIC

Dr. Morris Wessel defined a colicky infant as "one who is otherwise healthy and well fed, had paroxysms of irritability, fussing or crying lasting for a total of more than three hours a day and occurring on more than three days in any one week . . . and that the paroxysms continued to recur for more than three weeks." He told me that he added the criterion "more than three weeks" because many nannies left families after about three weeks of crying, and he thought that professional nannies, with their experience, knew that if babies cried for more than three weeks, then the crying was likely to continue. Because the mothers were now alone at night caring for their babies, they came to his office after three weeks, complaining that their children were always crying. About 26 percent of infants in his study had colic. Dr. R. S. Illingworth defined colic as "violent rhythmical, screaming attacks which did not stop when the infants were picked up, and for which no cause, such as underfeeding, could be found." Together, they studied about 150 infants.

The *age of onset* of these behaviors is characteristic. Both

Dr. Wessel and Dr. Illingworth found that the attacks were absent during the first few days after birth but were present in 80 percent of affected infants by 2 weeks and in about 100 percent by 3 weeks. Premature babies also start their attacks shortly after the expected due date, independent of their gestational age at birth. The *time of day* when these behaviors occur is another characteristic. During the first month, crying appears at any time of the day or night, but later it occurs predominantly in the evening hours. In 80 percent of infants, the attacks start between 5:00 and 8:00 p.m. and end by midnight. For 12 percent of infants, the attacks start between 7:00 and 10:00 p.m. and end by 2:00 a.m. In only 8 percent are the attacks distributed throughout the day and night. The *age of termination* of these spells is also characteristic. The attacks disappear by *2 months of age in 50 percent* of infants, by *3 months of age in 30 percent*, and by *4 months of age in 10 percent* of infants. The infant's *behavioral state* is associated with colicky behavior. Among colicky infants, 84 percent have crying spells that *begin when they are awake*, 8 percent have spells that start when they are asleep, and another 8 percent have spells under either condition. For 83 percent of infants, *when the crying spells end, they fall asleep.*

It is now known that persistent low-intensity fussing, rather than intense crying, characterizes infants diagnosed as having colic. In fact, to emphasize fussiness instead of crying, the title of a paper by Dr. Wessel was "Paroxysmal fussing in infants, sometimes called 'colic.'" Fussing is not a well-defined behavior, and although not defined in Dr. Wessel's paper, it is usually described as an unsettled, agitated, wakeful state that would lead to crying if ignored by parents. Because sucking is soothing to infants, some parents misattribute the "fussing" state to hunger and vigorously attempt to feed their baby. These parents may misinterpret their infants as having a "growth spurt" at 6 weeks because they were "hungry" all the time, especially in the evening. That is, they want to suck much more at this time. They view their child as hungry, not fussy. Even if they spend more than three additional hours a day, more than three days a week, for more than three weeks feeding them at night to prevent crying, these parents do not think their baby is colicky because there is so little crying.

Over a thirty-four-month period, at newborn visits in my office, I routinely asked every new parent who joined my general pediatric practice whether their child fulfilled Dr. Wessel's exact diagnostic criteria for colic (paroxysms of irritability, fussiness, or crying lasting for more than three hours per day for more than three days per week, and lasting for more than three weeks in an otherwise healthy child). All families had been followed by me since the child's birth and received counseling regarding the normal development of crying or fussing. There were 118 extremely fussy/colicky infants out of 747 (16 percent). However, the vast majority of infants had *little or no crying*. Instead, they fulfilled Dr. Wessel's criteria for colic because they had long and frequent bouts of fussing, which did not lead to crying because of *intensive parental intervention*.

Studies also show that between 2 and 6 weeks there is an increase predominantly in fussing, not crying. Furthermore, fussing and sleeping, but notably not crying, were found to be stable individual characteristics from 6 weeks to 9 months of age. The amount of crying during the first 3 months does not predict crying behavior at 9 months. Also, crying, alone, is not a prediction of sleep problems. Two separate and well-designed studies agree with Dr. Ian St. James-Roberts that "high amounts of early crying do not make it highly probable that an infant will . . . have sleeping problems at nine months of age." However, as discussed later, parenting style (either contributing to the crying or in reaction to the crying or both) does affect the likelihood that a child will be waking and crying at night when older.

What causes extreme fussiness/colic? A recent study showed that colicky infants had higher levels of serotonin, a chemical found in the brain and in the gut. This supported the theory of my wife, Linda Weissbluth, that some features of colic might be caused by an imbalance between serotonin and melatonin, another chemical found in the brain and in the gut. Concentrations of serotonin are high and present in infants during the first month of life and decline after 3 months. Immediately after delivery, concentrations of serotonin are higher at night and lower during the day. Melatonin, flowing across the placenta from the mother, causes high concentrations immediately after birth, but they rapidly fall to extremely low levels within several days. Melatonin increases slightly between 1 and 3 months, and only after 3 months is there an abrupt increase in melatonin levels, with higher levels at night and lower levels during the day.

Serotonin and melatonin have opposite effects on the muscle around the gut—serotonin causes contraction, melatonin causes relaxation. Linda Weissbluth's theory is that in some infants, high serotonin levels cause painful gastrointestinal cramps in the evening, when serotonin concentrations are at their highest. The high nighttime melatonin levels oppose the intestinal smooth muscle contraction caused by serotonin. On the other hand, melatonin and serotonin might be directly affecting the developing brain. For example, high levels of melatonin at night might cause night sleep to become longer.

Other hormones might be involved. In one study, extremely fussy/colicky infants had a blunted rhythm in cortisol production, while the control infants exhibited a clear and marked daily rhythm in cortisol that was not observed in the colicky infants. In addition, researchers in this study coded behavioral measures from video recordings made during the day and arrived at the same conclusion as have many other studies: the crying of these infants was not due to differences in handling by the mother, and the colic was not simply a maternal perception. While this supports a developmentally driven path regarding fussing and crying, more recent data, including video recordings made during the night (see Chapter 3), suggest that some parent behaviors also are important. Other studies have clearly shown that food hypersensitivity and gastroesophageal reflux are not linked to infantile colic.

Twenty percent of babies have extreme fussiness/colic, and the parents of these babies are unlucky. These babies require a lot of parental soothing. They tend not to be self-soothing, and they often appear intense, seem agitated, and have difficulty falling asleep and staying asleep.

Breast-feeding these babies is often difficult because the mothers tend to be exhausted or fatigued from sleep deprivation and the babies tend to be irregular. Feedings may be long and frequent because in addition to satisfying thirst and hunger, much of the nursing is non-nutritive sucking to reduce fussiness. When these babies are extremely fussy, methods of soothing other than breast-feeding often do not work. Frustration or despair is common because many of the popular techniques or strategies for soothing babies fail, even though many other mothers (80 percent) swear by them.

Some considerations going through the mind of the mother of a colicky infant are whether something is wrong with her breast milk, whether her breast milk is sufficient, and whether her diet or the current formula is causing the extreme fussiness/colic. Because soothing at the breast often seems to work when other soothing methods fail, the mother does not want to give it up. But painfully dry or cracked skin around the nipple, from prolonged non-nutritive sucking, may make breast-feeding an ordeal. The discomfort and pain associated with breast-feeding, plus unrelenting exhaustion from sleep deprivation, may conspire to cause so much stress that the breast milk supply becomes insufficient. Mothers who have enormous support—a dedicated husband who spends a lot of time soothing, housekeeping help, or baby care help—can get through this difficult time much more easily than mothers who lack a support system. Mothers who have other children to care for, pressure to return to work, medical problems, baby blues, or postpartum depression may find the additional stresses associated with breast-feeding these extremely fussy/colicky babies to be overwhelming.

Bottle-feeding these babies either formula or expressed breast milk can be a benefit to some mothers, but it can also create more stress in others. The benefits of complete or partial bottle-feeding are that the mother might get more rest because others can feed her baby, and the parents are calmer because, since bottle-feeding makes it easy to see how much the baby is swallowing, they can be certain their baby is not hungry. But in other mothers, giving bottles can create the feeling of having failed as a mother. Recognizing that bottles are not as soothing as the breast, these mothers feel guilty because they think they are causing their babies to fuss/cry more, and they worry that something in the formula may be causing the fussiness/crying.

If you want to breast-feed, a compromise position is to have someone else give a single bottle of expressed breast or formula once per twenty-four hours. This will not cause "nipple confusion" or interfere with lactation. It will give the mother a mini-break, will allow her to get a little more sleep, and will allow the parents a night out.

Before your baby is born, you might decide that you want to sleep with your baby (please see Chapter 1 regarding co-sleeping and SIDS) or that you want to use a crib or bassinet. But for the 20 percent of babies with extreme fussiness/colic, the plans that you made for sleeping with your baby might have to be altered, because these babies tend to be difficult to soothe and have difficulty falling asleep and staying asleep. Watching for drowsy cues is usually frustrating in these babies because they are not obvious, and even if you keep the intervals of wakefulness less than one to two hours, it is still difficult to soothe them. When they finally do fall asleep, they do not stay asleep for long. As a result, parents are often sleep deprived. Parents in this situation are at a high risk of feeling distressed, and I think that maternal depression is more likely to occur.

Because these babies are difficult to soothe, breast-feeding in the family bed may appear to be the best or only strategy that works. Although the mother's sleep may be fragmented by frequent feeding for both nutrition and soothing, this is probably the most powerful soothing method for these babies. During the first 4 weeks, these colicky babies are not really "sleeping like a baby." Placing a colicky baby in the crib is usually stressful. During weeks 4 through 8, the colicky baby may become even more wakeful and alert and have more evening fussiness, causing the parents to be at an even greater risk for distress. But about *50 percent* of these babies begin to settle down around *2 months* of age. About 27 percent of these infants, however, are at risk for becoming overtired 4-month-olds.

There is some research to suggest that parents who make the commitment to use the family bed from day one and stick with it will wind up with better-rested babies than those parents who initially wanted to use the crib but later brought their baby into their bed because it was the only way they could get any sleep. In the former group, proactive co-sleepers, sleep problems are less likely to develop as the children get older. But in the reactive group of co-sleepers, where the family bed was used only in response to soothing or sleeping difficulties, this short-term solution can create long-term sleep problems. What is happening is that parents, overwhelmed by the fussy/crying behavior, and with limited resources for soothing their baby, reluctantly use the family bed to gain relief, but the limited resources for soothing persist beyond the first months and may often cause sleep problems later in older children because those children have failed to learn self-soothing.

Sleep

I actually prefer the term "extreme fussiness/colic" instead of "colic" because fussiness is a bigger problem than crying. All babies have some fussing and crying, and for 80 percent of babies, I call this behavior common fussiness/crying. My idea is that extreme fussiness/colic is a sleep/wake disorder: the inability to sleep well or excessive wakefulness in about 20 percent of babies creates an agitated, uncomfortable state, especially in the evening or at night. I also suggest that post-colic sleep problems occur after 3 to 4 months of age because some parents experience difficulty in establishing age-appropriate sleep routines or fail to teach self-soothing after 3 to 4 months. Let's look at the facts.

Dr. Jarkko Kirjavainen asked parents to keep a daily diary, and he performed sleep recordings in the lab at night between 9:00 p.m. and 7:00 a.m. At about 4½ weeks, the total sleep time from the diary was significantly shorter in a colic group (12.7 versus 14.5 hours per day). The most dramatic decrease in sleep in the colicky babies occurred at night between 6:00 p.m. and 6:00 a.m. The diary data showed that by 6 months of age the extremely fussy/colicky infants slept slightly less than the non-colicky infants, but the group differences were small. Separate from the diary data, the first sleep lab recording was performed when the infants were about 9 weeks old. There were no differences in sleep characteristics between the groups in the night recordings. The second sleep lab recording was performed at about 30 weeks of age, and again, there were no differences in sleep characteristics between the infants formerly with and without extreme fussiness/colic.

Therefore, among infants with extreme fussiness/colic, parent diary data showed shorter total sleep times compared with the age-matched control group at 4½ weeks, but by 9 weeks there were no group differences in sleep lab data obtained during the night. Also, this report suggests that over time, between the ages of 5 and 9 weeks, sleep duration increased among extremely fussy/colicky infants. Based on the sleep lab data and ignoring the parent diary data, the authors concluded that infantile colic was not associated with a sleep disorder. However, Dr. Kirjavainen told me that the lab data were questionable because all children slept poorly in the lab setting.

Dr. Ian St. James-Roberts used the term "persistent criers" to describe extremely fussy/colicky infants. At 6 weeks of age, the extremely fussy/colicky infants slept significantly less than non-colicky infants (12.5 versus 13.8 hours per day, which is similar to the 12.7 versus 14.5 hours per day at 4½ weeks observed by Dr. Kirjavainen). There were no group differences regarding time spent awake or time spent feeding. Extremely fussy/colicky infants slept less throughout the twenty-four-hour diary record. The clearest group differences for sleep were during the day (in contrast to Dr. Kirjavainen, who found less sleep especially between 6:00 p.m. and 6:00 a.m.). In fact, there were no group differences regarding sleep at night. In addition, at night, there were no group differences for fuss/cry behavior. The clearest group differences for fuss/cry behavior were in the daytime. The groups were similar in the timing and duration of the infant's longest sleep period. This analysis of sleep cycle maturation led to the conclusion that the "chief difference between them lies in amounts of daytime fuss/crying and sleeping, rather than in the diurnal organization of sleep and waking behavior." In addition, at 6 weeks of age, the less a baby slept, the greater the amounts of fussing/crying observed. Because the authors observed no deficit in calm wakefulness, only sleeping, they felt that there was a specific trade-off between fussing/crying and sleep. In other words, more fussing/crying behavior reduced sleep time only, not calm wakeful time. The researchers concluded that persistent crying is associated with a sleep deficit.

Another study of extremely fussy/colicky infants using sensors embedded within a mattress to continuously monitor body movements and respiratory patterns showed that at 7 and 13 weeks of age, they slept less than common fussy infants. The extremely fussy/colicky infants had more difficulty falling asleep, were more easily disturbed, and had less quiet, deep sleep.

A separate study, at about 8 weeks of age, noted that colicky infants slept significantly less (11.8 versus 14.0 hours per day). The colicky infants slept less during the day, evening, and night; however, the big difference in sleeping was during the nighttime. Again, crying more was associated with sleeping less. The authors concluded that extreme fussiness/colic might be associated with a disruption or delay in the establishment of the circadian rhythm of sleep/wake activity.

Here is a summary of the data:

SLEEP AND FUSSINESS

Age (Weeks)	Average Total Sleep Duration from Parents' Diaries	
	Extreme fussiness/colic	Common fussiness/crying
4½	12.7	14.5
6	12.5	13.8
8	11.8	14.0

So at the six-week peak of fussiness/crying (the average being about three hours, in the evening, in Dr. Brazelton's study), the difference in total sleep duration is about one hour, but during the two weeks before and after the peak, the difference is closer to two hours. Almost half of all babies will fuss or cry more than three hours a day on more than three days in a week around this time. Sometimes this is called the "modified" Wessel's criteria for colic, because it leaves out Dr. Wessel's additional requirement that the behavior continue for more than three weeks. If this definition is used around 6 weeks of age, the difference in sleeping durations above is not great, but if the definition includes Dr. Wessel's original criterion that fussing/crying behavior continue for more than three weeks, and ages before and after 6 weeks are included, the differences in sleep durations are much larger. Colic is confusing to researchers as well as parents because there is no standard or universally accepted definition or diagnostic criteria.

My study showed that at about 16 weeks of age, the average total sleep duration, based on parental reports, of forty-eight infants who previously exhibited extreme fussiness/colic (using Dr. Wessel's exact definition) was 13.9 plus or minus 2.2 hours—much less than those with common fussiness/crying.

In my general pediatric practice, where all parents receive anticipatory advice regarding sleep hygiene at every visit, parents of extremely fussy/colicky infants say that development of early bedtimes, self-soothing to fall asleep at night, longer night-sleep periods, fewer night wakings, and regular, longer naps occur later in their babies compared to common fussy/crying infants. This suggests that while extreme fussiness/colic may be associated with a delay in maturation of sleep/wake control mechanisms at 4½, 6, 7, 8, 13, and 16 weeks, the diary data show that by 6 months there are no differences in *duration of night sleep* between extreme fussiness/colic and common fussy/crying groups.

However, *night waking* has been reported to be more common following extreme fussiness/colic at 4, 8, and 12 months. This might be interpreted as a persistent impairment of the learned ability to return to sleep unassisted (a failure to learn self-soothing) during a naturally occurring nighttime arousal from sleep in a post-colic infant.

Wakefulness

Parents of extremely fussy/colicky infants often report that daytime sleep periods are extremely irregular and brief. Also, some parents of extremely fussy/colicky infants describe a dramatic increase in daytime wakefulness and sometimes a temporary but complete cessation of napping when their infants approach their peak fussiness at age 6 weeks. I think that, before 3 to 4 months of age, the period of inconsolability in the evening hours, when the infant cannot sleep and cries, may reflect periods of high arousal similar to the circadian "forbidden zone." In adults, the forbidden zone is a time period during which sleep onset and prolonged, consolidated, and restorative sleep states do not easily occur. In this context, it might be more appropriate to describe colic not as a disorder of impaired sleep but as a disorder of excessive wakefulness in the evening. This view is supported by recent sleep lab investigations showing that, in infants, a circadian forbidden zone does exist between 5:00 and 8:00 p.m.

In summary, crying and fussing behavior is universal. Onset is around 1 week (or one week after the due date in a baby born prematurely). At 6 weeks, the behavior increases in duration and becomes focused in the evening hours. The behavior generally starts in a wakeful state and ends in a sleep state, and disappears around 2 to 4 months of age. Older studies failed to show substantial differences in daytime caretaking activities. All of this points to a biologically based or developmental basis for extreme fussiness/colic. In Wessel's report, about 49 percent of infants will behave this way for more than a total of three hours a day on more than three days in a week; 26 percent will behave this way for more than three weeks. In my study, 16 percent of infants fulfilled Wessel's exact criteria. So, although the prevalence varies with the definition, about 20 percent is a common ballpark figure in many studies.

Additionally, in a 2013 review of a developmental explanation for crying during the first 4 months, Dr. St. James-Roberts explained that except for a very small group of infants allergic to cow's milk, there was no good evidence that colic represents a gastrointestinal problem. Also, in a 2013 review by Dr. R. Shamir, the conclusion was that colic reflects brain maturation.

If this is true, then treatment should revolve around helping families *cope* with the stress of having a fussy/crying/wakeful baby. If instead, colic is viewed as a medical problem that needs *treatment,* then desperate parents will grasp at unproven treatments or treatments proven to be ineffective.

Treatment

Probiotics (organisms such as certain bacteria or yeast thought to improve health), prebiotics (nondigestible fiber compounds), and synbiotics (nutritional supplements containing probiotics and prebiotics) were studied in a 2012 review by Dr. Mary Mugambi. She concluded that they "had no impact on the incidence of colic." In another study, the conclusion of a double-blind, placebo-controlled randomized trial of a popular probiotic was that the results "do not support a general recommendation for the use of probiotics to treat colic in infants."

When studies of manipulative therapies (chiropractic, osteopathy, and cranial manipulation) for infant colic have a "low risk of performance bias [that is, parents are blind to whether the child actually received the treatment], the results did not reach statistical significance," according to a 2012 review by Dr. Dawn Dobson. Dr. Paul Posadzki, in his 2013 review of osteopathic manipulative treatment, agreed that effectiveness remains unproven.

Although popular, evidence for simethicone for "gassiness" as effective treatment for colic is lacking in the review by Belinda Hall in 2012. Also, there was a lack of evidence for effectiveness for acupuncture in a study by Dr. Holgeir Skjeie in 2013.

Drugs commonly used for gastroesophageal reflux are often given to fussy or crying babies under the mistaken notion that the problem is acid reflux. A 2011 review by Dr. Pamela Douglas showed that these drugs do not improve symptoms in irritable infants.

If an infant has a medical problem causing painful crying, such as a urinary tract infection, then by definition the infant does not have excessive fussiness/colic, because the definition always includes the notion that the baby is gaining weight well and is otherwise healthy.

There are several reasons parents have the false impression that these so-called treatments work. One is that parents often begin a treatment near the six-week peak of common fussiness/crying, and shortly thereafter the child becomes more settled. Another is that many individuals and companies profit by claiming that their treatments cure colic. A third is that one quick way for a pediatrician to shorten an office visit with a distraught sleep-deprived parent is to write a prescription or referral to a specialist. Please ask your pediatrician or child care provider whether he or she knows of any evidence that supports their recommendations.

The fundamental reason these treatments do not work for excessive fussiness/colic is that these children do not have a diagnosable medical problem. Excessive fussiness/colic is something some infants *do;* it is not a condition that they *have.* Think of *caring* for these infants and for yourself, not of searching for a *cure.* Caring involves getting help to take breaks without guilt and doing whatever you can to help prevent crying and fussing. Helping your baby sleep well during this difficult time has many benefits, including, as described in Chapter 2, preventing maternal depression. But some babies appear to be beyond help and are inconsolable.

Inconsolable Versus Consolable

Dr. Illingworth used inconsolability or unsoothability as part of his definition of colic. Is inconsolability or unsoothability a trait within the baby, a reflection of a parent's ability to soothe, or both? Let me share with you an observation I made in 1986. A mother with her colicky baby and her own mother came to my office. The mother had the baby on her lap; she was gently bouncing the baby up and down and patting the baby, but the baby was still crying loudly. The grandmother was reassuring and stroking the mother's hair. I asked the mother and grandmother if my nurse might take the baby outside the examining room so that we could talk without distraction for a few minutes, and they agreed. They passed the baby to my nurse, who then stepped out. Immediately, the baby stopped crying. My nurse, who was also a mother, was holding the baby chest to chest, with the baby's head resting on her right shoulder. The nurse's right cheek was gently pressed into the baby's right cheek, and the nurse gently rocked her body both from side to side and also with a slow and slightly rotational movement. It looked like my nurse was dancing with the baby in slow motion. The nurse was also whispering or shushing or humming directly into the child's right ear. Needless to say, we were all pleasantly surprised that the crying had abruptly stopped; in fact, we realized that the baby was now sound asleep. I clearly remember this event that happened more than twenty-five years ago, because it struck me that some mothers might have better soothing skills than other mothers and that the notion of inconsolability might, in part, reflect a mother's ability or inability to soothe. But at that time, I thought inconsolability was primarily a within-the-child trait, and in the absence of data I was strongly opposed to suggestions that mothers were responsible for or contributed to colic. Now we have data to consider a more nuanced view of the role of the mother and father.

Parent-Driven Path, the Role of the Parent (see Chapter 3)

Anxiety in the Mother

A 1965 study involving 103 mothers described a link between anxious mothers and colic. Dr. William Carey interviewed each mother within a few days after delivery. Forty of them expressed some anxiety. Dr. Carey compared their anxiety ratings with the presence or absence of colic in their children. He reported that only two of the colicky babies came from anxiety-free mothers, while eleven had mothers in the anxious category. This is a significant difference, and supports Dr. Carey's conclusion that maternal anxiety appears at least partly responsible for, or contributory to, colic.

However, there are a couple of fairly significant flaws in the research. The first is with Dr. Carey's diagnosis of colic. He quotes and claims to have followed Wessel's definition; however, he reports that "colic began in the first month for five [infants], the second month for four and the third month for four." Wessel's data, and almost every other study of colic, report the onset of colic within two or three weeks after birth. This discrepancy causes one to apply a degree of skepticism to Dr. Carey's diagnoses. Also, Dr. Carey did both the interviewing of the mothers and the diagnosing of their babies. This means the study was not "blinded"; what a mother told Carey about her anxiety may have colored his view of whether or not her baby's crying ought to be considered colic. He recognized that maternal anxiety cannot be the only factor causing colic, because most anxious mothers did not have colicky babies and at least two non-anxious mothers did. Because of the weaknesses of this study, I did not find it a credible challenge to my strong belief that extreme fussiness/colic resulted from developmental issues.

Now, about fifty years later, we have better data . . . and much of it supports Dr. Carey. In 2014, Johanna Petzoldt showed that "infants of mothers with anxiety disorders *prior to pregnancy* were at higher risk for excessive crying [colic as exactly defined by Dr. Wessel] than infants of mothers without any anxiety disorder *prior to pregnancy*. . . . Maternal depressive disorders prior to pregnancy were not significantly associated with excessive crying." Additionally, she speculated that "maternal anxiety might lead to *intrusiveness* that possibly intensifies infant crying" (emphasis added). Intrusiveness regarding unnecessary night feedings and attention at night is discussed in Chapter 3.

It should be noted that the mother's anxiety itself does not explain the observed typical onset (when awake) or cessation (when asleep) of colic or the six-week peak. But perhaps if the anxiety is worse at night, it may contribute to the evening clustering of infant crying. Although anxiety and depression may occur together in an individual, Professor Petzoldt did not implicate maternal depression as a statistically significant factor but suggested that with a larger number of subjects, depression would likely also be found to be associated with colic.

Dr. Joseph Lonstein observed that elevated postpartum maternal anxiety "is particularly prevalent in women who experienced pregnancy complications, gave birth prematurely, delivered a low birthweight infant, or are caring for an infant with a birth defect." These births represent about 10 percent of all births in the United States, but "the actual rate [of postpartum maternal anxiety] may be greater than 20–25%." It may not be coincidental that colic also occurs in about 20 percent of babies.

Depression in the Mother

Maternal depression may be caused by a child who is not sleeping well (Chapter 2) and may lead to unnecessary nighttime feedings or interventions that result in sleep fragmentation, causing a sleep-deprived baby to exhibit colic-like behavior (Chapter 3). Thus, maternal depression may be a cause of colic, a consequence of colic, or both.

Father

I surveyed many families of twins to find out what factors were important for sleeping well. For the entire group, maternal age was perhaps the most important variable, in part because young mothers are usually married to young fathers. Here are some data for the *entire group*, which was a mixture of identical and fraternal twins and those who did and did not use assisted reproductive technology (ART) such as in vitro fertilization. I compared families with younger mothers (at or under the median age for the group, which was 34 years) to families with mothers 35 years or older.

In the families with younger mothers, it was more common for both twins to sleep well, for the parents to start sleep training early (at 4 months or younger), and for there to be more success at breast-feeding. In addition, there was less baby blues or postpartum depression (BB/PPD), and the babies were less likely to have colic. These younger mothers were married to younger fathers (age 36 or younger). These younger fathers were more likely than older fathers to be involved in helping the twins sleep. I observed that when the younger fathers played an active role in caring for the twins and took an active part in sleep-training them, the sleep training went more smoothly and was successful at an earlier point in the process. Among the entire group, almost 30 percent reported that at least one of their twins had colic based on Wessel's exact diagnostic criteria.

No other report showed such a high (30 percent) prevalence of colic. To better understand why colic was so common, I looked at different variables separately. I first divided the entire group by whether or not ART was utilized, because ART is associated with infertility, stressful fertility treatments and sometimes multiple unsuccessful attempts, and fraternal twins and older mothers. Within the group not using ART, a further division was made between identical twins (similar sleep rhythms would make sleep training easier) and fraternal twins. The oldest mother with identical twins was 37 years. Within the group using ART, a further division was made based on the age of the mothers, using 38 years of age as the cutoff. Here are the data:

VARIABLES ASSOCIATED WITH COLIC

	Both Twins Sleep Well	BB/PPD	Colic	Breast-Feeding Only	Father's Involvement
No ART					
Group A: 37 yrs or younger Identical	60%	13%	9%	73%	92%
Group B: 38 yrs or older Fraternal	33%	20%	19%	33%	76%
ART, Fraternal					
Group C: 38 yrs or younger	28%	40%	32%	39%	88%
Group D: 39 yrs or older	22%	67%	40%	9%	70%

What puzzled me when I did this analysis in 2007 was that if colic was primarily a within-the-child characteristic, why would it be less common among younger mothers (a difference of 9 percent versus 19 percent or 32 percent versus 40 percent)? Younger mothers were more successful at breast-feeding (a difference of 73 percent versus 33 percent or 39 percent versus 9 percent), and their husbands were more involved in helping their babies sleep well (a difference of 92 percent versus 76 percent or 88 percent versus 70 percent).

From correspondence and conversations with all the mothers, it was clear to me that the stress of parenting increased with each group (from group A to group D). The dramatic trend of more colic from 9 percent to 40 percent may be a reflection of this increased stress of parenting. I understood how more colic might cause twins to sleep less well (from 60 percent to 22 percent) and mothers to have more BB/PPD (from 13 percent to 67 percent) and less ability to exclusively breast-feed (from 73 percent to 9 percent). In other words, colic might be causing these problems.

But mothers told me that fathers were highly involved or not involved at all in parenting *before the colic developed,* and the trend of fathers to be less involved in helping the child sleep well (from 92 percent to 70 percent) was a source of great stress for the marriage and for parenting in general. A common theme among older mothers, especially in group D, where 40 percent of the infants had colic, was that the lack of teamwork in the marriage between husband and wife continued to be an issue between father and mother after the babies were born.

I began to wonder whether the lack of involvement of the father in caring for the baby and his lack of teamwork in the marriage might be contributing to sleep deprivation in the baby and mother so that colicky behavior emerged. The important role of the father in helping children sleep well is discussed in Chapter 3.

Obviously, children's sleep issues reflect not only the mother's care for the baby but also the father's care and how well the parents cooperate or agree on parenting. An uninvolved, absent, abusive, or addicted husband or father may adversely affect a mother's mental health and a child's sleep. So studies that omit inclusion of the husband, father, or boyfriend may focus unwarranted blame on the mother or unwarranted attribution to the mother's mental health status. However, fathers are not usually mentioned in published scientific reports on maternal depression, maternal anxiety, or maternal mental health in association with children's sleep issues.

For example, in 2013, Dr. Jenny Radesky published a paper on a group of mothers, 89 percent of whom were married, that showed that "*inconsolable* infant crying may have a stronger association with postpartum depressive symptoms than infant colic." While this supports the notion that the baby's characteristics are the predominant factor (a baby-driven path), the father's role was not included in this study. Similarly, in Professor Petzoldt's 2014 study regarding maternal anxiety disorders prior to pregnancy being associated with colic (which supports the notion that the mother plays a significant role—a mother-driven path), no mention is made about the role of fathers or boyfriends. In Professor Petzoldt's study of mothers between 18 and 40 years old, those mothers who were younger and had only a tenth-grade education or less were more likely to have a colicky baby than older and more educated mothers. In her entire group, 61 percent were not married prior to the pregnancy, and among those reporting colic in their babies, 76 percent were not married prior to the pregnancy and 24 percent were married prior to their pregnancy. While marital status alone does not indicate the presence or absence of paternal support regarding parenting, it does appear that mothers who are younger, less educated, and single are more likely to have a colicky baby. Echoing the lack of teamwork described above in older mothers with colicky twins, Professor Petzoldt told me, "When we looked at social support and partnership characteristics, we find that perceived [by the mothers] social support and tenderness in partnership reduce the risk for excessive crying. However, these results are only preliminary." It seems to me that if the fathers are not included in the study, one should be cautious about attributing problems associated with sleep or crying in the baby to the mother.

In 2010, Dr. Douglas Teti studied a group of families in which 93 percent of mothers were married. He documented that fathers' involvement with infants at bedtime and at night was much less than the mothers'. Also in 2007, Joanna Martin showed that infant sleep problems "were associated with serious psychological distress and poor general health" in fathers as well as mothers. However, "relationship happiness and partner support showed strong evidence of a protective effect . . . reducing the odds of serious psychological distress on average by almost half." She concluded, "Fathers should be actively engaged in the assessment and management of child sleep problems because their health is also at risk." In the same year, Dr. Harriet Hiscock found that behavioral strategies designed to improve babies' sleep also improved the mothers' well-being (fewer depressive symptoms and better maternal sleep quality) and that "most mothers (80 percent) reported partner support with sleep strategies." Another 2007 study by Dr. Hiscock showed that "preventive strategies for infant sleep problems need to begin early . . . to improve mother's health. . . . Infant sleep problems were associated with parental disagreement about sleep management." I learned early on that for a sleep consultation to be successful I needed the active support or passive cooperation of the father, and therefore I do not begin a consultation without both parents present. The importance of having both parents present for a successful sleep consultation/intervention is discussed in Chapter 4.

Interaction Between Baby and Parent

Extreme fussiness/colic in babies, which appears to have a developmental component, along with the associated impairments in sleeping, may trigger depression in mothers. Furthermore, maternal anxiety or depression that is present before delivery might cause unnecessary feeding of or attending to babies at night (see Chapter 3). Because their sleep is fragmented, these babies become overtired and cry more. This in turn creates more sleep deprivation and emotional stress for the mother and father. The father may or may not be very involved in helping the child sleep (on his own or because the mother acts as a gatekeeper—either encouraging or inhibiting the father's involvement), be a partner in parenting in general, or be a team player in the marriage. So colicky behavior may have both a developmental and a parental component. Unresolved or unappreciated parent issues (see Chapter 3) may be the root cause of crying/fussing and sleep problems in the baby.

Living with and Soothing a Colicky Baby

My son, now 4 months old, had colic. He lacked the ability to fall and stay asleep. He would startle at the slightest noise and required darkness in which to sleep. Sleep, by the way, was only obtained by a very specific rocking/holding motion day and night for 3 months straight. When you mention "colic" to people, they immediately give you advice on symptomatic GI treatment. When I tried to explain how he was, nobody understood. Nobody. When I told our son's pediatricians that he would stay awake for 18 hours a day, they would just stare at me and make me take the Edinburgh Postnatal Depression Scale Test once again. It was so very isolating. People would say, "You are spoiling him by holding him so much," "All babies are difficult; get used to it," "Just put him down and let him cry." The degree of isolation and amount of criticism while caring for such a difficult baby cannot be understated. There is no way to describe how it feels to watch your new baby be so miserable. There are no words to fully explain this experience. I have a small but firm support system, and this experience pushed us to our limits. I had to leave my hard-earned career because I could not imagine how day care could put forth the effort of care our son required.

HOW TO SOOTHE A COLICKY BABY

I think ultimately parents have to experiment to find out what kind of soothing works best for their child at that particular time. I tried everything with my colicky child, who quickly became chronically overtired. We found that her preferred method of soothing changed as she learned to become a better sleeper over the course of one year. In the beginning, she seemed to like the "jiggle-sway." We would hold her and swing her side to side while simultaneously jiggling her. (I also think that I had an easier time using that method because I was frantic and nervous.) As time went on, she preferred to be held in a rocking chair with quick, jiggle-like rocking. Now she likes to sit in your lap with slow, long rocks while reading a story. Once she's ready for bed, she throws the book and starts to wiggle. You put her in her crib and she spends some time playing with her hair or pacifier and falls asleep. I also found that in the later stages of sleep training, Dad and Grandma had more success than me. Can't really explain it because we all use the same sleep routines. If I had to do it over again, I would have read Healthy Sleep Habits, Happy Child *before my daughter was born and not 4 months later. Then I would have understood that her extreme fussing was colic. I could have at least been armed with some tips and techniques to prevent or at least minimize the chronically overtired mess she became. I would also have made sure that I protected her naps and bedtime from day one. I also would have made sure that Dad was more involved and on the same page from day one.*

My first child was colicky, too, and we had to do an extreme amount of bouncing also. The rocking chair was absolutely useless! We had to swaddle him and walk around bouncing him. He also preferred the sideways, facing-out position. I definitely wonder if colicky babies need more motion—almost like they need some sort of distraction. I tried rocking with my second baby, non-colicky. But I quickly switched to walking and bouncing because that was what I was used to. I think she probably would have been fine with less motion, but I reverted to what I "knew" worked. With my third, we were able to rock in the rocking chair. She would just sit there in my arms and fall asleep. It was such a weird experience for me!

How Parenting Style Influences Crying

Dr. St. James-Roberts showed that carrying a baby more during the day will reduce common fussiness/crying, but carrying a baby more during the day does not make extreme fussiness/colic go away. To clarify what it means to carry a child more to reduce fussiness and crying, he also studied different approaches to infant care in three groups of parents: London, United Kingdom, parents; Copenhagen, Denmark, parents; and a "proximal care" group of parents who planned to hold their infants 80 percent or more of the time between 8:00 a.m. and 8:00 p.m., breast-feed frequently, and respond rapidly to infant cries. Proximal care is also called infant-demand care or attachment parenting. Here are his results:

> Proximal care parents held infants for 15 to 16 hours per 24 hours and coslept with them through the night more often than other groups. London parents had 50% less physical contact with their infants than proximal care parents . . . [and] abandoned breastfeeding earlier than the other groups. . . . Copenhagen parents fell in between the other groups in measures of contact and care. *London infants cried 50% more overall than infants in both other groups at 2 and 5 weeks of age. However, bouts of unsoothable crying occurred in all 3 of the*

groups, and the groups did not differ in unsoothable bouts or in colicky crying at 5 weeks. Proximal care infants woke and cried at night most often at 12 weeks. (Emphasis added.)

My interpretation is that while the near-constant holding and co-sleeping reduced the overall crying of babies in the proximal care group, it also interfered with their development of self-soothing skills, so that by 12 weeks there was substantially more signaling at night, which may persist, as Dr. St. James-Roberts noted: "Most [proximal care] infants continue to wake their parents at night when 10 months of age." In another study, Dr. St. James-Roberts pointed out that while most infants who cry a lot at 5–6 weeks of age do sleep well at night at 12 weeks of age, "four randomized controlled trials have found that 'limit-setting' parenting prevents continuation of night waking and signaling beyond 3 months of age. In contrast . . . 'infant-demand' care . . . increase[s] the number of infants who continue to wake and signal in the night at 12 weeks of age." As he stated, "Rather than one being better, [different parenting styles] are associated with different benefits and costs."

When to Allow Babies with Colic to Learn Self-Soothing

If you suspect that your baby has extreme fussiness/colic, do everything you can to maximize sleep and minimize crying during the first weeks. Parents who are able to put forth heroic efforts to soothe their fussy baby may note that there is really minimal or no crying, only fussing. But their baby would cry in the absence of heroic soothing efforts. The attempt to help your colicky baby may be mildly or overwhelmingly stressful to parents. You are likely to be in survival mode. Success or failure in your attempt to help your colicky baby sleep better by learning self-soothing may be based on factors within your baby and on your and the other parent's soothing skills, mental health, and resources. The most important thing to remember is that you will be more successful in soothing your baby and surviving your baby's colic if you *get help in order to take breaks*. Also remember: this, too, shall pass.

Teamwork and constant communication between parents is the bedrock that permits a family to cope with and emerge from colic well rested. Starting early and tolerating some crying is common in some situations, and no adverse effects occur: mothers of twins are much more willing to let a colicky baby cry to develop self-soothing skills because the reality of their situation is that they are not always available to soothe the crying twin. Mothers who have had a previous child are especially keen on having the colicky baby sleep so they can have some time with their older child, and mothers who had a previously colicky baby are more tolerant of letting their second baby cry as a means to the end of getting better sleep, because they are less likely to have a fear of crying it out or to worry about whether crying will hurt their child. I also think experienced mothers try hard to move the bedtime earlier after 6 weeks because they know that drowsy signs might not be very visible in their colicky baby. On the other hand, I think it is totally appropriate for some first-time mothers to have a go-slow approach and wait until colic passes.

All babies experience unexplained fussiness and crying in their first weeks of life, no matter what your ethnic group, no matter what birthing method brought your child into the world, no matter if your lifestyle is that of jet-setter or stay-at-home parent. All parents, too, tend to use the same techniques and strategies to successfully weather those first few months of life with their new baby, whether it's fair sailing for the most part or they feel storm-tossed by colicky waves of crying. Sleep problems arise after 3 to 4 months of age when some parents don't change their techniques for coping with crying and fussiness at bedtimes and nap times. That's when unhealthy sleep habits and their resulting problems begin.

Because colic winds down in 50 percent of babies at 2 months and 80 percent of babies at 3 months, you might try to help your baby sleep better before 4 months of age. Parents tell their stories of helping colicky babies sleep better at 8, 11, and 12 weeks in Chapter 4. Here are some more reports from mothers of babies with extreme fussiness/colic (or perhaps sleep deprivation masquerading as colic) who helped their babies sleep better:

> My baby was deemed colicky at 3 weeks old. I wasn't happy with that answer, and that is when I got the book Healthy Sleep Habits, Happy Child. This book changed my life. I really don't believe my child was colicky. I think she was just way overtired and completely strung out. She has always been a spirited baby and would never just fall asleep like typical babies. Ever since I started implementing Dr. Weissbluth's advice, she has become a totally different baby. Sometimes I wonder if a lack of sleep can cause colic or colic-like symptoms. I truly believe there are colicky babies, but sometimes I wonder if some are misdiagnosed.

> In retrospect, I think that my baby was colicky. He was terribly sensitive to light/noise—couldn't sleep anywhere but his quiet room by himself at 6 weeks, and would scream and scream to fall asleep even if I held him. Thankfully, my aunt had a colicky baby, and she recommended letting him cry. Starting at 4 weeks, I would just put him down in his room when he was tired [that is, drowsy but awake]. He would cry for five to ten minutes, and then sleep a full nap. If I had tried holding or rocking him, he would have screamed for a long, long time without sleeping. If it weren't for the fact that he got so much sleep (because I was willing to let him cry), he would have been full-blown colicky. As it was, he slept a lot! I am so grateful that I experimented with letting him cry to fall asleep. I can't even imagine how much screaming he would have done if I had insisted on holding him when he cried.

My maternity leave had ended, and I went back to work for the first full day. My 12-week-old daughter had "colic" (screamed for three to five hours every day) for the first 10 weeks, which I felt was 100 percent her being overtired. I did graduated extinction at 6 weeks to get her solid naps during the day, which helped her daytime crying/screaming immensely, but these naps were attained through use of a dark room, swaddle, and some quiet soothing.

We used extinction with a twenty-minute limit at 12 weeks. Our little guy would cry in our arms for two hours before he'd finally fall asleep. We'd take turns rocking him in our arms, swaying back and forth. When we finally decided to just try it, we were surprised at how little he cried before he fell asleep—eight minutes! The second day was equally easy, but then he quickly learned the twenty-minute time limit and would cry up to that point. We adjusted the bedtime from 6:30 to 5:30 [earlier bedtime] and removed the time limit [no cap]. First night, he cried for two hours. It was awful! But after four days, the crying stopped.

Our son was colicky and sleep was nonexistent in our house for three months. He refused to go in the swing or the bouncy seat, and hated the car even more (and still does!). If he did sleep, it was after being rocked for hours and he was put down in his crib in a dead sleep. At 12 weeks we did graduated extinction because he had no self-soothing skills. Our goal was four hours of sleep, and it worked. Within five nights, he was sleeping through the night! We were shocked to say the least. It was an absolute miracle and the best thing we ever did. Everyone in the house was much happier, and we started to really enjoy being parents. For the first 3 months he was definitely going to be an only child. ☺ Your book Your Fussy Baby helped us tremendously!

I have only one child, so my experience is limited to her. Based on our experience, at 6 weeks, all we were trying to do was survive. She was extremely fussy between 5 and 10 weeks. At the time, we felt that the best thing to do was soothe her and try to get the maximum sleep possible. Things were "messy" in the sense that we used swing, holding, the crib, extensive soothing—whatever worked that day/night. We made repeated attempts at drowsy but awake, but it never worked before 3½-4 months of age. Ultimately, we felt it was more important that she get some sleep in those earliest months, so we did what it took. From my perspective, parents of colicky children should be prepared to be somewhat flexible until about 4 months. You can attempt earlier bedtimes or some extinction, but if things are really disastrous, abandon the effort and try again later. We knew it was time around 3½ months because we were soothing more and she was sleeping less—it was like we were annoying her! I would add that dealing with colic is incredibly taxing, physically and emotionally. In the first 4 months, we were lucky to get four to five hours of consolidated sleep in a day. Most days, it was two to three hours. Add to that dealing with a fussy child almost around the clock, and you have a recipe for frazzled and distressed parents. I can certainly understand why many parents struggle with a postcolic sleep plan, as it can be hard to be resolute when you are completely burned out.

My baby was colicky and never slept. He did not take naps at all for the first 3 months of his life. At 4 months he started taking naps only in the car or in the swing. I feel like he was in the swing more often than not. As soon as the swing was stopped, he would wake right up. At 4 months I decided to do extinction; graduated extinction only riled him up and extended the crying. So we did extinction with no problems at night. He always went right to sleep, no crying and no night-waking problems. He wakes two times a night to nurse. The problems were his naps. He did not know how to self-soothe. So I taught him, and he caught on rather quickly. After two weeks he was going down every two hours for naps without much crying. At the beginning of this nap training there was a lot of crying. At first his naps were short, forty-five minutes or so. After a few weeks the midmorning nap lengthened to about an hour and a half, the midday nap went from forty-five minutes to an hour, and the third nap declined to about thirty-five minutes. I have been very happy with this! My family and friends think I am out of my mind because I schedule everything around his naps.

The hardest thing about dealing with colic was that we didn't know when it would end. People kept telling us, "Don't worry, it'll get better," but we had no idea whether that would be in a week, a month, a year. The need for twenty-four-hour intensive soothing efforts took a huge toll on me, emotionally and physically, and on my relationship with my husband. Almost a year later, I believe we are still dealing with the fallout from our very intense and difficult first few months. The turning point for us was when we discovered Healthy Sleep Habits, Happy Child and began sleep training at 4½ months. It was like suddenly we had our lives back. We knew that he would be in bed at 5:30 p.m., and while he would wake up to eat a few times during the night, he would go right back to sleep. Once we had naps under control it got even better. I believe that at a certain point, his natural colicky tendencies were fading, but still being exacerbated by his being horribly overtired. I will know for my next baby (won't be for a while!) that healthy sleep habits begin on day one, and that most babies don't just know when to sleep—they need us to help them.

The moment my daughter, Amanda, arrived home from the hospital, she exploded with a very bad case of colic. I took her to the pediatrician's office several times, only to be told there was "not a thing wrong, relax." I also received several suggestions about nursing and a pat on the back. All of these suggestions irritated me, and I felt as though I was being perceived as an anxious, first-time mother.

After twelve weeks of crying and screaming, Amanda was evaluated by two child development specialists. I decided we should work with one until my daughter's crying and screaming settled down. We also saw a psychiatrist, who recommended medication and also suggested that we continue to be followed by the development specialists. In the meantime, our lives had become a nightmare. Amanda cried most of the day and always screamed in the evening. To our horror, this behavior had worked itself into the night hours, too.

By 5 months, we were referred to Dr. Weissbluth for what we hoped was a sleep disorder. I say "hoped," because we were at the point of seeing a pediatric neurologist and having an EEG done. I was very frightened for my daughter, and my husband and I were exhausted. I was eager for the consultation. My daughter had definitely been cursed with colic. Could this now be wired exhaustion from a sleep disorder caused by the treatment for colic—rocking, swinging, motion all the time? It was.

Amanda was old enough now to try "crying it out." It was the most difficult thing I've had to do as a new mother.

The first night, Amanda screamed, choked, and sobbed for thirty-two minutes. I remember feeling sick to my stomach.

The first two days weren't too terrible. However, the third and fourth were almost intolerable. Amanda would cry through her entire nap time. Then I would get her up to keep

Dr. Weissbluth's time frame going. Her temperament after these episodes is known only to mothers who have been through the same ordeal! When she would scream for over an hour during nap time and in the evening, I felt cruel, insensitive, and guilty. Three things kept me going: my husband's support; Dr. Weissbluth's concern, encouragement, and compassion; and the fact that I knew it had to be done—Amanda had to learn to sleep.

It took Amanda about a week to catch on to the idea. The bags under her eyes faded, her sporadic screaming attacks stopped, and her personality was that of a predictable baby—a sweetheart when rested and a bear when past a nap time or her bedtime.

I would offer these suggestions to other mothers and fathers who have to take this measure in order to teach their babies to sleep. You, as parents, have to understand and believe intellectually that it is the right thing to do. Otherwise feelings of guilt will overpower you, and you will give in. You must have the support of your spouse, as it will be too much of a strain to bear alone.

You are doing what is best for your baby. It seems cruel and unacceptable, as a loving new mother, to let your baby cry. But it is a fact of parenting—many, many things will bring tears and protests in the years to come.

Enlist the support of a sympathetic friend as much as you feel the need to. I found close telephone contact a tremendous help. Some parents may not need this close interaction, but many of us do.

My son is now 5½ months. He was extremely colicky and also had reflux. My son cried pretty much all day and evening. He would only sleep fully swaddled in a swing in our bedroom, and even then he probably averaged six to eight hours of fragmented sleep in a twenty-four-hour period.

Needless to say, once the colic ended and his reflux turned into just being a "happy spitter," my husband and I were desperate to figure out how to get some sleep for all of us! After trying the gradual approach and graduated extinction with no success, we decided it was time for extinction. It was very hard to do, but luckily he didn't scream every night for as long as we had expected. I kept reminding myself that we weren't making him cry: we were allowing him to cry.

We decided that because our son had been premature, and so colicky and sick, we really needed to wait until he was closer to 5 or 6 months to start any kind of sleep training. So we did. My husband and I are both psychologists, and we both work with people who have been severely neglected or abused as children, so we are acutely aware of the importance of building a secure attachment in children. As such, we were also very nervous about trying any kind of cry-it-out method, fearing it might undermine our son's attachment to us. However, we were also desperate for sleep, and so was our son. I think the phrase that stuck out to me in Dr. Weissbluth's book (and that I still hang on to to this day) is that a sleepy brain is not an awake brain. When babies cry at night they are not lonely, afraid, and anxious or any of the other things they might be when they are awake; when babies cry at night, they are tired. So when our son was 6½ months old we laid him down for the night at his usual time (7:00 p.m.) after his bath and bottle and left the room [extinction]. He cried for almost an hour and then fell asleep, and he didn't wake up until five-thirty the next morning. I couldn't believe it. The next night we did the same thing, and I was sure the night before had been a fluke, that there was no way he could sleep that well two nights in a row. He did. He cried for forty minutes and slept until five-thirty the next morning. He is now almost 3 years old, and we still put him to bed between seven and seven-thirty at night. He talks to himself happily in his crib for about thirty minutes and then sleeps until seven the next morning. He naps for anywhere from an hour and a half to two hours a day. If our premature, sick, colicky son can learn to be a good sleeper, any baby can. It was the most difficult thing we've had to do as parents, letting our son cry, but it also taught us an important lesson—that even as babies what our children want and what they need are not the same thing. Teaching our son to sleep gave me the confidence to trust my instincts as a mother and to weather the criticisms I receive from others for "letting my baby cry." We firmly believe that tolerating or accepting some crying is worth the payoff of teaching our children to sleep. Refusing to allow them to develop this skill constitutes a form of selfishness of the part of my husband and me. I hope our experience can give other families who are suffering the confidence to succeed.

For many reasons (living in a one-bedroom condo, etc.), we did not sleep-train our daughter until 10 months old. We thought things would improve once we moved into a larger townhouse when she was 9 months old and had her own room. To our surprise, her sleep got worse. What we thought would take a few days to adjust went on for weeks of disastrous sleep for all of us. One day I sat down and wrote up our typical daily routine. To my surprise, I realized that I was spending up to two hours total per day just soothing her to sleep. I told Dr. Weissbluth our story. Although he said she might fight us pretty hard at her age (10 months), he assured us that we could still sleep-train her. He set us up with a weekend plan so my husband could help out. In just four nights we made it happen! Dr. Weissbluth followed up with me until we had reached success. Here's how it went:

> *First night: cried intermittently for seventy-five minutes*
> *Second night: twenty-five minutes*

Third night: forty-five minutes
Fourth night: fifteen minutes
Fifth night: done!

She goes down without a fight and sleeps like a baby—or, shall I say, like a baby is supposed to sleep! We wished we'd done this sooner. The many sleepless nights really took a toll on our new marriage, our health, and being able to enjoy our new baby. I think many new parents get stuck in the fog and can't bear to hear their babies cry. While it does take a degree of courage, my husband and I were astounded by how quickly our baby learned to soothe herself to sleep. So to all the parents out there who are sleep challenged, it doesn't get any easier the longer you wait. Educate yourself on the vital importance of sleep (not only for infants but adults, too). Start sleep training early, engage others to assist (Dad, partner, Grandma, best friend, etc.), and you'll be healthier, happier, find newfound freedom, and enjoy quality sleep where everyone wins!

A Final Note on Extreme Fussiness/Colic

Using the modified Wessel's criteria for colic (discussed above), researchers have studied how often colic occurs in different populations, and how colic is associated with sleep duration, night awakenings (signaling), temperament, parenting styles, maternal depression and anxiety, and subsequent sleep or developmental problems. The results of some of these studies are sometimes contradictory because the children studied represent a heterogeneous population of moderate and severely affected infants. However, when using a more restrictive, exact Wessel's definition, researchers are looking at a much smaller (26 percent in Wessel's report; 16 percent in my study) and more homogeneous group of children with more extreme fussiness/colic, and they are more likely to discover associations between these babies and the issues above. The associations described in this chapter and subsequent chapters are mostly supported by multiple studies, and I have taken into account different definitions of colic.

Summary and Action Plan for Exhausted Parents

THE FIRST WEEK

Begin to teach your baby self-soothing: many hands (enlisting the help of the father and others), putting your baby down drowsy but awake, and many naps (see Chapter 3). At this age, there are no established biological rhythms for night sleep, day sleep, or bedtime, so you need to watch for drowsy signs. Develop bedtime routines and avoid unnecessary feedings or interventions at night.

All babies become fussy and have some uncategorizable crying a few days after they are born, or a few days after the expected date of delivery if they are born early. About 20 percent of babies will develop extreme fussiness/colic. The exact cause is not known. But the effect is crystal-clear. When babies fuss or cry, they do not sleep. When they do not sleep, mothers do not sleep. Mind-numbing fatigue from lack of sleep is your main enemy!

WEEKS 2 TO 4

More fussing and crying will develop in all babies. Fussing occurs more than crying. Fussiness is a pre-cry state that will often change into crying if parents are unable to soothe their baby; some fussing leads to crying despite parents' soothing efforts. With increasing fussing and crying, your baby may sleep less. If you have not already begun, start to teach your child self-soothing, develop bedtime routines, and avoid unnecessary feedings or interventions at night. There are still no established biological rhythms for night sleep, day sleep, or bedtime, so you should continue to watch for drowsy signs.

As stated above, fussing and crying behavior can be expected to increase at this stage, and for about 80 percent of babies—the ones with common fussiness/crying—it peaks around 6 weeks of age and then decreases. About 20 percent of babies—those with extreme fussiness/colic—may not show a clear peak at 6 weeks, and for them the fussing and crying behavior lasts until about months 2 to 4. But at weeks 2 to 4, you do not know which path your baby will take, so to plan for the possible challenges ahead, arrange to get help from relatives, friends, and neighbors so that you can take breaks. Explore how parenting can be shared by both parents so that neither parent becomes totally exhausted.

If teaching self-soothing is not working, or if you think your child is developing extreme fussiness/colic, then temporarily abandon efforts to teach self-soothing. You cannot spoil your 2- to 4-week-old baby, so do whatever you can to maximize sleep and minimize fussing and crying.

> **Extreme fussiness/colic occurs in 20 percent of babies. It is not a medical condition requiring treatment. It is something babies do, not something they have. Remember: this, too, shall pass!**

Babies behave this way because of factors within the baby and within the family. Give your baby the opportunity to learn self-soothing if possible, or get help so that you can take breaks from the constant soothing your baby might require. But also review the parent issues (Chapter 3) that might make for a greater challenge to prevent fussing or crying.

CHAPTER 6

Healthy Sleep Habits in The Second Month

A main goal at this age is to encourage the development of self-soothing skills.

Weeks 5 and 6

Night sleep: More evening fussiness may be associated with less night sleep before 6 weeks; after 6 weeks, night-sleep rhythms emerge

Day sleep: Naps are brief and irregular; there may be many catnaps

Bedtimes: Bedtimes are irregular and may occur late, between 9:00 and 11:00 p.m.

For babies with common fussiness/crying, getting Dad on board, recognizing and respecting drowsy signs, allowing only brief intervals of wakefulness during the day, and establishing bedtime routines might help your baby sleep better. Try these items even if your baby has extreme fussiness/colic. And if they do not help, do whatever works to maximize sleep and minimize crying: swings, strollers, car rides, or sleep at Mom's breast or on Dad's chest. Exhaustion is your main enemy, so get help in order to take breaks.

Remember that the division line between common fussiness/ crying and extreme fussiness/colic is arbitrary, and these labels do not accurately describe all babies. At this age, it may or may not be clear to you that your baby has a little, a medium amount, or a lot of fussing/crying. And attaching a descriptive label to this behavior is less important than helping your baby sleep better and coping with the stress of sleep deprivation in the family.

Be experimental with different methods of soothing (see Chapter 3) and do not give up trying. Some methods that failed in the past might work now or in the future, or they might inconsistently help. For example, some but not all brief naps might be extended by reswaddling, a quick feeding, or replacing a pacifier. Swaddling and pacifiers might help; they will not harm your baby and should not be viewed as a "crutch" that somehow interferes with learning self-soothing.

Try to meet your baby's needs. If your baby is hungry, feed him. If he's tired, put him down to sleep.

COMMON FUSSINESS/CRYING PEAKS AROUND 6 WEEKS

About 6 weeks of age (counting from the due date), around the time your baby produces her first social smiles, night sleep becomes more organized, and the longest single sleep period begins to occur with predictability and regularity in the evening hours. This long sleep period is about four to six hours. If your baby has extreme fussiness/ colic, the longest sleep period might be less. This long sleep period may occur before or around midnight, and subsequent intervals of sleep may be much shorter. The maturation of the internal timing mechanism for night sleep rhythms takes time; please be patient.

Your baby will also start to settle down more and more. She will become more interested in objects such as mobiles and toys, she'll have more interest in playing games, and her repertoire of emotional expressions and social responses will dramatically increase.

Yet many parents find this time particularly frustrating, especially in the evening, since many babies reach a peak of fussing/crying and wakefulness at about 6 weeks. Even extremely fussy/colicky babies may be at their worst at 6 weeks of age, as shown by Dr. T. Berry Brazelton, and some may not appear to settle down much after their peak.

THE 6-WEEK PEAK
At 6 weeks of age, all babies are most fussy, cry the most, and are most wakeful.

One mother told me about her son at 6 weeks: "He's a little excited about all the living going on."

Here is a vivid description of the 6-week peak:

Antonio was born two weeks early and without difficulty. I remember thinking several hours after his birth that he was going to be a very easy boy, since my pregnancy and delivery were both routine and relatively easy. Three days after we brought him home, however, I realized that my expectations might have been a little off. Over the next three weeks we started to notice a pattern of crying that started at about 5:00 p.m. and usually lasted for about six hours. In addition to that, Antonio awakened every two hours to be fed during the night and didn't take daytime naps! During these early weeks, the only way Antonio would sleep, night or day, was if either my husband or I held him. My husband thought we must be doing something wrong, and I was afraid he might be right, although I didn't admit it at the time.

When Antonio was about 3 weeks old, I brought him to see Dr. Weissbluth. We discussed his sleep patterns (or lack thereof), and he advised me that Antonio's evening fussiness would get worse until he was 6 weeks old, and then it would start to improve slowly and hopefully end at about 12 weeks.

I was quite dismayed to also learn that since Antonio was born two weeks early, I had to count Antonio's age from his original due date, not his birth date. So instead of having only three more rough weeks, we would probably have at least five! That's an eternity when you're sleep deprived! I really didn't know how we were going to make it through that rough period! I think the biggest worry we had was that Antonio's fussiness would never end. We knew in our minds that he had to get better, but the big question was when.

Then, at about 6 weeks after Antonio's original due date, I couldn't believe it, but I actually started to notice that his evening fussiness was decreasing! In addition, at the same time, his nighttime sleep started becoming a little longer, and he started falling asleep in his crib instead of having to sleep with me! The improvements were small, but at that point I was just ecstatic to have four solid hours of sleep at night! At about 10 weeks I called the doctor and received encouraging advice. He suggested that I start putting Antonio to bed earlier at night, as this might help him feel less tired and make him fall asleep more easily. At the time, Antonio was going to bed between 10:00 and 11:00 p.m. So I moved his bedtime to around 8:00 p.m. for a few nights, and I could not believe how well this worked! I then started putting him in his crib even earlier, as I noticed that he actually became tired at around 6:30 p.m. Antonio is now almost 5 months old, and he has been sleeping from 6:30 p.m. through the night to about 7:00 a.m. He has been doing this since he was 12 weeks old. He does wake up occasionally at 4:00 or 5:00 a.m. if he's hungry, but for the most part he sleeps extremely well at night, and is even starting to form regular daytime naps! Antonio is such a joy to be with, I actually might want to have a second baby. Yikes!

This report eloquently describes the fear faced by many parents at this time: that the fussing/crying will never end. During this time, your baby may irritate and exhaust you. She may give up napping altogether around 6 weeks of age and, to make matters worse, when awake may appear to be grumbling all day. You may feel battered at the end of each day; you may be at your wits' end. This, too, is natural. Being annoyed with your baby does not make you a "bad" parent. Just understand why you're annoyed. Remember that your baby's immature nervous system lacks inhibitory control: your baby might have moments of tremulousness, quivering, or shaking of the arms or legs. The brain develops inhibitory capabilities as it matures, but this takes time; things will settle down after 6 weeks of age. This report also illustrates how an earlier bedtime, after 6 weeks of age, helps your baby sleep better.

> **A main goal after the 6-week peak is to ensure an early enough bedtime to prevent a second wind near the end of the day.**

Weeks 7 and 8

Night sleep: Becoming organized
Day sleep: Naps are brief and irregular; there may be many catnaps
Bedtime: Starting to be earlier

EARLIER BEDTIMES AND LONGER PERIODS OF NIGHT SLEEP DEVELOP

The major biological changes starting now are a tendency for your baby to go to sleep earlier at night and for longer periods of uninterrupted night sleep.

Watch for drowsy signs developing earlier in the evening, and if you do not see them, experiment with different earlier bedtimes. A pitfall is to assume that any bedtime in the time frame of 6:00–8:00 p.m. will work for your baby. Your baby might be developing a second wind or fatigue signs at 8:00 p.m., but you do not notice because of digital distraction or the demands of another child or responsibilities like preparing dinner. Or maybe drowsy signs are emerging at 6:30 p.m., but you don't get home from work until 7:00 p.m. and drowsy signs are masked by excited playtime.

Your baby will now develop longer blocks of night sleep. The single longest sleep period is now four to six hours long and will occur in the evening hours. Often this occurs before midnight, and after midnight the blocks of sleep might be shorter. Feed your child only when necessary and try to avoid unnecessary feedings, which might create a night-feeding or night-waking habit.

The failure to establish an early bedtime after about 6 weeks of age means that your baby might accumulate a sleep deficit from a bedtime that is too late. If this occurs, it will appear that common fussiness/crying continues longer or worsens, but what is really going on is the emergence of sleep-deprivation-driven fussy behavior. Help your baby sleep better after 6 weeks of age by moving the bedtime earlier to prevent a second wind. Sometimes parent issues (see Chapter 3) interfere with establishing an early bedtime, and this eventually causes an overtired family.

Every baby behaves a little differently during these first few weeks. Your baby most likely will fall somewhere in between the common fussy/crying baby and the extremely fussy/colic infant. And even if your baby has had mild fussing/crying, this may well be a period in which she becomes worse either because of the 6-week peak or because she begins to accumulate a sleep debt.

If social smiles are not already present, your baby will start to produce them shortly after 6 weeks of age (or 6 weeks after the expected date of delivery for preemies). Prepare yourself for changes resulting from your child's increased social maturation. The social smiles herald the onset of increased social awareness, and it may come to pass that your baby will now start to fight sleep in order to enjoy the pleasure of your company. This is natural!

During the day, when your baby appears slightly fidgety, ask yourself two questions. First, when did you last feed her? Second, how long has she been up? Sometimes you need to sleep her and not feed her. During the night, respond quickly to feed your baby when she is hungry, but when quiet, non-distressed-sounding vocalizations occur shortly after a feeding, try to delay your response to see if your child might return to sleep unassisted, or send Dad in promptly to check on your baby and do minimal soothing without feeding.

Here is an account of one mother's first weeks that describes how even colicky babies may be more settled after the 6-week peak:

Today my baby girl, Sophia, is 8 weeks old. I celebrated by taking my first uninterrupted bath since her birth. Of course, she woke up just as I was toweling off, but I have learned to be grateful for small pleasures.

Sophia doesn't sleep much, and when she's awake she's usually either crying or nursing. It's been a little better the past week, but she still sleeps very little: six to eight hours at night and two to four hours during the day. And since I can't bear to hear her cry, that means she spends most of her time on my breast, where, mercifully, she can always be soothed. I can't hold her and play with her; she's always squirming to get at my breast. So, anyway, she's on my breast ten to twelve hours a day.

Lately she's good for a couple of ten- to twenty-minute play periods (on the floor on her back, me leaning over her, or on the changing table while I change her diaper).

When I talked with the doctor, he said it did seem my baby was colicky, and I took his book home to read. Finally, I found descriptions by other mothers of babies like mine! I was not alone. I came to understand how sleep problems, like those of my baby, appear to be hunger but really aren't. I also learned that there's nothing I can do for my baby that I'm not already doing, and so I might as well turn some of my energy around and start taking care of myself. Truly, I be-

lieve that in the case of a colicky baby, who in most cases cannot be treated for her condition, it is the mother who "needs treatment" or help, and to this end I suggest:

1. *Get out of the house an hour or two a day, minimum.*
2. *When out of the house, try to get some physical exercise to burn off the tension.*
3. *Don't feel guilty about doing anything that makes you feel good.*
4. *Socialize as much as possible outside the home.*
5. *Keep a diary or log of your baby's sleeping/feeding habits.*
6. *When the baby is asleep, get some sleep yourself, unless you're doing something for your own peace of mind.*

And things are getting better. Yesterday afternoon Sophia woke up from a three-hour nap, nursed calmly, and wasn't fussy for several hours afterward. She didn't behave in her old way, but I got to hold her and play with her for over an hour; then she stayed calm in the swing for a while.

And I got my first bath in eight weeks this morning.

If you are lucky enough to have a baby with common fussiness/crying, at 5 to 6 weeks you may have already noticed her sleep patterns becoming somewhat regular. You can try to help your baby sleep better by putting her down drowsy but awake, or perhaps you want to lie down with her to sleep (see Chapter 1 regarding co-sleeping and SIDS) when she first appears tired, but in any case, you should put her down after no more than two hours of wakefulness. She may or may not drift into sleep easily. You do not need to let her cry at all, but some babies will fuss or cry in a mild fashion before falling asleep. If she quietly cries for five, ten, or twenty minutes, it will do her no harm, and she may drift off to sleep. If not, console her and try again at other times. Try to become sensitive to her need to sleep. The novelty of external noises, voices, lights, and vibrations will disrupt her sleep more and more, so try to have her in her crib or your bed when she needs to sleep. Go slowly and be flexible.

In summary, at or shortly after 6 weeks of age (counting from the due date) the brain matures predictably in three ways:

1. *Specific responsive social smiling.* When you smile at her, she returns your smile.

2. *Longer sleep periods (four to six hours) occurring predictably in the evening hours, usually before midnight.* This is part of the night-sleep circadian rhythm.

3. *The brain wants to fall asleep earlier in the evening.* The biological time of evening drowsiness dictates an earlier bedtime, about 6:00–8:00 p.m. It might be a little earlier or later for your child. This is part of the night-sleep circadian rhythm.

One parent described the early bedtime this way: "The early bedtime is a nonnegotiable component of healthy sleep training. If you want your child to sleep soundly and wake up well rested, you have to marry the idea of an early bedtime."

With two or more children, a common problem is that your older child distracts you early in the evening, so you miss signs of drowsiness in the baby and innocently keep her up too late. Cumulative sleepiness results and leads to major sleep problems. Also, sometimes it is hard to put an older child down at an earlier time than your baby, who needs a later bedtime because she has had a long midday nap. If so, begin the process of putting your older child to bed earlier when you have help, such as on a Saturday night, when Dad is home, so each child has one parent for soothing to sleep. Tell your first child, "Because you are a big boy, you do not need to nap like our baby. Our baby needs to nap, and that's why she can stay up a little later than you. Do you want to take naps?"

If you have only one bedroom and cannot sleep well because you find yourself awakened by or responding to every quiet sound your baby makes, consider temporarily giving your bedroom to your baby. Maybe you will have to camp out in your living room for a while until you or your baby sleeps better at night. If you have only one bedroom, temporary separation like this between parents and child is necessary for extinction, graduated extinction, and the check-and-console technique. If you have two bedrooms, consider moving her to her own room during this age range.

After 6 weeks of age, you might want to try to help your baby sleep better at night. The ease with which you can accomplish this is related to whether your child is currently well rested or overtired. And this is related to whether he had common fussiness/crying or extreme fussiness/colic and whether you were able to successfully soothe him during the first 6 weeks. Please see Chapters 3–5 for some parents' reports on helping their young babies, around 2 months of age and younger, get better sleep. For babies younger than 2 months of age, consider graduated extinction, extinction with a cap, or check and console. Extinction, even for extreme fussiness/colic, may also be considered and be successful at 2 months of age (see Chapter 4).

Alternatively, you may have no need or desire to try sleep-training strategies. Your baby might be sleeping well at night, and there is no reason to rock the boat. Or you are enjoying the family bed and do not wish to change or allow your baby to cry. This is fine for now, but eventually you probably will want to consider some changes in sleep routines to accommodate your baby's need for an earlier bedtime. The sooner you attempt an earlier bedtime, the more quickly the family will become better rested. These changes do not necessarily mean that your baby will cry. Always consider both your child's ability to self-soothe and your resources for prolonged daytime and nighttime soothing. Do what works best for you and your baby.

If you are considering helping your baby sleep better, usually start at *bedtime* with an earlier bedtime and/or by putting your baby down drowsy but awake, because night sleep develops around or after 6 weeks of age and this natural sleep rhythm will help your attempts succeed. You are using the developing internal timing mechanism for night sleep as an aid to get better quality sleep. At night, Mom might leave the house after feeding and let Dad do the soothing to sleep. In addition, or alternatively, try to help your baby sleep better for a nap in the *morning* by putting him down drowsy but awake and having Dad do the soothing. The reason you might see success here is that your baby is likely to be best rested from night sleep. In the morning, you might be even more successful if you try to put your child down drowsy but awake within only one hour after waking, to prevent a second wind. That is, you do changing, feeding, a little playing, and soothing all within one hour. Look at the clock when you think your baby awakens to start the day; this time may vary from day to day, but you should try to have him in his crib with lights out within one hour of that time. If the start-the-day hour is quite early, maybe this first "nap" is really a continuation of night sleep. Go for it anyway, and if you are successful with the drowsy-but-awake technique, celebrate your success even if this nap is frustratingly short.

Remember, early sleep training means starting to respect your baby's need to sleep by anticipating when he will need to sleep (within one to two hours of waking), introducing an earlier bedtime, learning to recognize drowsy signs, getting Dad on board, and developing a bedtime routine. Then your baby will not become overtired.

Encourage the development of self-soothing skills and bedtime routines as soon as possible.

Start helping your baby to sleep (see Chapter 4) at different ages, depending on the following circumstances:

- At a few weeks of age if you have to return to work or if you are totally exhausted and unable to function. This may work well for babies with common fussiness/crying.
- After 6 weeks of age for night sleep for babies with common fussiness/crying.
- Around 2 to 4 months of age at night for babies with extreme fussiness/colic. Success may be slow and difficult.

REMEMBER
Different children require different approaches.

Common challenges during the second month include:

- Sleep deprivation, excitement, and medical conditions push thinking about your child's sleep off your radar.
- Thinking that feeding directly causes sleeping makes you focus only on feeding, leading to unnecessary feeding at night.
- Unwarranted diagnosis of acid reflux is mistaken as the cause of not sleeping well.
- Distraction because an older child interferes with helping your baby learn self-soothing by causing you to miss drowsy signs in your baby, which results in a second wind.
- Extreme fussiness/colic interferes with learning self-soothing.

These common challenges may cause your child to become more parent-soothed than self-soothed. Don't necessarily worry now if your child is mostly or completely parent-soothed, but look forward or plan ahead to a time when your child is older and you can teach him self-soothing.

COMMON FUSSINESS/CRYING
Most babies with common fussiness/crying tend to be "easy" babies who are placid and easy to manage, quiet angels most nights. Sure,

they may have a fussy period in the evening, but it's not too long, intense, or hard to deal with. They appear to sleep well anywhere and anytime during the day and quite regularly at night. In fact, the early development of regular, long night-sleep periods—starting well before the age of 6 weeks—is a characteristic feature of "easy" babies. These kids are very portable, and parents bask in their sunny dispositions.

But shortly . . . dark clouds may gather. The baby starts to have some new grumbling or crabbiness that does not occur only in the evening. In fact, the quiet evenings might now be punctured by new, "painful" cries suggesting an illness. Or it might now take longer to put the baby to sleep. What has happened to your sound sleeper? Irregularities of sleep schedules, nap deprivation, and too late a bedtime are the chief culprits. Now is the time to become ever more sensitive to your child's need to sleep.

After your baby is about 6 weeks of age, the best strategy still is to try to synchronize your caretaking activities with her own rhythms. You should try to reestablish healthy sleep habits by removing the disruptive effects of external noises, lights, or vibrations. Although it may be inconvenient for you, try to have your baby back in her crib after no more than two hours of wakefulness. Consider this two-hour interval to be a rough guide to help organize the day into periods of naps and wakeful activities.

HINT
Be careful, but . . . no set schedules and no rigid rules.

Q: *How long can I keep my baby up?*
A: No more than two hours.

Two hours of wakefulness is about the maximum that most babies can endure without becoming overtired. Sometimes a baby may need to go to sleep after being up for only one hour or less. Often this brief wakeful period of just one hour occurs early in the morning. Try to soothe him to sleep *before* he becomes overtired—*before* he becomes slightly crabby, seems irritable, pulls his hair, or bats at his ears. Expect this type of behavior to develop within two hours of waking up if he is not put to sleep when he first shows signs of being tired. Look for drowsy signs (see Chapter 3). Please do not mistake this two-hour guide to mean that he should be up for two hours and then down for two hours. Rather, two hours is the time interval during which you should expect to put him to sleep.

When you have been out for a walk or running an errand with your baby, watch the clock and try to have him asleep within two hours after he wakes up. If upon returning home during this time interval you notice that he is becoming overtired, say to yourself, "I blew it this time; next time I'll return home sooner." Also, by paying attention a little to clock time, you will discover how much wakefulness your baby can comfortably tolerate.

Expect your overtired child to protest when he is put down to sleep. This is natural, because he prefers the pleasure of your soothing comfort to being in a dark, quiet, boring room.

Keep in mind the distinction between a protest cry and a sad cry. You are leaving your baby alone to let him learn to soothe himself to sleep; you are not abandoning him.

Q: *How long should I let him cry?*
A: Not at all if you want to lie down with your child in your bed and soothe him to sleep or soothe him to sleep at your breast. Or you might start with ignoring the crying for five, ten, or twenty minutes. Try to decide whether your child is tired, basing your judgment on his behavior, the time of day, and the interval of wakefulness (how long he has been up). See Chapters 3–5 for parents' reports about letting their child cry in this age range.

When you have decided your child is tired or overtired, consider putting him down to sleep—even if he doesn't want to sleep. Sometimes he'll fall asleep and sometimes he won't. When he doesn't, pick him up and soothe and comfort him. You may try again after several minutes to allow him to go to sleep on his own, or you may decide not to try again the next day or several days later. But remember, if your baby cries hard for three minutes, cries quietly for three minutes, and then sleeps for an hour, he would have lost that good hour-long nap if you had not left him alone for six minutes.

Also, when he needs to sleep but wants to play, then your playing with him is robbing him of sleep.

Keep a log or diary as you go through these trials to see if any trend or improvement occurs. Here's an account from Allyson's mother, who helped her baby make a dramatic—and permanent— improvement in her sleep habits at about *8 weeks* of age:

> Day 56: *Allyson woke up from an afternoon nap, and I thought she was ill—she was so calm! No jerky movements or agitated behavior, which I guess I'd assumed was just "normal" for her. About this time, though, she still cried a lot when not nursing, and she still had trouble falling asleep.*

On day 59, the mother decided to ignore some of the fussing/ crying.

> Day 59 (first day of extinction with a one-hour cap): *Let her fuss one hour—and she went to sleep for three and a quarter hours (5:45 to 9:00 p.m.).*
>
> Day 60 (second day of extinction with a cap): *Allyson fussed all morning and wouldn't sleep, but I kept her in her crib from 10:15 a.m. to noon, staying with her most of the time. Got her up to nurse at noon. That night she woke up at 2:30 a.m.—for the first time in several weeks. I nursed her until 3:00 and then put her down. She fussed off and on until 4:00, when she went to sleep.*
>
> Day 63 (fifth day): *Breakthrough! She went to sleep for*

forty-five minutes in the morning and took a really long nap in the afternoon (12:45 to 5:00). But she woke in the middle of the night again (3:20 a.m.). She went back to sleep at 4:30 and slept until 8:30. She was happy in her crib—no screaming as I changed her diaper, which was new behavior!

Review of this mother's records showed that up to day 59, the total sleep duration per twenty-four hours was about six to twelve hours. After day 63, the total sleep duration was longer—twelve to seventeen hours. The five-day training really helped her child sleep longer.

Day 64 (sixth day): Two wonderful things happened. First, Allyson took a midmorning nap (10:45 a.m. to 1:30 p.m.), and when I put her down for the night, with her eyes wide open, she did not fuss at all. I quickly left the room and heard no crying. She slept from 8:35 p.m. to 5:05 a.m.

Days 87-96: Allyson is just about perfect. If she starts to fuss, I know she is hungry, wet, or tired. If she's tired, I simply put her in her crib and within two minutes she is asleep. It's a miracle!

As this report and others in Chapters 3–5 clearly demonstrate, parents can help their children sleep better at around *2 months of age or younger,* and it often works quickly, especially if the child has common fussiness/crying. Extinction for babies with extreme fussiness/colic may also succeed quickly at 2 months of age, as described in Chapter 4. There is no compelling reason to wait until 3 to 4 months of age to help your child sleep better.

EXTREME FUSSINESS/COLIC

As previously discussed, 80 percent of babies exhibit common fussiness/crying, while 20 percent are extremely fussy or colicky.

Colicky babies are difficult to manage for the first 2 to 4 months because they are intense, wakeful, stimulus sensitive, and irregular when they do sleep, and they only sleep for brief periods. They have long periods of fussing and crying. And often a portion of their crying is inconsolable. Because of all this, many parents are reluctant to try to teach self-soothing at this time. These babies are hard to read. Most parents have difficulty telling whether they are hungry, fussy, or plain overtired. So leaving them alone to cry with the hope that they will sleep is potentially frustrating to everyone. The fear that the attempt will fail and that the crying will go on and on for hours and weeks inhibits many of these sleep-deprived parents.

So you might feel more comfortable waiting a little longer while you do whatever you can to maximize sleep and minimize crying. You might attempt an earlier bedtime after the 6-week peak. Try to get help so you can take breaks without any guilt. However, please note that some parents are successful with helping their babies with extreme fussiness/colic sleep better *before 4 months of age* (see Chapter 4). In Dr. R. S. Illingworth's review, colicky behavior ends in *50 percent* of afflicted babies by *2 months* of age, in an additional *30 percent* by *3 months* of age, and in an additional *10 percent* by *4 months* of age. So you might try to help your baby with extreme fussiness/colic sleep better with drowsy but awake, an earlier bedtime, and graduated extinction, extinction with a cap, or extinction for a four-to-five-day trial and be successful before 4 months of age. If the trial fails, abandon it and try again when your child is older. Of course you will be frustrated, and maybe angry with me, but I know that a trial this short will not harm your baby.

The reason that it is commonly believed that colic ends by 3–4 months is because it is true that 80–90 percent of infants have outgrown it by then. But you might be in the more fortunate group of 50 percent of infants whose colic is winding down at 2 months! There is no harm in trying to help your child sleep better with a five-day trial, even if you try graduated extinction, extinction with a cap, or check and console.

These first few months are rugged for many mothers because their baby's sleep/wake patterns are unpredictable, there may be lots of fussing and crying, and the mothers may not have fully recovered from the stress or complications associated with labor and delivery. Information in Chapter 5 and the following hints will help you get through these first few months.

Helpful Tips for Parents
>Pamper yourself; remember, this is smart for the baby, not selfish for you. If you feel better, you will be better able to nurture your baby.
>Forget errands, chores, housework.
>Unplug the phone.
>Ignore your baby's quiet vocalizations during sleep.
>Nap when baby sleeps.
>Hire help for housework or breaks when your baby is most bothersome.
>Plan pleasurable, brief outings without your baby (swimming, shopping, and movies).

Tips to Help Soothe Babies
>Definitely helpful in soothing:
>>Rhythmic rocking: in chair swing, arms, car rides
>>Sucking: pacifier, thumb, wrist
>>Gentle pressure: swaddling, massage
>>Gentle sounds: lullabies, music, singing, humming
>Possibly helpful in soothing:
>>Lambskin rug
>>Warm-water bottle placed on abdomen
>>Recordings of heartbeat sound, womb sounds, vacuum cleaner, running water, sounds of nature
>>Removal of stimulating toys from the crib or any bright night-lights
>>Some babies nap best in a pitch-black and/or very quiet

room (one family in a noisy city even used a large walk-
in closet with the door open for naps).
Placing a soft, tiny blanket in baby's hand
Putting the child's head against a soft crib bumper or laying
    a clean cloth diaper over the top of the head (not the
    face) like a scarf

Crying should not be thought of as a test for you. If your baby
has extreme fussiness/colic, don't feel that you are necessarily creating a crying habit because of your prolonged, complex efforts to
soothe her. Maybe your first test to help your baby sleep will come
around 2 months of age, or perhaps it will occur later, at 3 to
4 months of age, when almost all colic subsides.

You can't treat colic with smiles, but there will be less crying in a
home where there is a lot of social smiling. Practice smiling, smile
broadly, open your eyes wide, regard your child as you nod, and say
"Good boy" or "Good girl." Do all these especially when your baby
calms down or smiles at you. Even if your child does not always respond to your smiles, this practice, like a rehearsal, will pay off big-
time later.

Don't save your smiles until colic ends.

Summary and Action Plan for Exhausted Parents

WEEKS 5 TO 6: FUSSINESS/CRYING PEAKS

**A main goal at this age is to encourage the development of self-
soothing skills**

At 6 weeks of age, all babies are most fussy, cry the most, and are
most wakeful. At or after 6 weeks of age, the brain matures predictably in three ways:

1. *Specific responsive social smiling.* When you smile at her, she smiles back.

2. *Longer sleep periods (four to six hours) occurring predictably in the evening hours, usually before midnight.* This is part of the night-sleep circadian rhythm.

3. *The brain wants to fall asleep earlier in the evening.* This, too, is part of the night-sleep circadian rhythm. The biological time of evening drowsiness dictates an earlier bedtime, about 6:00–8:00 p.m. It might be a little earlier or later for your child.

A main goal after the 6-week peak is to ensure an early enough bedtime to prevent a second wind near the end of the day.

Parent issues (see Chapter 3) may get in the way of an early bedtime.

Encourage the development of self-soothing skills and bedtime routines as soon as possible:

- At a few weeks of age if you have to return to work or if you are totally exhausted and unable to function. This may work well for common fussiness/crying babies.
- After 6 weeks of age for night sleep for babies with common fussiness/crying.
- Around 2 to 4 months of age at night for babies with extreme fussiness/colic. Be patient: success may be slow and difficult.

REMEMBER
Different children require different approaches.

Common challenges around 5 to 6 weeks (see above) may cause your child to become more parent-soothed than self-soothed.

WEEKS 7 AND 8

For 80 percent of babies, those with common fussiness/crying, the worst is over, as long as you have established an earlier bedtime and taught your child some self-soothing skills. It's never too late, so if you have not yet begun, start now. "No-cry" or "maybe-cry" sleep solutions (Chapter 4) may work quickly.

For those 20 percent of babies with extreme fussiness/colic, consider a five-day trial with an earlier bedtime, putting the baby down drowsy but awake, permitting only brief intervals of wakefulness during the day, plus "maybe-cry" or "let-cry" sleep solutions (Chapter 4). If you see no benefit or would rather not try this now, then try it again in a few weeks or wait until your baby's extreme fussiness/colic naturally winds down at 3 to 4 months. Remember, though, that colic subsides in 50 percent of infants by 2 months, an additional 30 percent of infants by 3 months, and an additional 10 percent of infants by 4 months. Your child might be in the more fortunate group of 50 percent of infants whose colic is winding down at 2 months, so there is no harm in trying to help him sleep better with a five-day trial of the sleep solution of your choice at that time: also remember, however, that "no-cry" sleep solutions are less likely to work in babies with extreme fussiness/colic.

CHAPTER 7

Healthy Sleep Habits in Months 3-4

A main goal at this age is to encourage the development of self-soothing skills for night sleep and the midmorning nap.

MONTH 3: EXTREME FUSSINESS/COLIC WINDS DOWN

Fifty percent of all babies with extreme fussiness/colic will be more settled at 2 months of age. By 3 months of age, 80 percent have improved, and by 4 months of age, 90 percent have. So between 2 and 4 months, your baby should begin to appear calmer in the early evening and to sleep better at night. If you have not done so already, now is the time to practice letting your child learn more self-soothing (see Chapters 3 and 4). Your child's transition from being parent-soothed to learning how to self-soothe may be easy in a well-rested baby or difficult in an overtired baby.

I have examined many children who cry with such intensity and persistence at bedtime that their mothers are sure they're sick. During their crying, they may swallow air and become very gassy. If this happens, it is tempting to assume that their formula doesn't agree with them or that they have an intestinal disease—but only at bedtime or at night? These children are healthy but overtired. Not only do they cry hard and long when awake, they also cry loud and often during attempts to put them to sleep.

Your crying baby may be hungry, fussy, or over*tired*.

Let's consider the ways in which your child is changing. More smiles, coos, giggles, laughs, and squeals light up your life. Your child is now a more social creature. She is sleeping better at *night*, but *naps* may still be brief and irregular.

Become sensitive to her need to sleep and try to distinguish this need from her desire to play with you. If your child was previously or currently is primarily parent-soothed, she will naturally prefer the pleasure of your company to being left alone in a dark, quiet bedroom. Therefore, she may fight sleep to keep you around. This is in contrast to well-rested children with self-soothing skills, who usually go to sleep easily without protest.

In addition to your presence, which provides pleasurable stimulation, your baby's increasing curiosity about all the new and exciting parts of her expanding world may disrupt her sleep. How interesting it must be for an infant to observe the clouds in the sky, listen to the trees moving in the wind, hear the noise of barking dogs, or focus on the rhythms of adult chatter. When your baby needs to sleep, try to have her in an environment where she will sleep well. As she continues to grow, she will become more curious and social, and you will notice that she probably naps best in her crib.

Your child is becoming less portable. She cannot sleep equally well in any setting or situation, as she could when younger. Now you must become sensitive to the difference in quality between brief, interrupted daytime sleep and prolonged, consolidated naps. As your child's biological rhythms evolve for day sleep, your general goal is to *synchronize your soothing-to-sleep activities with her internal timing mechanism for sleep*. This is no different from being sensitive to her need to be fed or changed. Many children are overtired from not napping well or from going to sleep too late. They may not nap well because they're getting too much outside stimulation, too much handling, or too much irregular handling.

Sometimes at about 3 months of age, after the extreme fussiness/ colic has dissipated, or in a baby who had common fussiness/crying, a child who had been sleeping well begins waking at night or crying at night and during the day. The parents also may note heightened activity with wild screaming spells. These children have accumulated a sleep debt and decided that they would rather play with their parents than be placed in a dark, quiet, and boring room. Parents who do not recognize the new sleep debt might believe that this new night waking represents hunger due to a "growth spurt" or insufficient breast milk. But when these parents begin to focus on establishing a healthy night-sleep schedule, when they put these babies in their cribs when the babies need to sleep, and when they shield their babies from overstimulation, the frequent night waking stops. If the children had developed irritability or fussiness, this disappears, too.

REMEMBER
The more rested a child is, the more she accepts sleep and expects to sleep.

NAPS

After she's been awake for no more than about two hours, plan to put your 3- or 4-month-old child somewhere semi-quiet or quiet to nap.

Q: *When I put my child to sleep after no more than two hours of wakefulness, how long should he sleep?*

A: At this point, the naps may be either short or long, without any particular pattern. This variability occurs because the part of the brain that establishes regular naps has not yet fully developed. By learning to recognize *drowsy signs,* you will be able to determine the best time to give your child the opportunity to nap. An awareness of *sleep inertia* will help you decide whether a particular nap was long enough. And sensitivity to the *witching hour* will help you determine whether naps on a particular day were long enough (see Chapters 1 and 3).

The two-hour limit on wakefulness is an approximation. Often there is a magic moment of tiredness when the baby will go to sleep easily. She is tired then but not overtired. If you go past this point in time, expect fatigue to set in. When your baby is up too long, she will tend to become overstimulated, overaroused, irritable, or peevish from a *second wind* (see Chapter 1). Please don't blame changes in weather—it's never too hot or too cold to sleep well.

Many parents misunderstand what overstimulation means. *A child becomes overstimulated when the duration of wakeful intervals is too long.* Overstimulation does not mean that you are too intense in your playfulness. It occurs once your baby has been awake for too long, regardless of what actions are taking place or not taking place. Your baby is a sponge; she soaks up input from the world around her whenever she is awake. And like a sponge, she will quickly reach an oversaturation point. That point is what we call overstimulation.

Do not think of overstimulation as excessive intensity in play with your child; rather, think of it as too long a duration of the baby's normal period of wakefulness. It's not too much of a good thing; it's just being up too long.

The Midmorning Nap Develops Between 9:00 and 10:00 a.m.
Watch the clock a little, but watch your baby more during the day, and expect your baby to need to sleep within two hours of wakefulness. Use whatever soothing method or wind-down routine works best to comfort and calm your baby. This may include a scheduled feeding, non-nutritive ("recreational") nursing, a session in a swing or a rocking chair, or a pacifier.

After a while you may notice, in the morning, a partial or a rough pattern of when your child's day sleep is best. Based on your child's behavior, the time of day, and how long she has been awake, you may reasonably conclude that she *needs* to sleep at any given time. However, she may *want* to play with you instead. Please try to distinguish between your child's needs and her wants. Have the confidence to be sensitive to her need to sleep, and lie down with her (see Chapter 1 regarding co-sleeping and SIDS) or leave her alone a little to let her sleep. How long should you leave her alone? Maybe five, ten, or twenty minutes; there's no need for a rigid schedule. Simply test her once in a while to see whether she goes to sleep after five to twenty minutes of protest crying. When you put your baby down drowsy but awake, you are giving her the opportunity to develop *self-soothing skills,* to learn how to fall asleep unassisted. Some children learn this faster than others, so don't worry if your child seems always to cry up to your designated time. If this approach fails, pick her up, soothe her, comfort her, and then either try once more to get her to go to sleep or play with her for a while and try again later or the next day. Perhaps she was too young; wait a few weeks and try again. Never letting your child cry might reflect confusion in your mind between the healthy notion of allowing her to be alone sometimes and your fear that she will feel abandoned. But you are not abandoning your child by allowing her to learn self-soothing skills! You are protecting her. Always going to your child when she needs to sleep actually robs her of sleep.

Why focus on the midmorning nap? Simply because it develops before the midday nap. Try to teach self-soothing for the midmorning nap and then do whatever works to maximize sleep and minimize fussing/crying for the remainder of the day (being mindful to limit wakefulness to short intervals). Success or failure to achieve a regular midmorning nap depends on how well rested your child is when she wakes up to start the day; thus, a prerequisite for a good midmorning nap is good-quality night sleep.

This lack of rigid scheduling is appropriate for children a few months old, who are biologically immature. However, as the child gets older, extreme inconsistency will produce unhealthy sleep habits. Be flexible, but also become sensitive to your child's need to sleep. Remember, it's your responsibility as a parent to provide structure for your child: she cannot do it on her own. That doesn't mean imposing some arbitrary sleep regimen on her. It means being aware of the signals your child is sending about when she needs to sleep, and then acting on those signals in a firm but loving way to help her sleep better now and in the weeks, months, and years to come. Here's an account from the mother of a 3-month-old infant who successfully accomplished the midmorning nap and helped her baby sleep better at night:

> It started at just 12 weeks. Katie was so fatigued she would cry for hours, screaming completely out of control, scratching her head, pulling her ears. Holding her didn't help, so it wasn't hard not to pick her up—she screamed anyway.
>
> Instituting a new day schedule was easy. As soon as she started getting cranky, I rushed her to her crib to sleep. She would watch her mobile, and then sleep for hours at a time. The first week, she was so tired that she only stayed up thirty to fifty minutes at a time and slept three to four hours in between. The key for me was to get her down before she got really upset.
>
> The afternoon was when she was awake the longest, and then it was hard getting her to sleep at night. The first few nights under our new regime were the worst. Positive reinforcement from my doctor was important then. I had to hear several times that this "cure" was the best thing to do.
>
> The first night under our new strategy, my husband lay on the floor in her room (I guess to make sure she didn't choke) while I sat crying in our living room. Finally, after forty-five minutes, Katie was quiet! Hurray! Each night she cried less and less, and I handled it better and better. After a week, her hysteria was gone! Sure, she cried a little sometimes, but now she was on a schedule. She napped two or three times a day, two to four hours at a time, and slept twelve to fifteen hours a night. Sleeping promotes more sleep, and makes it easier to fall asleep. It's a catch-22.

Writing down the sleep patterns helped, too. For one week I kept track of every time I put her down and every time I picked her up from her nap. At the end of the week I noticed a distinct pattern. She fell into it herself!

Reports from other mothers with children at even younger ages can be found in Chapters 3–6.

MAJOR POINTS

Letting your baby "cry it out" is *not* the only way your baby will learn to nap. Babies and children learn to nap well when parents focus on timing, motionless sleep (sleep in a crib or stationary stroller, as opposed to sleep while in a moving car or stroller), and consistency in soothing style.

As Katie's mother noticed, sleep begets sleep. This is a true statement. Even though it is not logical, it is biological!

Q: *My 3-month-old used to take very long midmorning naps, but now, at 4 months, they are shorter. What happened?*

A: Between 3 and 4 months, your child went to sleep later at night. He now goes to sleep earlier and wakes up better rested in the morning, so he no longer needs a very long midmorning nap.

Timing of Naps

Sleep periods for naps develop as the brain matures. This means that there are times during the day when your baby's brain will become drowsy and less alert. These "windows of opportunity" for sleep occur when the sleep process begins to overcome your baby. They are the best times for him to be soothed to sleep, both because it is easier to fall asleep at these times and because the restorative power of sleep is greatest when your baby's brain is in a drowsy state. Yes, of course your child is able to sleep at other times, but going to sleep is more difficult at such times, and the restorative power of sleep is much less. Unfortunately, your baby's brain may not be drowsy when you want him to sleep. You cannot control when he will become drowsy any more than you can control when he will become thirsty. As your infant's brain matures, these biologically determined periods of drowsiness will become more predictable and longer.

Here is a quick recap of the developmental timeline for sleep. After your baby is born, there is a quiet and calm honeymoon during which he is very sleepy, when your baby really will "sleep like a baby." This ends when he is a few days old (or a few days after his due date if he was born early). You may not even have a honeymoon if your baby was born several days late! After a few days of life, the sleepy brain wakes up, and during the first 6 weeks of life infants display increasing amounts of fussiness, crying, or agitated wakefulness, during which they swallow air and become gassy. At 6 weeks (or 6 weeks after the due date) the duration of these periods peaks, and they become more common in the evening hours. During these first weeks, the longest single sleep period is not very long and can occur at any time: this is day/night confusion. At about 6 weeks of age, something dramatic occurs naturally: your baby begins to produce social smiles, and the evening fussiness begins to decrease in most babies. One mother asked me if she could "fast-forward to 6 weeks" and skip the hard part. Sorry! But from 6 weeks, a more predictable and longer midmorning nap will emerge.

REMEMBER
Night-sleep periods will develop first, so you will notice longer sleeping at night before you will notice longer naps.

The onset of social smiles followed by a decrease in fussiness in the evening reflects maturational changes within your baby's brain. In addition, the brain becomes more able to inhibit the stimulating effects of sights, smells, sounds, and other sensations. Your baby is more able to console herself—she is becoming more capable of self-soothing. As a result of these biological changes, at 6 weeks of age your baby develops *night-sleep organization*. This means that her longest single sleep period now occurs at night. This is the end of day/night confusion. This longest night-sleep period may be only four to six hours, but it regularly occurs at night. You cannot control the exact time when this long sleep period will occur, but at least you now know that you will get a little more rest at night!

Night sleep usually develops without problems at 6 weeks of age because:

1. Darkness serves as a time cue.
2. We slow down our activities and become quieter at night.
3. We behave as if we expect our baby to sleep.

These three factors may be absent during the day, and so the major way to *prevent* sleep problems from developing now is to focus your efforts on *helping your baby nap during the day*.

There are three factors that will help your baby sleep well during the day: timing, motionless sleep, and consistency in soothing style. If you have experience already because you have more than one child, or if you have a child with common fussiness/crying, you may start your efforts early; if you have a colicky baby, you might have to start later.

Keep the intervals of wakefulness short. Look at the clock when your baby wakes up in the morning or after a nap. Within one to two hours after your baby wakes, begin a soothing process *before* your child appears grumpy, crabby, or drowsy. Usually the total duration of wakefulness, including the time of soothing, should be *less than two hours*. This does not mean that you keep your baby awake for about two hours before trying to soothe him to sleep. The point is that young infants cannot comfortably tolerate long periods of wakefulness. In fact, some babies go to sleep after being awake for only *one* hour or less. You want to catch the approaching wave of drowsiness as it is rising, to enable your baby to have a long, smooth ride to deep, refreshing slumber.

MAJOR POINT
Perfect timing produces no crying.

If your timing is off and your child's sleep wave crashes into an overtired state, then the ride to slumber is bumpy and sleep itself brief. If your timing is off, your child will become overtired, and then there will be some crying. This you may safely ignore. Such crying is the consequence of your having accidentally allowed your child to become overtired.

Think of how your baby behaves when she becomes overly hungry. She twists, turns, and may dive-bomb at the breast for a few minutes before she settles down to suck well. Similarly, the overtired baby takes a few minutes to settle down to sleep. I repeat: crying is the consequence of becoming overtired. At this particular time, your efforts to soothe—hugging, rocking, talking—may be stimulating and interfere with the natural surfacing of the sleep process. After all, your baby does not fall asleep immediately in the same way a light switch is turned off. Rather, the sleep process takes time. Remember, it is easier for her to fall asleep before she becomes grumpy, because when she becomes overtired—from nap deprivation or any other reason—her body produces stimulating hormones to fight the fatigue. This chemical stimulation interferes with sleeping well. This is why sleeping well during the day will improve night sleeping and why, conversely, *nap deprivation causes night waking.*

One mother told me that her child had been extremely fussy/colicky but that he began to slip into a better night-sleeping routine at 12 weeks of age and began taking longer naps during the day between 12 and 16 weeks of age. She was breast-feeding and used the family bed; her child went to sleep at about 10:00 p.m. around 12 weeks of age. Her 2-year-old son was not sleeping well at night either and distracted her, and this allowed the baby to become overtired. The predictable result: the baby's naps were a mess. He was "napping" between 5:00 and 6:00 p.m. and asleep for the night between 7:00 and 8:00 p.m. The mother recognized that her baby should be falling asleep for the night around 6:00 p.m., not napping then. Here was the solution that eventually corrected the overtired state:

Temporarily, her baby was put to sleep at a very early time, between 5:30 and 6:00 p.m. The plan was to help the child get more sleep at night and be asleep before a second wind developed. The mother was to soothe her baby at night and then either lie down with him or put him in his crib. She wanted to use the crib because the hour was so early and she had a 2-year-old to deal with. Because of the baby's age, and because he had been extremely fussy/colicky, and because he had become accustomed to sleeping with his mother in her bed at the breast, we knew he would protest our plan. We decided that we would ignore his protest crying at the onset of sleep and would use the father to soothe him at night when he might cry but was not hungry. During the day, the mother would do whatever worked to maximize sleep and minimize crying to keep him as well rested as possible. The 2-year-old made this part of the plan a little difficult. But within eight days, there was substantially less crying at night, and longer and fewer naps were occurring during the day. Now that the baby was better rested, he was able to stay up a little later at night. However, he still needed to go to sleep between 6:00 and 6:30 p.m.

EARLY BEDTIMES

A common complaint is "We don't get to eat dinner as a family." Or, "How can we play outside as a family after dinner?" My answer is that what is most important is a well-rested family.

Consistency in Soothing Styles for Naps

Parents often assume that there is a right and wrong way to soothe a baby to sleep. This is not the case. Falling asleep is simply learned behavior, a habit. The important thing is that the behavior is learned, not how it is learned. Your child will learn best if you are consistent in how you soothe him to sleep for naps. Below are two popular ways to soothe a baby to sleep. Either will work as long as you are consistent.

> Method A: *At nap time your baby sometimes soothes him-self to sleep unassisted.* After soothing your baby for sev-eral minutes, you *always* put him down to sleep *whether or not he is asleep.* You are practicing putting him down for a nap *drowsy but awake.* The soothing is a winding down, a transition from active to quiet, from alert to drowsy. Soothing may include breast- or bottle-feeding. Contrary to popular belief, your child will not develop night-sleep problems if you include breast-feeding as part of the soothing process. Also contrary to popular belief, it is not necessary that you always put him down fully awake. The key is that you consistently spend a relatively brief period of time soothing your baby to sleep for naps. Because he is not necessarily always asleep when you put him down, he eventually learns how to soothe himself to sleep without being held. In other words, you are always attempting to put your baby down for naps drowsy but awake, but sometimes he falls asleep during your soothing. If when the child is put down there are some vocalizations or low-level, quiet crying, some mothers will ignore it and other mothers, knowing from experience that with this child it will always escalate into hard crying, will resume soothing for a few more minutes. Also, if there is hard cry-ing upon being put down, some mothers will ignore it for a while to see whether their child will soon fall asleep,

while other mothers, again knowing from experience with their individual child that this always means there will not be a nap, will immediately pick up their baby for more pre-nap soothing or attempt the nap at some other time. Method A may be viewed positively (creating independence, learning self-soothing skills, acquiring the capacity to be alone) or negatively (creating insecurity, neglecting or abandoning your baby, selfishness in the mother). There is no benefit in being judgmental of yourself or others. Choose a method that is comfortable for you and be aware of how your behavior affects your child.

Method B: *Your baby always begins naps with your help.* You *always* hold and soothe your baby *until she is in a deep sleep state, no matter how long it takes.* You are not practicing putting him down for a nap drowsy but awake. You may lie down or sit down with your baby, nap with her, or perhaps put her down only after she is in a very deep sleep state. Your child learns to associate the process of falling asleep with the feel of your breast, your breathing and heart rhythm, and your body's scent. Contrary to popular belief, this association, in and of itself, does not automatically lead to a night-waking problem (signaling). A night-waking problem sometimes occurs when the mother indiscriminately responds to normal arousals, misinterprets them to reflect hunger, and, because of unnecessary feeding, inadvertently fragments the child's sleep. Perhaps this situation at night occurs more often in those mothers who choose method B for naps, but that is not because of the method itself but because of psychological factors that cause certain mothers to prefer method B over method A. Like method A, method B may be viewed positively (providing more security, is more natural) or negatively (creating dependence, spoiling). Method B is often what works best for babies with extreme fussiness/colic and is often a component of attachment parenting.

One method is not better than another; both method A and method B can help your child sleep well. There is no reason to be judgmental about soothing styles or brand other parents as "bad" simply because they do not agree with you. Different methods will seem more natural or more acceptable to different parents, and different methods work better for different children.

Be decisive; choose a soothing style and *be consistent*. Consistency helps your baby sleep better, because, as noted above, the process of falling asleep is a learned behavior. Please review "Resources for Soothing" and "Parent Issues" in Chapter 3 to help you decide which method is best for you. Grandparents and babysitters should handle your baby just as you do. Sometimes grandparents are a major problem because they interfere with the baby's sleep schedule. They want to come over to play with their grandchild when it is convenient for them, or they see their role as being more permissive than the parents. This is a difficult problem without a simple answer, because, in addition to wanting your child to be well rested, you want to maintain family harmony. If the grandparents are the primary caregivers during the day, consistency may be difficult. Try to teach them how important sleep is for their grandchild.

Q: *When should I start to try to establish regular naps? When should I start to become consistent in how I soothe my baby before naps?*

A: Day-sleep organization develops at 3 to 4 months of age. A regularly occurring midmorning nap appears first, followed by a regularly occurring midday nap a few or several weeks later. The age when you start nap training depends on your experience and your baby's degree of fussiness/crying.

Regardless of when you begin to start nap training, the sooner you develop a consistent approach, the easier it will be for the family. Please begin to be consistent around 6 weeks of age, when your child is clearly becoming more social and everyone is getting more rest at night. For babies born before their due date, these changes occur about 6 weeks after the due date, and that is when you should start.

I encourage fathers to become as involved as possible for naps—for example, on weekends. With either method A or B, sometimes the mother breast-feeds the baby and then passes the baby to the father to be soothed to sleep (see Chapter 3). As I said, either soothing method works well, but my observation is that for well-rested babies whose parents have consistently used method B and sometime later decide to switch to method A, the transition is made with very little or no crying. However, the children of parents who use method B *inconsistently* (because of real-life events that often interfere with prolonged soothing for naps) may never develop regular naps; they then become overtired, and when the parents switch to method A, the overtired child cries a lot. For some parents, then, it is simply easier to be consistent using method A.

If you have more than one child, it is very difficult to consistently use method B, even with full-time help, because an older child's time demands may make it impossible to devote sufficient time to getting your younger child into a deep sleep before putting him down. Therefore, it is more practical to use method A. In addition, because of your experience, you can begin helping your younger child sleep well as soon as you get home from the hospital. With two children, starting sleep training early for your newborn is especially important. Here, too, fathers need to help out more. As one basketball fan told me after the arrival of his second son, "Now I have to shift from one-on-one to zone defense!" Here is an account from a mother who started early with her second child using method A:

> As patients of Dr. Weissbluth, we were ready to commit our-
> selves to promoting good sleep habits in our children. When

our first son, Hayden, was born, it was easier said than done. Being new parents and not knowing what the different cries meant, we would pick Hayden up at the slightest whimper. We were quick believers when at 4 months we were a bit more seasoned and decided not to rush in at the first cry. The cry lasted fifteen minutes, and then it was smooth sailing; he gradually went to bed earlier and earlier until we reached a 6:00 p.m. bedtime with a 6:30 a.m. wake-up, and then naps at 9:00 a.m. and 1:00 p.m. This pattern still holds true minus the first nap, and bedtime is at 6:30 p.m. at almost 3 years old. He is social, happy, sweet, and most of all well rested.

With the birth of our second child, a girl, Lily, we were busy with Hayden, now a toddler, and were quite the experts on all the "signs" babies give out. We had a rule: If she was sleepy and not crying (even at a few days old), she was to be put in her bassinet. We still played with her and enjoyed her, but we were not walking around the house with her twenty-four hours a day. We also provided Lily with the same nighttime routine we give Hayden: dim the lights and give a massage, bath, bottle, book, and bed. This prompted Lily to develop a quicker sleep schedule, and we found by 2½ months she was sleeping through the late night feedings. By 3 months she was going to bed at 5:00 to 5:30 p.m. and sleeping until 6:30 a.m. Also at 3 months we began putting her down for her midmorning nap two hours after she woke up, and that began her nap schedule. Now Lily, almost one, wakes up at 6:30 a.m., takes her first nap at 8:15 a.m., takes her second nap at 12:30 p.m., and is in the bathtub by 5:00 p.m. and asleep by 5:30 p.m.

We are vigilant about not letting either child nap in the car, strollers, or for that matter miss naps or have delayed naps. Once our children are in their cribs for the night, we don't hear from them until the morning ... no night waking or games! We greet them each morning with a smile on their faces.

We are committed to having well-rested children and will defend our decisions with any naysayer suggesting we don't get to be with our children at night or we are too strict with the daytime schedule. We find too often it is the parent who is putting the child on their schedule instead of vice versa.

Babies yearn for routines and respond unbelievably to them. Again, we feel that we have two of the happiest, sweetest children, and knowing that teaching them good sleep habits and, more important, the ability to fall asleep unassisted is the best gift you can ever give!

Your goal is to synchronize your caretaking with your baby's needs: feed her when she's hungry, change her when she's wet, play with her when she's awake, and help her sleep when she's tired. Because of the irregularity with which these events occur, it's hard for first-time parents to "read" their baby's needs, but experienced parents should trust their instincts and put their baby to sleep when she appears tired.

If you have an extremely fussy/colicky baby, one who is more irritable, wakeful, harder to soothe, and harder to read, you may find that only method B will help this kind of baby sleep at nap time without crying. Later you will want to make a transition from method B to method A in the colicky baby so that learning self-soothing for naps will occur.

Here are some common nap mistakes:

Keeping the intervals of wakefulness too long
Using swings, cars, or strollers during naps too much with
　older children
Inconsistency in methods used to soothe your baby to sleep

Q: *Doesn't this mean I have to become a slave to my baby's nap schedule?*

A: Not at all. Simply respect his need to have good-quality naps. Try to distinguish between routine days and exceptional days. On routine days, try to partially organize your activities around the naps. On exceptional days, naps may be lost because of special events: for example, birthdays, holidays, and family vacations. Well-rested children tolerate not sleeping well if such episodes occur once or twice a month, but not if they are happening once or twice a week. A reset (see Chapter 4) might be needed after a special event.

If you are suffering from the inconvenience of hanging around your house on routine days when you think your baby will need to nap, perhaps it will help to keep in mind that between 12 and 16 weeks (or maybe somewhat later in colicky babies) your child will start taking fewer and longer naps, and longer periods of wakefulness between naps will develop during the day. There will be no late afternoon fussiness, and your baby will have longer periods of night sleep. So while it is socially *limiting* to plan ahead and protect naps, it is *liberating* to have a well-rested child who never fusses or cries during the day at home or in public. An early bedtime with consolidated night sleep is also liberating for parents, who can enjoy calm private time together early in the evening and overnight. Isn't all that worth a little temporary inconvenience?

Remember that healthy sleep depends on different but interrelated elements (see Chapter 1):

Sleep duration
Naps
Sleep consolidation
Sleep schedule, timing of sleep
Sleep regularity

When all the pieces are considered, healthy sleep will be accomplished. It won't happen overnight, but it will happen, and sooner than you think, if not as soon as you may desire.

MONTH 4: PREVENT POST-COLIC SLEEP PROBLEMS

A main goal at this age is to encourage the development of self-soothing skills for night sleep, the midmorning nap, and the midday nap.

If your baby has self-soothing skills and is sleeping well at night without bedtime or nighttime problems, and if naps are going well, consider skipping or skimming the following section and resume reading about naps on page 413.

How to prevent post-colic sleep problems? The discussion that immediately follows assumes that infant-driven influences are most important. Later I will give equal weight to the idea that mother-driven influences are most important. Finally, I will discuss how both infant- and mother-driven influences interact with each other. The reason I say "mother-driven" instead of "parent-driven" is because all research on this subject focuses on the mother, but obviously the role of the father, or lack thereof, may be equally or even more important in some families (see Chapter 3).

The Baby-Driven Path: The Role of the Baby

What is meant by infant-driven influences? Studies by Dr. C. Anderson Aldrich have shown that all babies have some uncategorizable crying: that is, they cry for no apparent reason. From studies by Dr. Ian St. James-Roberts, we know that no matter what the parenting style, bouts of inconsolable crying can occur. Also, Dr. T. Berry Brazelton showed that fussing/crying behavior increases around 6 weeks and then decreases. These facts (universality, occurrence independent of parenting style, and predictable time course) strongly suggest that there is a developmental component underlying the behavior called extreme fussiness/colic during the first few months of life. Later this developmental feature may be expressed at 4 months of age as a difficult temperament. After 4 months of age, the developmental issue might cause the child to have sleep problems that persist despite the parents' efforts. With this developmental framework in mind, let's consider what we know about temperament and how we might prevent post-colic sleep problems.

After extreme fussiness/colic winds down around 4 months of age or sooner, your child may be overtired, not sleeping well, and difficult to manage. The observation that brief and interrupted sleep often follows extreme fussiness/colic might suggest that some congenital, biological factors lead initially to extreme fussiness/colic, and that they are still present in the baby after the colicky period has passed. This is supported by the observation that despite successful drug therapy that eliminated or reduced colicky crying, brief sleep periods were still the norm at 4 months of age (see Chapter 5). In addition, some, but not all, post-colic infants continue to behave as if they had heightened activity levels and excessive sensitivity to environmental stimuli.

Night Waking, Sleep Duration, Sleep Problems

I studied 141 infants between *4 and 8 months* of age from middle-class families and showed that the history of extreme fussiness/colic was associated with the parents' judgment that night waking was a current problem. The frequency of awakening was a problem in 76 percent of infants, the duration of awakenings a problem in 8 percent, and both frequency and duration a problem in 16 percent. The more often a child woke up, the longer were the durations of the night wakings.

Other studies also reported more night waking at *8 and 12 months* and ages *14 to 18 months* in post-colic children compared to babies who did not have colic. Also, among those post-colic infants, the total sleep duration was less (13.5 versus 14.3 hours). So post-colic infants tend to have, for several months, brief sleep durations and more frequent or longer night awakenings (signaling). These group differences in night waking and sleep durations between previously not-colicky and post-colic babies *decrease* as children become older.

There are studies suggesting that both infant irritability and sleep deficits are moderately stable individual characteristics during the first year of life and beyond. One study showed that children with extreme fussiness/colic had more sleep problems and the families exhibited more distress than a control group at age 3 *years*. But the trend of decreasing group differences between colicky and non-colicky infants with age, at least on the measures of night waking and sleep as these were measured by parent diary reports or sleep lab recordings of colicky infants at 9 weeks of age, suggests that the biological differences diminish over time and/or parenting practices become more influential.

However, it may be difficult for parents of post-colic infants after 4 months of age to eliminate frequent night wakings and lengthen sleep durations. Because of parental fatigue, parents may unintentionally become inconsistent and irregular in their responses to their infant. As a reminder, one mother wrote:

Dealing with a fussy child almost around the clock, you have a recipe for frazzled and distressed parents. I can certainly understand why many parents struggle with a post-colic sleep plan, as it can be hard to be resolute when you are completely burned out.

I would like to emphasize that soothing a fussy or crying child is something both parents can do (see Chapter 3). Even if she is breast-feeding, it is not solely the mother's responsibility. Fathers can, and in my opinion should, help with their children. If a father can be at home to help the mother for a time after she arrives home from the hospital and again for a period when the baby is about 6 weeks old, then the mother will be able to adjust to the changes in her baby. One father called this "tag-team parenting" because whenever one parent became exhausted, the other one took over for car rides, walks, or trips in the stroller to let the other get some much-needed rest. Two exhausted parents don't make a good couple!

Treatments such as simethicone drops, probiotics, and chiropractic spinal manipulation have been proven to be completely ineffective (Chapter 5). Gastroesophageal reflux disease is the newest popular diagnosis in fussy and crying babies, but research has shown it to be a coincidental finding and not the cause of irritability in babies. Although many remedies have been suggested for extreme fussiness/colic, including catnip or herbal tea, papaya juice, peppermint drops, recordings of heartbeat or womb sounds, hot-water bottles, or trying new baby formulas, three main maneuvers have been found to calm fussiness and crying. The three maneuvers are:

1. *Rhythmic motions:* rocking chairs, swings, cribs with springs attached to the casters, cradles, carriages, and strollers; walking, "taking ceiling tours," using your baby as a weight for biceps curl exercises, and taking car rides. However, avoid water beds, which are dangerous because they may cause suffocation (see Chapter 3). Other dangerous colic "treatments" include certain herbal remedies, which have caused poisoning; beanbag pillows, which have caused suffocation; and trampoline-like devices suspended in the crib, which have caused strangulation. Tryptophan was once used to help babies sleep well, but we now know that this is dangerous; similarly, melatonin should not be given to babies.

2. *Sucking:* at breast, bottle, fist, wrist, thumb, or pacifier.

3. *Swaddling:* wrapping the child in blankets; snuggling, cuddling, and nestling. After the first few weeks, however, this maneuver is often less effective.

You should avoid trying gimmick after gimmick; it will only make you feel more frustrated or helpless as the crying continues.

You may also feel resentment or anger if your child, perhaps unlike your friend's child, doesn't seem to respond well to home remedies.

Feelings of anger toward your crying child are frightening—and normal. You can love your baby and hate her crying spells. All parents sometimes have contradictory feelings about their baby.

Take breaks when your baby is crying. This will enable you to better nurture your child; it's a smart strategy for baby care, not a selfish idea for parent care.

You may feel during the first few months that you are not influencing your extremely fussy/colicky child's behavior very much. And you are right, but consider this period to be a rehearsal. Your hugs, kisses, and loving-kindness are expressing the way you feel. Practice showering affection on your baby, even when he's crying. This loving attention is important for both of you.

However, unceasing attention showered on a fussing or crying baby, whether he is extremely fussy/colicky or just showing common fussiness during the first few months *can* have complications if you continue this strategy of intervention for the older, post-colic child at bedtime and nap times. Thus, after the extreme fussiness/colic passes, if the older child is never left alone at sleep times, he is deprived of the opportunity to develop self-soothing skills. These children never learn to fall asleep unassisted. The resultant sleep fragmentation or deprivation in the child, driven by intermittent positive parental reinforcement, leads to fatigue-driven fussiness long after the biological factors that caused the extreme fussiness/colic have been resolved.

It cannot be overemphasized that, as stated by Dr. A. H. Parmelee, "parents are never truly prepared for the degree to which the babies' sleep/wake patterns will dominate and completely disrupt their daily activities."

Temperament

When the extreme crying and fussiness of your baby's first few months have passed and your child seems more settled, what next? After about 4 months of age, most parents have learned to differentiate between their child's *need* for consolidated sleep and the child's *preference* for soothing, pleasurable company at night. Most parents can learn to appreciate that prolonged, uninterrupted sleep is a health habit they can influence; they can quickly learn to stop reinforcing night wakings and irregular nap schedules that rob kids of needed rest. A process of "social weaning" from the pleasure of a parent's company at nap times and bedtimes is under way. As one young mother said, "I see—I should now forget the company she [the baby] wants."

But parents of post-colic babies still have a few challenges to face. That's because babies who have had extreme fussiness/colic appear more likely than other babies to develop shorter sleep durations and more frequent night wakings between 4 and 8 months of age. My research also has shown that parents of post-colic babies are more likely to view frequent (instead of prolonged) night wakings as a problem.

Additionally, around 4 months of age, a difficult temperament might occur. The term "temperament" refers to the behavioral style or the manner in which the child interacts with the environment. It does not describe the motivation of an action. The reason it is important to understand temperament in detail is that the behavior of a post-colic and/or sleep-deprived child is predictably stressful to parents, and recognizing how these children appear allows parents to better understand their behavior and to institute healthier sleep habits. All parents naturally make their own assessment of their babies' temperaments, but there is a standardized system for evaluating infant temperament, and although it is not absolutely objective, it has proved over the years to be very useful.

Dr. Alexander Thomas and his wife, Dr. Stella Chess, both pioneers in child development, described temperament differences among babies. In a study based on both his own careful observations and parent interviews, Dr. Thomas noted interrelations among four temperament characteristics: *mood, intensity, adaptability,* and *approach/withdrawal.* Infants who were moody, intense, slow to adapt, and withdrawing in Dr. Thomas's study were also rated as *"irregular"* in all bodily functions. Thus, they were diagnosed as having "difficult" temperaments because they were difficult for parents to manage! We don't know why these particular traits cluster together, but we do know that infants with "easy" temperaments have opposite characteristics. In Dr. Thomas's study, four additional temperament characteristics were described: *persistence, activity, distractibility,* and *threshold.* Threshold means how sensitive or insensitive the child appears to be to noises or changes in lighting. These four temperament characteristics were not part of either the easy or difficult temperament clusters.

The researchers who developed this system did not have extreme fussiness/colic anywhere in their minds. There is not even a specific crying dimension in their system. But the mood rating does include the notion of fussiness and crying, and the mood rating is highly correlated with the traits of intensity, adaptability, and approach/withdrawal (these four traits are used to define a "difficult" temperament), so the construct "difficult temperament" would be expected to be linked to extreme fussiness crying. Yet no one connected temperament, as rated on this scale, with extreme fussiness/colic until much later. However, as you will see, the connection proved to be striking. Below are the nine infant-temperament characteristics described by Drs. Thomas and Chess.

1. *Activity (general motion, energy).* Does your baby squirm, bounce, or kick while lying awake in the crib? Does she move around when asleep? Does she kick or grab during diapering? Some infants always appear to be active, while others only appear active in specific circumstances, such as bathing. Activity

levels in infants have nothing to do with "hyperactivity" in older children

2. *Rhythmicity (regularity of bodily functions)*. Rhythmicity is a measure of how regular or predictable the infant appears. Is there a pattern in the time when he is hungry, how much he eats at each feeding, how often bowel movements occur, when he gets sleepy, when he awakens, when he appears most active, and when he gets fussy? Some babies are very regular at age 2 months, while others seem to be irregular throughout the first year. As infants grow older, they tend to become more regular in their habits.

3. *Approach/withdrawal (first reaction)*. Approach/withdrawal is a temperament characteristic that defines the infant's initial reaction to something new. What does he do when meeting another child or a babysitter? Does he object to new procedures? Some infants reach out in new circumstances—accept, appear curious, approach—others object, reject, turn away, appear shy, or withdraw.

4. *Adaptability (flexibility)*. Adaptability is measured by observing such activities as whether the infant accepts nail cutting without protest, accepts bathing without resistance, accepts changes in feeding schedule, accepts strangers within fifteen minutes, and accepts new foods. It is an attempt to measure the ease or difficulty with which a child can adjust to new circumstances or a change in routine.

5. *Intensity*. Intensity is the degree or amount of an infant's response, either pleasant or unpleasant. Think of it as the amount of emotional energy with which the child expresses her likes and dislikes. Intense infants react loudly, with much expression of likes and dislikes. During feeding they are vigor-

ous in accepting or resisting food. They react strongly to abrupt exposure to bright lights; they greet a new toy with enthusiastic positive or negative expressions; they display much feeling during bathing, diapering, or dressing; and they react strongly to strangers or familiar people. One mother described her extremely fussy/colicky baby's intense all-or-nothing reactions: "Her mood changes quickly; she gives no warning—she can go from loud and happy to screaming." Intensity is measured separately from mood. Infants who are not intense are described as "mild."

6. *Mood.* If intensity is the degree of response, mood is the direction. It is measured in the same situations described above. Negative mood is the presence of fussy/crying behavior or the absence of smiles, laughs, or coos. Positive mood is the absence of fussy/crying behavior or the presence of smiles, laughs, or coos. Most intense infants also tend to be more negative in mood, less adaptable, withdrawn (difficult temperament). Most mild infants also tend to be more positive in mood, more adaptable, and approaching (easy temperament).

7. *Persistence.* Persistence level, or attention span, is a measure of how long the infant engages in activity. Parents may value this trait under some circumstances but not under others. For instance, persistence is desirable when the child is trying to learn something new, like reaching for a rattle, but it is undesirable when the infant persists in throwing food on the floor. Unfortunately, some babies persist in their prolonged crying spells and their prolonged wakeful periods. One father described his persistently crying baby as follows: "We have a copper-top, alkaline-battery-powered baby, and we're powered by regular carbon batteries. He outlasts us every time."

8. *Distractibility.* Distractibility describes how easily the baby may be distracted by external events. Picking up the infant

easily consoles a distractible infant's fatigue or hunger; soothing can stop fussing during a diaper change. New toys or unusual noises easily distract the infant. Distractibility and
persistence are not related to each other, and neither trait is
related to activity or threshold levels.

9. *Threshold (sensitivity)*. Threshold levels measure how much
stimulus is required to produce a response in the infant in specific circumstances, such as loud noises, bright lights, and
other situations previously discussed. While some infants are
very reactive or responsive to external or environmental
changes, other infants barely react.

Difficult Temperament

As previously mentioned, while observing many children and analyzing many questionnaires, Drs. Thomas and Chess noticed that
four, and only four, of these temperamental traits tended to cluster
together: *intensity, adaptability, mood,* and *approach/withdrawal*.
In particular, infants who were extreme or "intense" in their reactions also tended to be slowly adaptable, negative in mood, and
withdrawn. This appeared to be a personality type.

According to their parents' descriptions and direct observation
by the researchers, these infants seemed more difficult to manage
than other infants. Consequently, a child whose temperament scores
fall into this pattern is said to have a difficult temperament. One
mother referred to her infant jokingly as a "mother-killer." Infants
with the opposite temperamental traits are said to have easy temperaments. These are sometimes called "dream" babies. One father
described his "easy" infant as a "low-maintenance baby." The difficult temperament and the easy temperament are only descriptions
of a behavioral style. Temperament research usually does not ask
why a child behaves in a particular way. There is no scientific basis
for labeling a child with a difficult temperament as a "high-needs"
child. In fact, there is no scientific support for labeling a child a

"high-needs" child under any circumstances. Many so-called high-needs children are really very overtired children or children with a difficult temperament.

Of the original group of infants Thomas and Chess studied, about 10 percent fell into the difficult-temperament category. These infants also tended to be irregular in biological function such as sleep schedules and night awakenings. They were more likely to have behavioral problems—particularly sleep disturbances—when they grew older. One of the most interesting differences between difficult and easy babies is the way they cry when they are past the extreme fussiness period—that is, when they are 3 or 4 months old. Published research found that mothers listening to the taped cries of infants rated difficult (but who were not their own babies) described the crying as more irritable, grating, and arousing than the crying of easy infants. They said that the difficult-temperament group sounded spoiled and were crying because of frustration rather than hunger or wet diapers. An audio analysis of cries helped explain why this should be. The crying of the difficult-temperament infants was found to have more silent pauses between crying sounds than that of the easy babies. These silent pauses caused the listener to repeatedly think that the crying spell had ended. Also, at its most intense, the crying of difficult-temperament infants was actually pitched at a higher frequency. These two differences can make the crying seem much more frightening, piercing, and annoying.

What causes the difficult temperaments? Temperament is usually thought to be an expression of your nature. As we will see, nurture may also play a role.

Here's how child development specialist Laya Frischer described a post-colic baby:

> Jane is difficult and unpredictable, with less than average sleep and cuddling and more than average crying. Observations over five weeks have revealed an extremely sensitive infant. For a period of time, she could not even

tolerate touches on her abdomen. Swaddling helps a little, and the rhythmic swing movement gives her some relief. If these things fail, the parents walk her around. Sometimes these efforts quiet her fussiness, but at other times it escalates to panic crying. Jane seems to have no capacity to console herself, and very little capacity to be consoled by usual methods of touch. The pacifier has been helpful, but not always successful. Jane does not have good state regulation. *She can be in a panic cry state when she seems to be asleep.*

Jane goes from sleep to distress in seconds. She becomes overtired and cannot sleep, which contributes to her irritability. She does not habituate easily to sensory stimulation of light and touch. Jane requires a very protective environment, which puts great stress on her parents, particularly her mother. Her cries are very hard to read; her parents feel she is unpredictable, and often uncommunicative.

Here is another example of sensitivity to environmental stimuli from my own experience. When my first son had colic, I had to keep the crib railing up and locked in place, because the clunk of the spring lock would always awaken him. That made it awkward for me to place him in his crib, but fortunately I was limber from college gymnastics. For my wife, it was an impossible situation until we got a sturdy stool for her to stand on—but it still hurt our backs!

Interestingly, two temperament characteristics (high activity and high sensitivity) are not part of the diagnostic criteria for babies who fall into the difficult-temperament category. But some post-colic infants are exquisitely sensitive to irregularities in their nap or night-sleep schedule. Disruptions of regular routines due to painful ear infections or holidays and trips subsequently caused extreme resistance to falling asleep and frequent night waking, lasting up to several days after the disruptive event. These prolonged recovery periods might reflect easily disorganized internal biological rhythms caused by enduring congenital imbalances in arousal/inhibition or sleep/wake control mechanisms. Alternatively, parents who put their baby to sleep slightly too late, or who often cause their children to skip naps after 4 months of age, keep their post-colic infant close to the edge of overtiredness. What happens when some natural disruptive event occurs is that the child falls into the abyss of severe agitated wakefulness and irritability and is unable to easily get back into a regular sleep pattern.

Some post-colic kids are extremely active; they appear to have boundless energy. "She crawls like lightning" was how one mother described her baby. These babies are constantly on the move. They would rather crawl up Mom's chest to perch on her shoulder than sit quietly in her lap. But once having reached the shoulder, they immediately want to get down and check out that dust ball or some equally exciting object off in the corner. They appear easily bored; they also seem very stimulus-sensitive, especially to mechanical noises such as those of a vacuum cleaner, hair dryer, or coffee grinder (which may have seemed to calm them down during colicky spells when they were younger). It's as if they have a heightened level of arousal, activity, and curiosity. When overtired, they are always crabby and socially demanding, needing Mommy's presence and wanting to be held all the time. They also are quick to fuss when Mom leaves the room for only a minute. But when they are well rested, it's a different story. They may remain very active but less frantic, and this suggests that whatever biologic process may be contributing to high activity behavior, lack of sleep is also part of the picture. When they've had enough sleep, these same babies appear to have boundless curiosity, actively seeking opportunities to learn.

Some pediatricians, in their attempt to shorten the discussion of colic in the office, simply tell parents not to worry, because nobody dies of colic; it will pass, and anyway, colicky babies turn out to be smarter kids. They suggest that these post-colic babies who are so alert, curious, and bright that they have difficulty controlling their impulses to explore or investigate the world are unusually intelligent. No data support the conclusion that post-colic kids in general are more intelligent, but there may be a small number who are so exceptionally bright that they gave birth to this myth. One study of infants published in 1964 connected increased crying (induced by snapping a rubber band on the sole of the foot at age 4 to 10 days) to increased intelligence at 3 years of age. Whether this artificially induced crying and its link with intelligence can be generalized to colicky crying is an open question.

Association Between Temperament and Sleep

Continuous recordings of sleep patterns during the *second day of life* were linked with temperament assessments at *8 months:* it was observed that infants with the most extreme values on all sleep variables were more likely to have difficult temperaments. Observations on such young babies tend to support a developmental or biologic basis for this association as opposed to parenting.

In my study of sixty 4- to 5-month-old infants, the infants rated as difficult had average sleep times substantially less than the infants rated as easy (12.3 versus 15.6 hours). Although nine infant-temperament characteristics were measured, only five are used to establish the diagnosis of a difficult temperament. And four of these (mood, adaptability, rhythmicity, and approach/withdrawal) were individually highly associated with total sleep duration.

When this study was extended to include 105 infants, those infants with difficult temperaments slept 12.8 hours and those with easy temperaments slept 14.9 hours. This observation was subsequently confirmed in a Chinese American group with different parenting practices. It thus appears that infants who have a difficult temperament have briefer total sleep durations when assessed at *4 to 5 months* of age regardless of differences in parenting practices. While this might suggest a developmental link between sleep duration and temperament, it is also possible that despite differences in parenting practices, the difficult temperament at 4 to 5 months simply represents an overtired infant whose parents were unable to establish healthy sleep.

Support for an association between sleep and temperament is also based on a study by Dr. Marcia Keener in which objective measures of sleep/wake organization, derived from time-lapse video recordings, were compared with parental perceptions of infant temperament at 6 *months* of age. Dr. Keener stated that "infants considered [temperamentally] easy have longer sleep periods and spend less time out of the crib for caretaking interventions during the night." Her analysis also led her to the conclusion that night waking is caused by environmental (parental) rather that biological factors. This observation of increased time out of the crib for temperamentally more difficult children at 6 months is similar to the observation that increased night waking occurs in formerly extremely fussy/colicky infants at 4, 8, and 12 months, and it is also similar to the observation that mothers with depressive symptoms unnecessarily attend to their babies by removing them from the crib more often than mothers without these symptoms.

Utilizing a computerized movement detector, it was observed that for *12-month-old* children, those with the temperament trait of increased rhythmicity went to sleep earlier and had longer sleep durations, and by *18 months* of age there was again the observation that both subjective and objective improved sleep measures were associated with easier temperament assessments.

At several ages during the first year of life, using sleep diaries and objective measurements, more recent research by Dr. Karen Spruyt also confirmed that increased sleep is correlated with an easy temperament.

Association Between Temperament and Extreme Fussiness/Colic

When parents performed a temperament assessment when their child was 2 *weeks* of age and kept a twenty-four-hour behavior diary at 6 *weeks* of age, it was observed that more difficult temperaments at 2 weeks predicted more crying and fussing at 6 weeks. At 4 *weeks* of age, infants who were temperamentally more difficult in general, and more intense and less distractible (less consolable) in particular, cried more during their second month of life than other infants.

Another prospective study performed temperament assessments at the ages of 3 and 12 *months*. At 3 *months,* the extremely fussy/ colicky infants were more intense, more persistent, less distractible, and more negative in their mood. However, at 12 *months,* ratings on the temperament questionnaire showed no group differences between the formerly extremely fussy/colicky infants and the control group, but the general impression of the mothers of the colicky group was that they were more difficult.

Infants who had extreme fussiness/colic, using Dr. Wessel's exact criteria, are more likely to have a difficult temperament than noncolicky babies when the temperament assessment is performed at 4 *or 5 months* of age. Furthermore, this progression occurs even when extreme fussiness/colic is successfully treated with the no longer used drug dicyclomine hydrochloride. Similar results were observed in another study: while behavioral management significantly reduced evening fussing and crying, successful treatment had no effects on later temperament ratings—the infants were still described as difficult. This suggests the possibility that some developmental feature causing extreme fussiness/colic before 4 months was suppressed by the drug, but when the drug was stopped at 4 months, this developmental feature, no longer suppressed, expressed itself as short sleep durations, night wakings, and a difficult temperament.

The Mother-Driven Path: The Role of the Mother

What is meant by "mother-driven influences"? Dr. Aldrich showed that all babies have some uncategorizable crying, or crying for no apparent reason. But in my study, I found that babies that fulfilled Wessel's exact criteria for colic did so because of lots of fussing *but not crying.* These mothers were my patients from the time they gave birth, and at each office visit I gave them information regarding fussing/crying, soothing, and sleeping. This strongly suggests that there is a mother-related component underlying the behavior called extreme fussiness/colic, because when mothers were armed with more information on how to soothe their babies, there was less crying.

Situations in which the mother might find parenting more challenging and thus be associated with extreme fussiness/colic in her baby include young single mothers with anxiety issues, older mothers of twins, mothers with baby blues or postpartum depression, and mothers who used assisted reproductive technology. These challenges might impair the mother's ability to calm a fussy baby and prevent crying. Later, when the baby is 4 months of age, the mother's influence may be expressed in an overtired infant who is difficult to manage. After 4 months, this child might have sleep problems that persist because of a failure to learn self-soothing or a continuation of parent issues that interfere with healthy sleep (see Chapter 3). With this mother-driven framework in mind, let's consider what we know about night waking and temperament and how we might prevent post-colic sleep problems.

Night Waking

Previously, the infant-driven pathway emphasized developmental changes with the baby. An alternative view is that instead of or in addition to biologic factors, parenting practices, such as unnecessary feedings at night, contribute to sleep fragmentation during the first few months (see Chapter 3). And these parenting practices may continue to cause fragmented night sleep even after the biologic factors subside around 3 to 4 months of age.

We know that different parenting styles influence crying and soothing, and we know, too, that differences in mothers' confidence in their role as a parent and differences in discipline style influence when and how babies learn self-soothing. Also suggestive of the important role of the mother is the fact that in industrial societies attachment-parenting practices reduce fussing and crying in some babies during the first few months, but later these same babies are more likely to be unable to sleep well during the night—possibly because they did not learn self-soothing skills (see Chapter 5).

Parents may become overindulgent and oversolicitous regarding night wakings and not appreciate that they are inadvertently depriving their child of the opportunity to learn how to fall asleep unassisted. Some mothers have difficulty separating from their child, especially at night, while other mothers have a tendency toward depression, which might be aggravated by the fatigue that results from struggling to cope with a colicky infant. In either case, simplistic suggestions to help the child sleep better often fail to motivate a change in parental behavior. If a child fails to learn to fall asleep unassisted, the result is sleep fragmentation or sleep deprivation driven by intermittent positive parental reinforcement. This causes fatigue-driven fussiness long after the colic has resolved, which ultimately creates an overtired family.

Support for this view comes from research on infants at 5 *months* of age who were followed to 56 *months* of age. Dr. Dieter Wolke showed that crying alone was not the problem, writing, "Long crying duration and having felt distressed about crying during the first five months were significant predictors of night waking problems at twenty months" but not at 56 months. In other words, the combined factors of long infant crying or fussing plus parental distress at 5 months of age make it more likely that a night-waking problem will develop. Even more significantly, crying with sleep problems at

5 months, rather than crying alone, predicts sleep problems when older. Sleep problems at 5 months remain the best predictor of sleep problems, especially night waking, at 20 months. Dr. Wolke concluded that post-colic "sleep problems are likely to be due to a failure of the parents to establish and maintain regular sleep schedules. . . . This conclusion does not blame parents for sleep difficulties. Rather, it recognizes why many parents adopt strategies to deal with night waking in the least conflictual manner by night feeding or cosleeping. This may be especially true of parents who are dealing with a temperamentally more difficult infant." Thus long crying in and of itself at 5 months is less predictive of a future night-waking problem than the association of long crying plus parental distress or long crying plus sleep problems.

Although the night waking disappeared between 20 and 56 months in this study, children continued to not sleep well, with unhealthy consequences. In another study, Dr. Wolke examined sixty-four children, ages 8 to 10 years, who as infants had "persistent crying," defined as fussing or crying more than three hours for three days or more each week. The author concluded that they were at risk for hyperactivity problems and academic difficulties. In addition, at 8 to 10 years of age, the previous persistent criers took a longer time to fall asleep, suggesting that "they were less effective in controlling their own behavioral state to fall asleep."

Therefore, it appears that the increased crying/fussing behavior in infancy is associated with less infant sleep and more signaling at night (fragmented sleep), but the crying/fussing alone does not directly cause later sleep problems. Although the post-colic child's family may be stressed, it appears that it is the failure to establish age-appropriate sleep hygiene that specifically leads to later disrupted sleep and behavioral problems.

Here is a story of a child who probably had extreme fussiness/colic, even though the parents wanted to call him sleep deprived. Remember, these labels might be interchangeable and are far less important than your child's behavior. There was no quick sleep solution, but improvement did come slowly. Patience is always re-warded if you are reasonably consistent.

When Jackson was 4 months old, he had never been on any kind of sleep schedule. He seemed to cry all the time and would only sleep about four hours at a time (if we were lucky!). My husband and I would spend hours on end, hold-ing, rocking, bouncing, singing, playing, and doing anything we could think to do to get him to stop crying. Our pediatri-cian said that he had colic and there was nothing we could do about it but to wait it out. Looking back on it all now, I am convinced that he didn't have colic at all, but was just plain sleep deprived. At first we were hesitant to allow Jackson to cry without holding him. Given that we are both psycholo-gists, we were scared that leaving him alone to cry would be emotionally scarring and would affect his attachment and self-esteem. But we were both sleep deprived ourselves, stressed out, and desperate to try anything. Dr. Weissbluth's belief that to not allow him to learn to soothe himself to sleep was damaging in and of itself was what allowed us to finally take the plunge. The first time I put him to sleep in his crib for a nap, I left the room and he screamed bloody mur-der. I sat at the top of the stairs and just cried and cried. I was convinced I was the worst mother in the world. After twenty minutes (which felt like an eternity), he finally fell asleep and slept for two hours. Unfortunately, later naps did not prove to be so easy. There were times in which he screamed for the whole hour (and I cried for the whole hour) and we would get him and try again later. Jackson was a bit resistant to the whole idea, and even though we were very consistent, he always put up a good fight. Even now, at 9 months old, Jackson will still cry before most naps and bedtime. Sometimes it's thirty seconds, sometimes it's thirty minutes. He sleeps so much better and longer than he ever did. We calculated that before he was averaging ten hours of sleep per day, and after just a few weeks he was sleeping around seventeen hours a day. The best part of all was that he learned how to sleep through the night. Now he goes to bed most nights between 6:00 and 7:00 p.m., and he wakes up usually between 6:00 and 7:00 a.m. He takes two naps per day, one around 9:00 a.m. and the other in the early afternoon. My husband and I finally got the sleep we needed, and the stress level went down dramatically. We have our evenings together back, which we desperately needed. And Jackson's temperament is dramatically improved. I would still say he is a highly active baby, but would no longer say he is fussy. Before, I was certain we would never have another child because it was just too much on us emotionally. But now we are planning to conceive again within the next year.

When you become your child's timekeeper and program her sleep schedules, she will be able to sleep day and night on a regular schedule. For most parents, this is a relatively easy adjustment to make. But for post-colic infants, expect to put forth a greater effort to get them to be regular and consistent. Your effort to keep the child well rested will be rewarded by a calmer, happier, easier temperament child. Improvement in temperament with better sleep, as mentioned in the story above, is discussed a little later in this chapter. One family that was finally able to permanently "de-crab" their baby with better sleep explained, "The 'other' baby is back!"

Without your effort to maintain sleep schedules, your child will have a tendency to sleep irregularly and become unmanageably wild, screaming out of control with the slightest frustration and spending most of the day engaged in crazy, demanding, and impatient behaviors. The majority of post-colic infants do not fit this extreme picture, but they do require more parental control to establish healthy sleep schedules, compared to non-colicky infants. Thus it appears that after about 3 to 4 months of age, poor sleep habits are learned, not developmentally driven.

For all post-colic infants over 4 months of age, my clinical observations are that frequent night wakings may be eliminated and sleep durations lengthened if, and only if, parents establish and maintain healthy sleep schedules for their child.

From the perspective of a mother-driven path, it appears that most post-colic sleep problems are not caused primarily by a biological disturbance of sleep/wake regulation; rather, the problem is the parents' failure to allow their baby to learn self-soothing between 2 and 4 months or to establish regular sleep patterns when the colic dissipates. Both obvious and subtle reasons can be cited as to why parents have difficulty in enforcing sleep schedules when colic ends.

Two or more months of crying sometimes adversely and permanently shapes parenting styles. An inconsolable infant triggers in some parents a perception that their baby's behavior is out of their control. They observe no obvious benefit to their young extremely fussy/colicky child when they try to be regular according to clock times or to be consistent in bedtime routines. Naturally, but falsely, they then assume that this handling will not help their post-colic child, either. Unfortunately, they do not observe the transition, at around 2 to 4 months, from colicky crying to fatigue-driven crying.

Alternatively, some parents may unintentionally and permanently become inconsistent and irregular in their responses to their infant simply because of their own fatigue. The constant, complex, and prolonged efforts they use to soothe or calm their extremely fussy/colicky baby are continued. But these ultimately lead to an overindulgent, oversolicitous approach to sleep scheduling when the colic has passed. Their nurturing at night, for example, becomes stimulating overattentiveness. In responding to their child's every cry, the parents inadvertently deprive her of the opportunity to learn how to fall asleep unassisted. The child then fails to learn the important skill of self-soothing, which she will need her entire life.

Effective behavioral therapy to establish healthy post-colic sleep patterns by teaching the child how to fall asleep and stay asleep may or may not be acceptable to you, depending on your ability to perceive and respond to the sleep needs of your infant (see Chapter 3).

Some parents, usually mothers, have extreme difficulty separating from their child, especially at night, as was discussed in Chapter 3. They may have some difficulty themselves being alone at night because their husband's work requires frequent or prolonged absences, or because nights have always been lonely times for them as a result of anxiety. They perceive every cry as a need for nurturing. These women are wonderful mothers, but they may be too good. The infant's every need is anticipated and met before it is experienced; in doing so, the mother unintentionally thwarts the development of her child's capacity to be alone. For example, she may block her infant's attempts to provide herself with a substitute (such as thumb sucking or use of a pacifier) for her physical presence.

These parents perpetuate brief and fragmented sleep patterns in their children. Their infants become, according to Dr. Thomas Ogden, a child psychiatrist, "addicted to the actual physical presence of the mother and [can]not sleep unless they are being held. These infants are unable to provide themselves an internal environment for sleep." Although the *child* has disturbed sleep, here the focus of the problem and the key to its solution lies with the *parent*.

WARNING
Persistent sleep problems in children have been linked to
hyperactivity in children, psychiatric symptoms in adolescents,
and depression in their mothers.

Extreme fussiness/colic is the most obvious example of extreme crying, but please remember that any painfully overtired infant or child might cry. In some nonindustrial societies and among parents practicing proximal care (attachment parenting), babies rarely cry, because they are always held close to the mother in a soft carrier, highlighting the role of the mother. However, even where there is constant holding and unrestricted breast-feeding throughout the day and night, babies still cry and fuss, which supports the notion of a baby-driven path. Here, too, the crying and fussing peak at about 6 weeks of age! Of course, the babies in nonindustrial cultures are less likely to have any tendency toward fussiness caused by overtiredness. These mothers do not drive cars, wear watches, text, check email, or keep many daily appointments to which they must drag their infants. Also, there is less environmental stimulation during the day, so the baby might sleep well outdoors when the mother is planting rice or cooking. Our lifestyles are different, and may cause our children to become overtired more often.

Temperament

Early temperament research suggested to me that biological factors primarily or exclusively caused increased fuss/cry behavior during the first 3 to 4 months of age and subsequently led to difficult-temperament assessments. I recognized that colic-induced parental distress or fatigue occurred, but I thought that parenting behavior was a much less important factor. Now I have a slightly different view that includes parenting practices both in reaction to the baby and independently contributing to the baby's behavior. The mother's mental health may be a cause of, a reaction to, or both a cause of and a reaction to infant fussing/crying and sleeping issues. For example, Dr. Jordana Bayer found that mothers reporting infant sleep problems in their 4-month-olds "had poorer mental and physical health compared with those not reporting sleep problems. . . . [Those infants with sleep problems] were more likely to be 'exclusively breast fed and perceived by their mothers as temperamentally difficult.'" This topic and the contributing role of the father are also discussed in Chapters 4 and 5.

To further confuse the contributions of nature and nurture, some researchers have suggested there is no connection between extreme fussiness/colic and a difficult temperament. According to Wessel, irritability, fussiness, or crying lasting more than three hours a day and occurring more than three days in a week occurs in 49 percent of babies. As described in Chapter 6, these arbitrary criteria of more than three hours a day and more than three days in a week are sometimes used to describe Wessel's "modified" criteria for colic. Using these modified criteria, researchers have concluded that colic is not an early manifestation of a difficult temperament. However, Dr. Wessel defined colic as having the additional characteristic of lasting more than three weeks, and this led to the conclusion that about 26 percent of babies had colic. Looking at this smaller and more severely affected group, an opposite conclusion might be drawn: there is a strong association between extreme fussiness/colic before 4 months of age and difficult temperament at 4 months of age. So much depends on how researchers define colic.

But even when Wessel's strict criteria are used, the reason that extreme fussiness/colic should be viewed perhaps as a risk factor but not as an inevitable path to a difficult temperament is that at 4 months of age about 40 percent of children with a difficult temperament did not have extreme fussiness/colic and about 73 percent of infants with excessive fussiness/colic do not develop a difficult temperament. So while there are developmental features contributing to fussing/crying behavior during the first 4 months and temperament at 4 months, these developmental features are not destiny. Parenting matters!

Also, the good news for parents is that extreme fussiness/colic does not appear to be an expression of a *permanently* difficult temperament. In one study of extremely fussy/colicky infants, subsequent measurements of temperament at 5 and 10 months did not show group differences between formerly extremely fussy/colicky and common fussy/crying infants. So by practicing healthy sleep habits when extreme fussiness winds down, you may increase the chances that your baby's temperament might dramatically improve. I will discuss how sleep modulates temperament below.

Interaction Between Baby and Mother

Dr. Douglas Teti wrote, "There is general agreement that infant sleep patterns are complexly determined, and coregulated, with ongoing contributions from both infant and parent. . . . It is very likely that both mother- and infant-driven influences are at play in terms of linkages between maternal depressive symptoms and infant night waking."

Night Waking

Extreme fussiness/colic certainly does not necessarily cause the parents to have difficulty separating from their child. But it is more than a sufficient stimulus to cause some parents to regress toward the least adaptive level of adjustment: they respond and interact too often with their child at night. The result is severe, enduring sleep disturbance in the child. In this setting, simplistic suggestions to help the child sleep better often fail to motivate a change in how the parents approach the problem. Thus, while it is the wakeful child who may be brought for professional help, it may be the parent who has the unappreciated problem.

Temperament

Temperament assessments, performed at an average age of 3.6 months, showed an association between problems of sleep/wake organization, difficult temperament, and extreme crying. Mothers of crying infants scored high on depression, anxiety, exhaustion, anger, adverse childhood memories, and marital distress (see Chapters 3 and 4). The authors concluded that factors related to parental care, while not *causing* persistent crying, did function to *maintain or worsen* the behavior. The persistence of parental factors may explain why at 1 year there is reported to be more difficulty in communication, more unresolved conflicts, more dissatisfaction, and greater lack of empathy in families with an extremely fussy/colicky infant, and after 4 years formerly extremely fussy/colicky children have been reported to be more negative in mood on temperament assessments.

The exact same sixty infants that I examined at 4 to 6 months of age were restudied at 3 years. Again, temperamentally easy children had longer sleep durations compared to children with more difficult temperaments. However, there was *no individual stability of temperament traits (except for adaptability) and no individual stability of sleep durations between the ages of 5 months and 3 years.* Thus, except for adaptability, temperament ratings and associated sleep patterns at age 5 months do not predict temperament or sleep patterns at 3 years. Infants who were ranked as having brief sleep periods and difficult temperaments at 5 months and who were ranked as sleeping longer at 3 years had easier temperaments. But for 5-month-olds with brief sleep durations and difficult temperaments who also had brief sleep durations at age 3 years, the difficult temperament persisted. Similarly, individual infants who were ranked as having long sleep periods and easy temperaments at 5 months and who later, at 3 years, were ranked as sleeping for shorter durations had more difficult temperaments. But for those 5-month-olds with long sleep durations and easy temperaments who also had long sleep durations at age 3 years, the easy temperament persisted. Sleep modulates temperament!

Dr. John Bates agrees with my hypothesis that sleep modulates temperament and told me that "parenting responses to [sleep] issues would be involved in the continuity/discontinuity of temperament. . . . If parents make the effort to manage their kids' sleep schedules consistently, I would think that over the years they are going to see less difficult and unmanageable behavior."

It appears that both nature and nurture contribute to sleep, temperament, and fussing/crying. I believe that how babies sleep does influence the development of temperament *at 5 months* of age. And how babies sleep during the first few months is a combination of factors within the child and the parents' ability and skill at soothing. I also believe that *at 5 months* of age, the difficult temperament represents an overtired baby and the easy temperament represents a well-rested baby. However, temperament at 5 months of age is not like a fingerprint; it is *not* a permanent marker of your baby's personality.

Over time, temperament changes as babies develop and parents change how they soothe their children. Individual temperament measures become more stable during the second year of life or shortly after the second birthday. If you are reading this book before you have had your baby, be prepared to invest enormous efforts in soothing and consider yourself unlucky if your child is among the 20 percent of extremely fussy/colicky babies. However, if you have already had your baby and you are in the midst of suffering through 4 months of extreme fussiness/colic, reevaluate some of your decisions, if necessary, regarding how you soothe your baby and what is best for your baby and family. Be optimistic, because everything settles down at about 4 months. Everyone gets a second chance at about 4 months to help their child sleep better.

DIFFERENT DECISIONS FOR DIFFERENT BABIES

Research—both my own and others'—has shown that about 80 percent of babies develop common fussiness/crying and 20 percent develop extreme fussiness/colic. What happens to these babies over the first 4 months? At 4 months of age, some children are supercalm, regular, smiling all the time, and good sleepers, while other babies are the opposite. The good sleepers are described as having an "easy" temperament; the opposite have a "difficult" temperament. Some children are more in-between and are described as having an "intermediate" temperament. Remember that the measurements of sleeping, crying/fussing, and temperament are graded or continuous, like your weight in pounds on a scale, and not discrete measurements, like positive or negative results on a pregnancy test. Also, the definitions of common fussiness/crying (or extreme fussiness/colic) and easy temperament (or difficult temperament) are arbitrary. So labels are far less important than your baby's actual behavior. The main message is to watch your baby and pay attention to your own behavior, because how you care for your baby influences your baby's sleeping, crying/fussing, and temperament.

For now, I wish to lead you through a numerical exercise involving a hypothetical group of *one hundred babies*. Skip or skim this numerical exercise if you already have strongly held convictions or if you find it not useful for you. The reason this exercise might be useful is because it might:

1. Help you set your expectations on what you will need to do with your baby, both during the first several weeks in terms of soothing and over the following several months to prevent sleep problems.

2. Help you decide whether you will breast-feed or bottle-feed.

3. Help you decide whether you will use a family bed, sleep with your baby (see SIDS warning, Chapter 1), use a co-sleeper, or use a crib.

Out of a group of one hundred babies, during the first 3 to 4 months, 80 percent (eighty babies) will have common fussiness/crying and 20 percent (twenty babies) will have extreme fussiness/colic. My research has shown that these two groups of babies differ in how their temperaments develop.

Consider the *eighty* common fussy/crying babies at 5 months of age:

A. 49 percent, or *thirty-nine* babies, are temperamentally easy.

B. 46 percent, or *thirty-seven* babies, are temperamentally intermediate.

C. 5 percent, or *four* babies, are temperamentally difficult.

Consider the *twenty* extremely fussy/colicky babies at 5 months
of age:

D. 14 percent, or *three* babies, are temperamentally easy.

E. 59 percent, or *twelve* babies, are temperamentally intermediate.

F. 27 percent, or *five* babies, are temperamentally difficult.

Another way to look at this is to note that out of our original
hundred babies, at 5 months of age:

Among all 42 temperamentally easy babies, 39, or 93 percent,
had common fussiness/crying.

Among all 49 temperamentally intermediate babies, 37, or
76 percent, had common fussiness/crying.

Among all 9 temperamentally difficult babies, 4, or 44 percent, had common fussiness/crying.

A point of view that emphasizes a developmental perspective
might argue that a baby with extreme fussiness/colic is five times
more likely to develop a difficult temperament than a baby with
common fussiness/crying (27 percent versus 5 percent). But obviously, the status of fussing/crying during the first few months is not
destiny, because 73 percent of babies with extreme fussiness/colic
do *not* develop a difficult temperament, and the role of the parent in
modulating temperament is discussed above. It is informative to understand that at 5 months of age, most babies are neither easy nor
difficult but somewhere in between.

Of the original hundred babies, the largest temperament group at age 5 months is "intermediate." Forty-nine babies (49 percent) are in this temperament category. Because temperament measurements form a gradation, and the temperament categories represent arbitrary cutoff points, it is possible that the thirty-seven babies in group B, who had common fussiness, tend toward being temperamentally easier than the twelve babies in group E, who had extreme fussiness/colic. I suspect that the parents of the twelve babies in group E had to put forth much more soothing effort into this intermediate temperament group than the parents of the thirty-seven babies in group B. So the biggest temperament group at 5 months of age is in between easy and difficult temperament. It is a mixed group, and within this group some babies may tend to be easier or more difficult but not extremely so in either direction. Enjoy your baby and try not to compare your baby with other babies who may have different temperaments.

Of the original hundred babies, the next largest temperament group at 5 months is "easy." Forty-two babies (42 percent) are in this temperament category. Of these, thirty-nine babies in group A were born mellow, self-soothing, and calm, and/or their parents were unusually skillful in soothing and/or had vast resources to help them soothe their babies. This was not the case with the three babies in group D. These babies had extreme fussiness/colic at birth. They were not born mellow, self-soothing, or calm. I think these lucky three babies had superhero parents who put forth enormous effort to soothe and probably also had lots of other resources to help them maintain this effort over a period of several months. For these families, it should be smooth sailing ahead regarding sleeping.

The smallest temperament group at 5 months is "difficult." Only nine babies of the original hundred are in this temperament category. The four babies in group C had common fussiness/crying, but they may have been almost, but not quite, extremely fussy/colicky. Alternatively, for these four common fussy babies, maybe something went wrong with the parents' ability to soothe or teach self-soothing. Why might parents be unable to effectively soothe their baby? As we have seen, reasons may include maternal depression, an unsupportive husband, too many other children to care for, illness, financial problems, stress from an extended family, and marital problems between husband and wife (see Chapter 3). The five babies in group F may have overwhelmed all the resources that the parents could bring to bear on soothing their baby. This implies that factors within the baby were so powerful that no matter what the parents did, the baby's extreme fussiness/colic led to a difficult temperament at 5 months of age. It is also possible that the difficult temperament evolved because a combination of factors within the baby and problems within the parents or family conspired to create an overtired child. Preexisting problems such as marital discord, stress from an unsupportive husband/father/boyfriend, or maternal anxiety or depression only get worse when parents are trying to cope with an extremely fussy/colicky baby. Parents' inability to soothe may grow out of, or be a response to, the fatigue, frustration, and exhaustion of trying, without much success, to soothe an extremely fussy/colicky baby. For these few families, it might be rough or very stormy seas ahead regarding sleeping.

As previously stated, the largest temperament group *at 5 months,* comprising 49 percent of the total, is the intermediate temperament group. Some of these babies will closely but not quite resemble easy-temperament babies or difficult-temperament babies. Therefore, for almost half of all babies, advice regarding common fussiness/crying and extreme fussiness/colic (and their respective links to easy and difficult temperaments, and a correspondingly low and high risk of sleep problems) fits only approximately. So please read the entire following section and take out of it only that which applies to your baby.

The risk of developing sleep problems *after 4 months* of age probably looks something like this:

RISKS FOR SLEEP PROBLEMS AFTER 4 MONTHS

LOW RISK (42%)

39 percent of common fussy/crying babies who develop easy temperaments

3 percent of extremely fussy/colicky babies who develop easy temperaments

MEDIUM RISK (49%)

37 percent of common fussy/crying babies who develop intermediate temperaments

12 percent of extremely fussy/colicky babies who develop intermediate temperaments

HIGH RISK (9%)

4 percent of common fussy/crying babies who develop difficult temperaments

5 percent of extremely fussy/colicky babies who develop difficult temperaments

Different temperaments and perhaps different paths to these temperaments will lead to different sleep strategies for each child. It appears to me that the difficult temperament at 5 months mostly represents an extremely overtired baby, while the easy temperament represents an extremely well-rested baby. But keep in mind that biological factors within the baby, such as elevated serotonin levels or immature development of sleep/wake rhythms, may contribute to a baby's behavior during the first 4 months. It is equally necessary to remember that there is enormous variability regarding the resources with which parents are able to soothe their babies, as previously discussed (see Chapter 3). So it is important to look at the big picture: your baby, your ability to soothe, and the support structure and resources available to you. What will work for one family may not work for you. As Cindy Crawford says in the foreword, "The most important thing is a well-rested *family*." The goal is to develop a *caring* environment for the family, not a *cure* for extreme fussiness/colic.

Common Fussiness/Crying: Low Risk for Sleep Problems Developing

Breast-feeding becomes much easier around 4 months of age or sooner for babies exhibiting common fussiness/crying because everyone is better rested and life is more predictable. At 3 to 4 months, your baby will start to show drowsy signs earlier in the evening. Instead of becoming sleepy at 8:00 to 10:00 p.m., she will become sleepy at 6:00 to 8:00 p.m. Respect her need to sleep and *begin the soothing-to-sleep process at the earlier hour*. If you are using a crib, simply put her to sleep earlier. But if you are using a family bed, you have to make some choices. The first is to go to bed much earlier yourself, but this is not usually practical. The second would be to lie down with your baby in your bed and create a safe nest or use a co-sleeper where she will sleep, and then leave her after she has fallen asleep. One danger here is that she might roll off the bed and injure herself. (See Chapter 1 on co-sleeping and SIDS.) The third is to transition her to a crib for the beginning of night sleep and until she awakens for her first night feeding, and then bring her to your bed for the remainder of the night. Because these are well-rested 4-month-old babies, they are more adaptable and easy to transition to a crib. One strategy is to breast-feed at night and then pass your baby to his father, who soothes him in his arms and then puts him down in the crib. This breaks up the previous pattern of mother/breast-feeding/sleep in parents' bed. If your baby cries, soothe him without picking him up. But if this fails, pick him up and, after soothing, try again.

If you are bottle-feeding (formula or expressed breast milk) or breast-feeding and using a crib around 4 months of age, expect to feed your baby about four to six hours after her last evening bottle and again early in the morning around 4:00 to 5:00 a.m. until about 9 months of age. Some bottle-fed babies are fed only once, around 2:00 or 3:00 a.m. If you are breast-feeding and using a family bed, you might feed your baby many times throughout the night.

If you are using a crib, there is more social stimulation as you pick up your baby and more handling as you put the baby down to sleep again. Under these circumstances, after 4 months of age, feeding your baby more than twice at night is likely to create a night-waking or night-feeding habit. If you are breast-feeding, the obvious question is whether the awakenings at night, other than the two times mentioned, are due to hunger. If your breast milk supply has not kept pace with your baby's needs or has decreased, then your baby will awaken more at night because of thirst or hunger. One clue suggesting inadequate breast milk is that you are thirsty throughout the day. If so, you are not drinking enough fluid. Or maybe there are some unusual stresses in your life, such as an important trip that you have to take. Are you worried about balancing child care and working, or worried about returning to work and continuing to breast-feed? Is your baby producing less urine? Has the volume of your expressed breast milk decreased? When offered a bottle of expressed breast milk or formula, does your baby now quickly take a much larger feeding? Does he now sleep better or longer after taking a bottle? If you think your child is hungry and you want to continue breast-feeding, contact a lactation consultant through your pediatrician or maternity hospital.

If you are using a family bed (see SIDS prevention, Chapter 1), feeding often throughout the night is not likely to create a night-waking habit. This is because your baby is partially asleep or barely awake when fed. Therefore, the risk of sleep fragmentation for both mother and baby from too much social stimulation is low. With early bedtimes in place, the family bed does not create any sleep problems, and in fact, the family bed may have been part of the soothing solution during the first few months.

After the development of an earlier bedtime, the next sleep

change is the evolution of a regular midmorning nap around 9:00 to 10:00 a.m. This nap may initially be about forty minutes, but it will lengthen to one or two hours. The rest of the day may be snatches of brief and irregular sleep periods. After the midmorning nap develops, when the baby is a little older, the next regular nap occurs around noon to 2:00 p.m. This nap will also lengthen to become about one to two hours. There may be a third mini-nap that is irregular and brief in the late afternoon.

These sleep rhythms are maturing for night sleep and day sleep. A common mistake is to approach the timing of naps and night sleep by strictly enforcing a "by the clock" (BTC) routine. A temperamentally very regular baby might appear to be sleeping BTC, but watching your baby's behavior for sleepy signs is more important than watching the clock.

Consider our original group of one hundred babies. At 5 months, of the forty-nine babies in the intermediate temperament group, thirty-seven babies (about 76 percent) had common fussiness when younger. Also, at 5 months, of the forty-two babies in the easy-temperament group, thirty-nine babies (about 93 percent) had common fussiness when younger.

So, out of the original *eighty babies* with common fussiness/crying before 4 months of age, the vast majority, seventy-six babies (thirty-nine babies with an easy temperament plus thirty-seven babies with intermediate temperament), or 95 percent, are at a low risk or medium risk at 4 months of age for developing sleep problems because:

Parents are not likely to be stressed.
The infant is likely to be well rested.
The infant is likely to be able to self-soothe.
At night, consolidated sleeping (long sleep duration) develops early.
During the day, regular and long naps naturally develop early, without parental scheduling.

If sleep problems exist, "no-cry" or "maybe-cry" solutions
usually work.

Another way to look at this is that out of our original hundred
babies, at 4 to 6 months of age, this low- or medium-risk group represents 91 percent of temperamentally easy and intermediate babies.

Extreme Fussiness/Colic: High Risk for Sleep Problems Developing
Out of the original *twenty babies* with extreme fussiness/colic before 4 months of age, the majority of babies (fifteen, or 75 percent)
are at a low or medium risk for developing sleep problems, because
they develop easy or intermediate temperaments. But five babies, or
25 percent, develop a difficult temperament and are at a high risk for
developing sleep problems because:

Parents are likely to be stressed.
The infant is likely to be overtired.
The infant is likely to be only parent-soothed.
At night, fragmented sleep (night waking) persists.
During the day, irregular and brief naps persist.
If sleep problems exist, "let-cry" solutions might be neces-
    sary.

Another way to look at this is that out of our original hundred
babies, at 4 to 6 months of age, the high-risk group represents 9 percent of temperamentally difficult babies. These nine infants might
represent two somewhat different groups of children. The first group
with a difficult temperament comes from the large group (80 percent) of infants who previously had common fussiness/crying. Only
about 4 percent of these children, or about four infants out of a hundred, fall into this category. I think they are less overtired than the
second group of five infants who previously had extreme fussiness/
colic.

For the first group of infants who had common fussiness/crying and now have a difficult temperament, there is relatively fast improvement when parents put forth great effort to help them sleep better. Such infants are more adaptable, and it is easier to change their sleep routines. "No-cry" or "maybe-cry" sleep strategies are likely to work well. Perhaps these parents simply failed to establish an early bedtime after 6 weeks of age or provide timely opportunities for naps after a few months of age, and their child developed cumulative sleepiness during the first 4 months. On the other hand, there may be parent issues (see Chapter 3) that contributed to the development of a difficult temperament, and these same issues, if they persist, may interfere with helping the child sleep better. Perhaps these babies reflect mainly a mother-driven path.

The second group with a difficult temperament comes from a small group (20 percent of all infants) who previously had extreme fussiness/colic. About five infants out of a hundred fall into this category. I think they are more overtired than the first group. When parents put forth great effort to help them sleep better, there is relatively slow improvement. They are less adaptable, and it is more difficult to change their sleep routines. "No-cry" or "maybe-cry" sleep strategies are not likely to work, and these parents have to consider "let-cry" sleep strategies. Perhaps these babies reflect mainly a baby-driven path. This group represents the majority of children that are referred to me for a sleep consultation.

I believe this small percentage (9 percent) of all babies have the most severe and hard-to-solve sleep problems. There are two reasons for this. The first is that for five of the nine babies, the biological factors that led to extreme fussiness/colic in the first place might persist and frustrate the parents' best efforts to solve sleep problems. The second is that for four of the nine babies who started off with common fussiness/crying, something occurred that led to the children developing a difficult temperament, and whatever social, emotional, or family factors occurred during the first 4 months might persist thereafter.

However, this explanation is incomplete, because for the group of five babies with extreme fussiness/colic, maternal anxiety (or depression) may cause the behavior and/or maternal depression may result from this behavior; this suggests that baby-parent interaction is the main path. Also, for the group of four babies who had common fussiness/crying, the fact that measurements of fussiness and crying are graded or continuous means that they might have been close to but just did not quite meet the criteria for extreme fussiness/colic. So it might be an error to overly dwell on nonbiologic factors such as the mother.

My idea that at 4 to 6 months of age there are two groups of overtired children who appear to have a difficult temperament is supported by research on an initial group of 1,019 mothers. Many mothers dropped out of the study, but the 560 mothers who stayed were more likely to be married, have completed more formal education, have higher household incomes, be nonsmokers, breast-feed, and have "higher levels of social support." The researchers noted that at 3 months of age there were thirty-five children (6 percent of this selected population) who were crying enough to be called colicky. Of these thirty-five colicky infants, eighteen (51 percent) had been this way at 6 weeks of age (called "typical colic"), but seventeen (49 percent) had not (they were called "latent colic"). The researchers felt that typical colic and latent colic represented two groups of colicky infants. They went on to describe a third group (14 percent of all colicky infants) that continued to cry substantially past 3 months of age. The authors called this a "persistent mother-infant distress syndrome."

Interestingly, in Dr. William Carey's work with anxious mothers (see Chapter 5), he noted the time of onset of colic among thirteen babies: for five, or 38 percent, it was in the first month; for four, or 31 percent, it was in the second month; and for another four, or an additional 31 percent, it was in the third month. Maybe these three groups are similar to the three groups described above: typical colic, latent colic, and "mother-infant distress syndrome."

Maybe the typical colic infants were what I refer to as extreme fussiness/colic and reflect a mainly baby-driven pathway, while the latent colic infants may have started out as common fussiness/crying and reflect a mainly mother-driven pathway, so after 6 weeks these overtired infants (from sleep fragmentation or a late bedtime) exhibited colicky behavior. In other words, comparing the above study on 560 families to my analysis, I would say that at 4 months of age there are about 9 percent of overtired children with difficult temperaments, falling into two groups: the first, five out of nine children (56 percent), were formerly extremely fussy/colicky babies (similar to the 51 percent with typical colic); the second, four out of nine (44 percent), had common fussiness/crying (similar to the 49 percent with "latent colic"). I believe that those families with limited resources for soothing or persistent parent issues (see Chapter 3) are more likely to have babies who are at greater risk for the overtired/fussy/crying state to persist. The term "mother-infant distress syndrome" is similar to the notion of mother-baby interaction issues, discussed above. But this term and the general notion of a mother-driven path are objectionable because of the blame they direct solely to the mother. Obviously, fathers, grandparents, financial factors, and so forth can stress a family independent of the mother's capabilities to nurture her child.

UNDERSTANDING YOUR BABY

Before 4 months: Was there extreme fussiness/colic or common fussiness/crying?

At 4 to 6 months: Is there a difficult or easy temperament?

After 4 months: Will there be a high or low risk for sleep problems?

UNDERSTANDING YOUR FAMILY

Consider the behavior of both parents and any parent issues.

Consider your resources for soothing.

Living with and soothing a baby who has extreme fussiness/colic is discussed in Chapter 5. Here is some more information on how common fussiness/crying/easy temperament versus extreme fussiness/ colic/difficult temperament may affect some parenting decisions.

HOW AND WHEN TO MOVE YOUR BABY OUT OF YOUR BED

If you decided that you wanted a family bed before your child was born (see Chapter 1 regarding SIDS), and if your child has common fussiness/crying, you might decide to continue the family bed for a long time. Then, when you move your baby out, the transition might be very easy if your baby now develops an easy temperament. But if your decision for a family bed was in reaction to extreme fussiness/ colic and your child now has a difficult temperament, the transition might be very stressful for the entire family because your child may not have learned self-soothing.

Q: *I am breast-feeding and my child sleeps with us, but I want to move him out of our bed. How do I do this?*
A: There is no one right way to do this, but if your child has learned self-soothing, you can do this quickly at any age. However, if your child lacks self-soothing skills, you probably will do it gradually and slowly over several weeks or a few months. Make the move when both parents agree that it is the right time. Always be mindful of your baby's safety. Initially, respond promptly when your baby calls for you. Later, you might delay your response. A baby might be placed in a crib close to the side of your bed. Later, the crib is moved a few inches from your bed. Gradually the crib is moved farther away until it is in baby's room. An older child might sleep on a mattress on the floor in your room, with or without the parent. Later, the mattress is moved to the child's room, with or without the parent. Sometimes you might just want your child to be in her crib or bed but in your room. If you are going to use a separate room and your child is older, announce the planned move in advance, and make the room very attractive or let her help decorate her room. Alternatively,

move your baby into the room or bed where the siblings are sleeping. Some parents will begin the night with the child in the parents' bed and then move the child to a crib after she has fallen asleep.

Q: *Do I have to wean my baby from breast-feeding before I move him out of our bed?*

A: I think the answer depends on your resources for soothing other than breast-feeding, especially the assistance of the father, plus your desire to continue or to discontinue breast-feeding. I see no reason why weaning from breast-feeding has to precede or accompany your moving the baby. But if non-nutritive breast-feeding is the only way your child will fall asleep, you probably will want to teach your child some self-soothing before discontinuing completely the non-nutritive breast-feeding and moving him out of your bed.

BREAST-FEEDING

Breast-feeding babies with extreme fussiness/colic/difficult temperament may be difficult because everyone is tired. As the biological need for an earlier bedtime develops, the best strategy is to temporarily try to put your baby to sleep earlier, but the main theme is to do whatever it takes to maximize sleep and minimize crying. The plan is to keep your child as well rested as possible in order to buy time for the development of more mature sleep/wake rhythms. Once these rhythms are developed, they may be used as an aid to help your child sleep better. For example, the breast-feeding mother of an infant with extreme fussiness/colic/difficult temperament might want to take the baby into her bed and nurse him to sleep at the earlier bedtime and then, once he is asleep, move him to a co-sleeper or crib or use a family bed (see SIDS warning, Chapter 1). However, real-life events, such as returning to work or caring for other family members, might not permit the luxury of always sleeping with your baby whenever he appears to be sleepy.

ATTACHMENT PARENTING

You may have wanted to practice attachment parenting before your baby was born. If your baby has common fussiness/crying/easy temperament and is at low risk for sleep problems, then it is more likely that caring for your baby will not be exhausting and both mother and baby will have opportunities for sleep, making attachment parenting attractive and easy to execute. The opposite scenario occurs with a baby with extreme fussiness/colic/difficult temperament and a high risk for sleep problems. With these babies, a proactive decision to practice attachment parenting or a decision made reactively to the child's behavior may succeed if there are enormous resources for soothing, but in their absence the result might be an extremely overtired family.

Can you change your lifestyle so that your child will receive the soothing to sleep at those times when your child needs to sleep? Can you avoid too much social stimulation from interfering with sleep even if it means ignoring your child's crying at those times when your child needs to sleep? These are difficult questions that challenge about 20 percent of families during the first 2 to 4 months because of extreme fussiness/colic and about 9 percent of families at 4 months because of overtired/difficult temperament. Successfully dealing with these challenges will prevent sleep problems in the future.

MAJOR POINT
To help children sleep better, most families never have to let their child cry, if they start teaching self-soothing early.

SLEEP MODULATES TEMPERAMENT

Understanding temperament allows you to more clearly identify specific features in your baby's personality. Sleeping better makes for an easier temperament (see page 395 and Chapter 2), and healthier sleep is something that parents can accomplish.

I believe that the quality of your baby's sleep influences the development of temperament at 4 to 6 months of age. And how babies sleep during the first few months is a combination of factors within the child and the parents' ability and skill at soothing. It is also my belief that at 4 to 6 months of age the difficult temperament represents an overtired baby and the easy temperament represents a well-rested baby. Remember: the temperament that your baby has at 4 to 6 months of age is *not* permanent. Temperament changes over time as babies develop and parents modify how they soothe their children.

Additionally, as described by parents on pages 366 and 389, children's personality may be severely and adversely affected when they are short of sleep, but the good news is that these changes are reversible!

NAPS

The Midday Nap

After the midmorning nap develops, a midday nap rhythm evolves that will have your baby sleeping best between 12:00 and 2:00 p.m. Some caveats are in order, however. The evolution of nap rhythms is not the same in all children, as mothers of fraternal twins can attest! Additionally, the window when naps are easily obtained varies among children in terms of being wide (for example, anytime between 12:00 and 2:00 p.m.) or narrow (for example, between 12:30 and 1:30 p.m.). There will be some trial and error to find the best times when your child's brain goes into nap mode, so be patient and do not compare your child with other children.

Children who had common fussiness/crying and later an easy temperament might slip effortlessly and early into two long naps, while parents of children with extreme fussiness/colic who later have a difficult temperament might struggle longer with the challenge of establishing regular and predictable naps—and be frustrated because the naps are somewhat short! The foundation for the midday nap is the midmorning nap, just as the foundation for the midmorning nap is night sleep. Gradually, for all children, naps will become more predictable and longer. Attempts to extend naps by reswaddling, replacing a pacifier, or offering a quick feeding may help.

A third, brief, late afternoon nap is common, but this nap does not occur in all children, and among children who take this nap, some do not take it consistently.

Transition from Brief Intervals of Wakefulness to Clock Time

As nap rhythms mature, the naps will become more predictable and longer if and only if they are in sync with biological nap cycles. Although they will not occur at exactly the same clock time every day, you will be able to watch the clock a little more. If you have good timing, you might not see drowsy signs, because you are perfectly catching the sleep wave. Because drowsy signs might be absent and because the naps are now getting longer, you want to move away from the notion of brief intervals of wakefulness and focus more on the clock-time window when your child takes his or her nap best. (Naps are also discussed in Chapters 1, 2, and 3.)

SLEEPING THROUGH THE NIGHT

What does the phrase "sleeping through the night" mean? You might be surprised that there is no standard or widely accepted definition. In 2010, Dr. Jacqueline Henderson studied three different definitions of "sleeping through the night":

1. Sleeping uninterrupted from midnight to 5:00 a.m.
2. Sleeping eight hours uninterrupted between sleep onset and waking time in the morning, without regard to the clock time when the sleep occurred
3. Sleeping uninterrupted between 10:00 p.m., or earlier, and 6:00 a.m.

Sleeping uninterrupted means that there is no feeding or soothing.

Here are her data:

INFANTS SLEEPING THROUGH THE NIGHT

Age	Definition of "Sleeping Through the Night"		
	12:00– 5:00 a.m.	8 Hours Straight	10:00 p.m.– 6:00 a.m.
3 months	58%	Less than 50%	Less than 40%
4 months	Almost 70%	58%	Less than 50%
5 months	More than 70%	About 60%	53%

So at 3 months of age, 58 percent of babies are able to sleep uninterrupted for 5 hours between midnight and 5:00 a.m. By 4 months of age this number is almost 70 percent, and 58 percent of babies are able to sleep uninterrupted for 8 hours. By 5 months of age, more than half of all babies (53 percent) sleep uninterrupted for 8 hours or more when their parents are likely to sleep. So by any definition, more than half of all babies are sleeping through the night by age 5 months. The data about sleeping through the night describe a population of children. But what is most important for you is your own child's behavior and mood in the late afternoon and early evening, which can guide you toward a reasonably early bed-time and help you avoid unnecessary soothing and feeding in the middle of the night.

Dr. Henderson wrote, "The most rapid consolidation in infant sleep regulation occurs in the first 4 months. . . . [This] reflects the emergence of infant's self-regulation and self-soothing capacities." A 2015 report showed that about 70 percent of 3-month-olds were described by parents to sleep continuously for five hours or more, but video evidence showed that about a quarter of them actually "resettle"—they awaken and return to sleep unassisted (see "Arous-als" in Chapter 1). These reports support the idea of using the child's natural internal sleep regulation machinery as an aid to help your child sleep better during the first 4 months. Because this pro-cess of sleep regulation is developing during the first 4 months, there is no reason for most parents to delay and begin to think about help-ing their child sleep better only at 4 months of age. Starting earlier is easier.

As discussed in Chapter 4, my research shows that with extinc-tion in children *younger than 4 months* the average amount of cry-ing is as follows:

Night 1:	Crying lasts 30–45 minutes
Night 2:	Crying lasts 10–30 minutes
Night 3:	Crying lasts 0–10 minutes
Night 4:	No crying

In children *4 months of age* and older the usual pattern is:

Night 1:	Crying lasts 45–55 minutes
Night 2:	A little more or a little less crying than night 1
Night 3:	Crying lasts 20–40 minutes
Night 4 or 5:	No crying

If the bedtime is too late or naps are not going well, the process might take longer or not work.

Therefore, because children may cry less and for fewer days when younger, parents should respect and take advantage of their baby's capabilities to sleep longer at night during the first 4 months of life and not wait until their child is older to help their baby sleep well. The earlier you start to teach self-soothing, the better. It is never too early to start—but it is also never too late to begin.

Summary and Action Plan for Exhausted Parents

MAJOR POINT

To help children sleep better, 91 percent of families never have to let their child cry, provided that they start helping their baby learn to sleep early.

During the first 4 months, colicky infants, by definition, exhibit more fuss/cry behavior. Extremely fussy/colicky infants sleep less than common fussy/crying infants at 4 months of age, but group differences disappear by 6 to 8 months. Also, by 6 months of age, researchers are more apt to describe parents contributing to sleep problems, especially night waking or signaling.

Infant crying alone does not predict the development of sleep problems. Rather, the combination of crying plus parental distress or crying plus sleep problems at 5 months predicts night waking at 20 months, but not at 56 months.

Assessments at 2 and 4 weeks of age showed that infant-temperament difficultness predicted increased crying/fussing at about 6 weeks of age. Infants with extreme fussiness/colic are more likely to have a difficult temperament when assessed at 4 months of age, but not at 12 months. A difficult temperament is associated, at many ages, with problems in sleeping, such as shorter sleep durations and night waking, but this association is not predictive of later sleep problems.

Despite successful treatment of colic, a difficult temperament and sleep problems may emerge after 4 months. This led to my original view that emphasized the baby-driven pathway. We now know that maternal behavior during the night (unnecessary feeding and attending to the baby) causes sleep fragmentation, which in turn may contribute to or cause sleep problems such as night waking.

It is important for parents to help post-colic infants establish healthy sleep habits.

After extreme fussiness/colic winds down around 4 months of age or sooner, a child may be overtired, not sleeping well, and difficult to manage. But not all difficult-to-manage 4-month-olds had extreme fussiness/colic. I think there are two groups of children at 4 to 6 months of age, both of whom have difficult temperaments.

The first group with a difficult temperament comes from the large group (80 percent) of infants with common fussiness/crying. Only about 4 percent of the children with common fussiness/crying fall into this category. "No-cry" sleep strategies are likely to work well with these children.

The second group with a difficult temperament comes from a small group (20 percent) of infants with extreme fussiness/colic. About 27 percent of children with a difficult temperament fall into this category. "No-cry" sleep strategies are not likely to work with these children, and parents have to consider "let-cry" sleep strategies.

Difficult-temperament children in both groups have trouble falling asleep and staying asleep. At about 4 months they have not developed self-soothing skills, perhaps because parents invested constant soothing to prevent their child's fussiness from developing into crying; because anxious mothers caused sleep fragmentation; or because the inability to self-soothe is an integral component of colic. A successful intervention effort to help families cope with infant crying during colic will reduce parental distress. Continued age-appropriate sleep hygiene after colic ends is likely to prevent sleep problems persisting beyond 4 months. Unsuccessful intervention increases the likelihood that temperament issues, family stress, and sleep problems will persist beyond 4 months.

Intervention with extinction is effective, fast, and safe, but some parents are unable or unwilling to use this method. For these parents, graduated extinction or fading may offer a more palatable and still effective alternative (see Chapter 4).

CHAPTER 8

Healthy Sleep Habits in Months 4–12

The main goals at this age are:
To encourage the development of self-soothing skills for night sleep,
the midmorning nap, and the midday nap
To synchronize the time when you put your child to sleep with the
onset of your child's biologic sleep rhythms

Routines that comfort your baby, including rocking, soft blankets, lullabies, stroking, patting, and cuddling for bedtime (see Chapter 3), may also be used intact or modified for nap time. Maintain these routines so your child learns to associate certain behaviors occurring at certain times in a familiar place with the behavior called "falling asleep."

Helpful Hints for Comforting Routines
Soft, silky, or furry-textured blankets, dolls, or stuffed animals in crib
A small soft blanket over the top of the head, like a scarf
Dim night-light
Nursing to sleep

Nurse to sleep? Isn't that contrary to the advice to always put your baby down drowsy but awake? There are many well-rested

4-month-old children with self-soothing skills who often fall asleep with nursing. Some of the parents of these children had practiced putting them down drowsy but awake when their children were younger so their baby could achieve self-soothing skills. If this is the case with your family, there is nothing wrong with nursing your baby to sleep. Most nursing mothers in my practice do this all the time. But if you have difficulty letting your child learn to fall asleep unassisted, if your child *always* falls asleep at the breast, and if your child has disturbed sleep, then nursing to sleep might be part of the sleep problem. It may reflect the kind of separation problems discussed in Chapter 3.

Many mothers nurse their babies for soothing and comfort as well as feeding, and their babies may or may not fall asleep at the breast. In either case, the key is to place your baby in the crib when there is a *need* to sleep. I think that this intimacy between mother and infant is beautiful, and nursing to sleep, in itself, does not necessarily cause sleep problems.

Here are some common questions in this age range:

Q: *Do I roll my older child over to his favorite sleeping position when he wakes up during the night? Do I help him get down when he stands up and shakes the crib railings?*

A: No. I doubt that you like playing these games with your child at night. Think, too, about what you teach him when you go to him at night to roll him over to his favorite sleeping position or help him down. But if he rolls over only once at night or gets stuck in the railings of the crib, then help him go back to sleep.

Q: *Won't he hurt himself if he falls down in his crib? He can't get down by himself.*

A: No, he won't hurt himself. He may fall into an awkward heap . . . and sleep like a puppy.

Try to be reasonably regular: watch the intervals of wakefulness in babies 4 months of age or younger, and when your baby is over

4 months, watch both him and the clock. However, try not to get locked into a fixed or unvarying bedtime or nap time hour; vary the times a little depending on the wake-up time, the duration of naps, when the second nap ended, and indoor versus outdoor activities. Often babies between 9 and 12 months need to go to bed earlier because of increased physical activity in the afternoon and the absence of a third nap. Remember, too late a bedtime causes disturbed sleep just as nap deprivation does.

When you are somewhat organized regarding sleep schedules, the child accepts and expects sleep. But don't feel you have to be so organized for feeding or other infant care practices! Probably the opposite is true for feeding. When parents are creative, free-spirited, and permissive regarding wholesome foods, feeding solid foods usually goes well. So respect the biological basis for regular sleep, and accept or reject popular practices for feeding wholesome solid food as you see fit. But sleeping and feeding are similar in that just as junk food is bad for the body, junk sleep is bad for the brain (see Chapters 1 and 2).

Our goal is to establish sleep habits, so we don't want to get sidetracked at this stage by worrying too much about crying. When your 2-year-old cries because he wants to play instead of having his diaper changed or your 1-year-old cries because he wants juice instead of milk, you don't let the crying prevent you from doing what is best for him. Establishing healthy sleep habits does not mean that there will always be a lot of crying, but there may be some in protest. If you find this to be unacceptable when your child is 4 months old or younger, then by all means consider waiting until he is older to help him sleep better. But also consider that it may be harder to achieve when older.

As discussed in Chapter 4, my research shows that with extinction in children *younger than 4 months,* the average amount of crying is as follows:

Night 1:   Crying lasts 30–45 minutes
Night 2:   Crying lasts 10–30 minutes

Night 3:   Crying lasts 0–10 minutes
Night 4:   No crying

In children *4 months of age and older,* the usual pattern is:

Night 1:   Crying lasts 45–55 minutes
Night 2:   A little more or a little less crying than night 1
Night 3:   Crying lasts 20–40 minutes
Night 4 or 5: No crying

If the bedtime is too late or naps are not going well, the process might take longer or not work.

Therefore, because children may cry less and for fewer days when younger, parents should respect and take advantage of their baby's capabilities to sleep longer at night during the first 4 months of life and usually not wait until their child is older to help their baby sleep well at night. The earlier you start to teach self-soothing, the better. It is never too early, but it is also never too late to begin.

It will become more difficult to change your baby's sleep patterns after about 6 months of age because of the development of *self-agency.* Self-agency means that your child can express likes and dislikes with greater energy and persistence than previously. If your infant wants to reach a desired toy, she may persist longer in trying to get it into her grasp. Your infant might protest at being changed or being put down to sleep, and she can now express her protest more loudly and longer than when she was younger. This increased ability to express intentional behavior may be described as persistence, drive, or determination.

Self-agency becomes stronger over time. During the first few months, you could change the diaper whenever you wished, and there was no protest. Distraction was an effective method to help get the job done when she became squirmy. After 6 months, distraction is now less effective because your infant has a stronger sense of self-agency. Your baby thinks that she can do whatever she wants to do, whenever she wants to do it. This independence leads to persistence, which may be desirable ("My son is determined to walk") or undesirable ("He is so stubborn all the time"). We welcome some efforts, but willful opposition makes the daily ordinary chores of parenting much harder. Some infants are more strong-willed than others. This is their nature, and you cannot change this feature of their personality. Being strong-willed may have a negative ring to it, but maybe the trait of being persistent as an infant will turn into the desirable trait of ambition or grit as an adult.

Self-agency might lead your child to protest naps because he would rather play than sleep or stay up late for more soothing company with parents. If you allow him to not nap or to stay up late, then he will become fatigued. The adaptive response to fatigue is to fight it with stimulating hormones, which allow your baby to maintain more wakefulness. However, this heightened state of alertness or arousal creates an inability to easily fall asleep or stay asleep for subsequent naps or night sleep. Not only does a vicious cycle of sleep problems begin, but as a by-product, your child may develop emotional lability (swift, sharp changes in mood) or an impaired attention span.

Total Sleep Duration Trends over Time

A review by Lisa Matricciani found that "over the last 103 years, there have been consistent rapid declines in the sleep duration of children and adolescents." A study by Dr. Ivo Iglowstein showed that total sleep durations have decreased steadily from 1974 through 1979 and 1986. This trend was confirmed in studies by Dr. Anna Price and me for middle-class or middle-socioeconomic-status (SES) families.

AVERAGE TOTAL SLEEP DURATION, 1979–80 AND 2004

1979–80	2004
14.1 hours (4–11 months)	14.0 hours (4–6 months)
	13.6 hours (7–9 months)
	13.4 hours (10–12 months)

This trend was also noted for higher-SES families in the early part of the twentieth century by Dr. Josephine Foster and at the beginning of the twenty-first century by Dr. Avi Sadeh:

AVERAGE TOTAL SLEEP DURATION, 1927 AND 2006

1927	2006
14.0 hours (6–11 months)	13.3 hours (3–5 months)
	12.9 hours (6–8 months)
	12.8 hours (9–11 months)

We do not know why children are currently sleeping less than in the past. Here are three possible explanations:

1. Center-based day care became more popular when mothers entered the workforce in large numbers between the 1970s and 1990s. Center-based day care is associated with shorter naps according to two studies, one conducted by Dr. Price and the other by Dr. Janet Lam. In 2011, the Institute of Medicine published specific recommendations for center-based day care with the expectation that they would be included in state regulations for licensing child care centers: (1) encourage practices that promote child self-regulation of sleep (putting infants to sleep drowsy but awake), (2) create an environment that ensures sleep, such as no screen media in sleeping rooms and low noise and light levels, and (3) encourage sleep-promoting behaviors and practices, such as calming nap time routines and avoiding stimulating children just before nap time. A 2014 re-

view by Dr. Sara Neelon documented that only eleven states recommended both of the first two suggestions and no state recommended the third. Additionally, in my experience, the long drive home from the child care center, along with the natural desire of parents who did not see their child during the day to want to play with their child in the evening, causes the bedtime to be too late. Even with an early bedtime, some families have to awaken their child in the morning to get to the center on time.

2. Having a television in the child's bedroom became more popular after the 1980s. Dr. Judith Owens and others have documented that this is associated with less sleep and more sleep problems. Modern screen-based media use at night has only made matters worse.

3. More women are delaying the time when they have their first child. There was a sixfold increase in the rate of first births among women in the age range 35–39 years between 1973 and 2006, and a fourfold increase for the rate among women 40–44 years between 1985 and 2002. As previously discussed (see Chapter 5), helping children sleep well is more challenging for older mothers and fathers.

Night Sleep

SLEEPING THROUGH THE NIGHT

What does the phrase "sleeping through the night" mean? You might be surprised that there is no standard or widely accepted definition. In 2010, Dr. Jacqueline Henderson studied three different definitions of "sleeping through the night." Uninterrupted sleeping means that there is no feeding or soothing.

1. Sleeping uninterrupted from midnight to 5:00 a.m.
2. Sleeping eight hours uninterrupted between sleep onset and waking time in the morning, without regard to the clock time when the sleep occurred
3. Sleeping uninterrupted between 10:00 p.m., or earlier, and 6:00 a.m.

Here are her data:

INFANTS SLEEPING THROUGH THE NIGHT

Age	Definition of "Sleeping Through the Night"		
	12:00– 5:00 a.m.	8 Hours Straight	10:00 p.m.– 6:00 a.m.
3 months	58%	Less than 50%	Less than 40%
4 months	Almost 70%	58%	Less than 50%
5 months	More than 70%	About 60%	53%
7 months	—	—	About 60%
8 months	About 80%	About 70%	—
11 months	—	About 80%	About 70%
12 months	87%	86%	73%

By 5 months of age, more than half of all babies (53 percent) sleep uninterrupted 8 hours or more when their parents are likely to sleep. So by any definition, more than half of all babies are sleeping through the night by age 5 months.

Dr. Henderson wrote, "The most rapid consolidation in infant sleep regulation occurs in the first 4 months. . . . [This] reflects the emergence of infant's self-regulation and self-soothing capacities." This supports the idea of using your child's natural sleep regulation machinery as an aid to help your child sleep better during the first 4 months.

In her study, the average bedtime at 12 months was 8:30 p.m. Based on my research and experience, at 12 months, 8:30 p.m. is too late for many children (see below), especially those who are taking a single nap (17 percent of children) and those who have total nap duration of less than two hours (whether in one nap or two). A bedtime that is too late would likely produce a second wind that interferes with easily falling asleep and staying asleep. In my experience, all children who are napping well and have early bedtimes are sleeping uninterrupted through the night by 9 months or earlier. The data about sleeping through the night presented above describe a population of children. But what is most important for you is your own child's behavior and mood in the late afternoon and early evening, which can guide you toward a reasonably early bedtime and help you avoid unnecessary soothing and feeding in the middle of the night.

BEDTIME HOUR TRENDS OVER TIME

The shift in children's bedtimes toward later hours has run in tandem with advances in night illumination. On a historical scale, it is only fairly recently that more illumination at night has become available. The industrial production of candles began in the 1850s, the wide use of kerosene lamps in the 1860s, and the commercialization of lightbulbs in the 1880s. Shortly thereafter, physicians began to blame modern life and, more pointedly, late bedtimes for causing sleep problems.

The following quote from an editorial in the *British Medical Journal* in 1894 titled "Sleeplessness" is typical: "The subject of sleeplessness is once more under discussion. The hurry and excitement of modern life is quite correctly held to be responsible." Today, because keeping our children up at night is so common, we might give little thought to the consequences of late bedtimes. But that does not mean those consequences are nonexistent or benign. As discussed previously, threats to our children's health may go largely unnoticed for generations before slowly beginning to become known. It is the same with late bedtimes.

So, how late are our children staying up?

Data collected by Dr. Iglowstein, Dr. Price, and me over many years show that the bedtime hour has shifted to later times. The cause of this shift is not known.

BEDTIME HOUR (P.M.) BY YEAR

Age	1974	1979	1979–80	1986	2004
6 months	7:18	7:41	8:00 (4–11 months)	8:16	8:00 (4–9 months)
1 year	7:08	7:35	8:00	7:46	8:00 (10–12 months)

After about 1980, the trend toward a later bedtime plateaued in young children, perhaps because increasingly later bedtimes would eventually be significantly disruptive to the child and the family. Although the wake-up times were a little later—for example, three minutes later in 1-year-olds—the later wake-up times failed to fully compensate for the later bedtimes. This means that children today are getting less night sleep than in the past. It is important to note that research has shown that just a *nineteen-minute* decrease in total sleep time may cause significant impairments (see Chapter 4).

In this discussion of a trend over the years of later bedtimes (and of trends over time for less night sleep, less day sleep, and less total sleep, to be discussed later), the general conclusions appear to be sound because they represent large numbers of children in many studies. Some caution is warranted regarding these conclusions, however, because at every specific age for every specific year, only the average value is reported, and the range in values around this average is often very wide. Therefore, small differences between reported values over a short period of time may occur by chance alone (for example, the difference between 7:08 and 7:35 p.m. bedtimes in 1-year-olds between 1974 and 1979). On the other hand, larger differences over a longer period of time and fairly consistent trend data in between from multiple sources suggest that the overall trend is real (for example, the difference between 7:08 and 8:00 p.m. bedtimes between 1974 and 2004).

Television and other electronic screen-based devices in the bedroom have recently become more popular. These intrusive objects cause later bedtimes, and they are associated with less sleep and more sleep problems (see Chapter 10).

BEDTIME

Remember, you are establishing an orderly home routine and enforcing a bedtime hour. You are not forcing your child to sleep. When your child starts to seem tired and needs to sleep, you try to begin his bedtime routine, whether he likes it or not. The bedtime routine should be regular in terms of *what* you do: bathing, massage, reading a story, lullaby, rocking, or other soothing efforts. Approximately the same sequence each night, at approximately the same time, helps signal to the child that it is time for night sleep. Your child begins to associate the bedtime routine, which includes your leaving him, with falling asleep in the same way that you associate a yellow traffic light with slowing down before stopping on red. But don't be rigidly regular in terms of *when* you do it; there is enough normal irregularity in napping to produce some variability in bedtime. However, in much older children, extreme variability in bedtimes has been shown to be unhealthy.

Sometimes parent issues (see Chapter 3) interfere with a reasonably early bedtime or with consistency in bedtime routines and need to be directly addressed.

A parent who keeps a baby up past his natural time to sleep may be using this playtime with the child to avoid unpleasant private time with the other parent.

Some parents make the mistake of always putting their baby down to sleep at exactly the same time every night. For a few months this may work well, but when naps are irregular or your child stops taking the third nap, parents should learn to be more flexible in the timing of soothing to sleep at night, especially in the direction toward an earlier bedtime!

Method A and method B for soothing to sleep (see Chapter 7) apply only to naps. At night, adopt whatever style seems comfortable to you. For example, at nap time you may wish to put your baby down drowsy but awake after soothing, and at night you may prefer to sleep with your baby (see co-sleeping and SIDS prevention, Chapter 1). No problem. It appears that different parts of the brain are responsible for day and night sleep, so simply be consistent in how you soothe to sleep for daytime naps and in how you soothe to sleep at night, even if the two routines are different. You are "training" different parts of the brain at different times.

If it is your desire to put your baby down for the night after soothing and he is *overtired,* then there may be some crying. During the day, limiting the amount of crying to one hour, in the hope of getting a nap at a time that will not mess up the rest of the schedule, is reasonable. But at night, if you chose to do extinction, the crying that occurs as you put your overtired child down should not be time-limited unless you decide to do extinction with a cap. If you go to him after a brief bout of crying or if you choose a short cap, you may train your child to cry to your predetermined time limit. If you do not check on your baby, he will eventually fall asleep. He may cry more the second night, but each subsequent night he will cry less. This assumes that the bedtime is early, naps are in place, and night sleep is not fragmented. Alternatively, you might use graduated extinction, check and console, or a fade procedure (see Chapter 4). If a sleep solution involves establishing an earlier bedtime and your child is taking long and late midday naps, a part of the solution will be to not allow her to sleep past 4:00 p.m., by awakening her if necessary.

This may be the first time you will ignore your child's protests, but it certainly will not be the last. As he becomes mobile, you will protect his physical safety by not allowing unreasonable risks involving playground equipment. At some future point you will teach your child other health habits such as hand washing and tooth brushing. Later still, you're not going to risk brain damage by letting him ride his bike without a helmet. In each of these cases, you won't let protest crying discourage you from implementing healthy practices and safety rules. Starting early and being consistent are the keys to establishing good habits.

Now is the time to let your child learn to fall asleep at night by himself, to return to sleep at night by himself, and to learn that being alone at night in slumber is not scary, dangerous, or something to avoid. Keep everything calm and not too complicated as you go through a bedtime ritual. Fathers should be helping out at bedtime and nighttime, especially if the child is breast-fed, because babies know dads cannot nurse them, and so any protest crying is likely to be less intense or shorter.

If you are using the extinction method, once your child is in bed, he is there to stay, no matter how long he cries. Please do not return with curtain calls. Little peeks, replacing pacifiers, or reswaddling may be relatively harmless for some babies when they are 4 months old or younger, but they will eventually sabotage your efforts to help your older child sleep well because intermittent positive reinforcement has enormous teaching power.

HELPFUL SUGGESTION

When your child is crying and she is not hungry or ill, say to yourself: "My baby is crying because she loves me so much she wants my company, but she needs to sleep. I know the value of good sleep, and I love my baby so much that I am going to let her sleep."

NIGHT WAKINGS FOR FEEDING

Your child may awake at night to be fed four to six hours after his last feeding. Some children do not get up then. Others are actually hungry at this time, and you should promptly respond by feeding.

You may say, "But when my baby was younger, he slept through the night." Remember, in a child under 4 months, maybe the bedtime and the last feeding at bedtime were both much later. Now your baby is going to bed earlier, is fed earlier in the evening at bedtime, and may need a middle-of-the-night feeding; this is normal. This bedtime feeding, and an early morning feeding, may be needed until your baby is about 9 months of age.

As you may recall, partial awakenings or light sleep stages, called arousals, occur every one to two hours when your child is asleep. Sometimes your child will quietly call out or cry during these arousals. Quiet, nondistressed vocalizations during arousals are normal and should be ignored. If your child is not sleeping with you in your bed, going in to him at the time of these partial awakenings will eventually lead to a night-waking or night-feeding habit. This is because picking up, holding, and feeding your baby will eventually cause him to force himself to a more alert state during these arousals for the pleasure of your company. He will learn to expect to be fed or played with at every arousal. He will learn to more loudly and persistently call out for your company.

However, if you are sleeping with your baby (see co-sleeping and SIDS warning, Chapter 1) and breast-feeding, you might promptly nurse at all of these arousals while you and the baby are still in a somewhat deeper sleep state, and then there is no real sleep fragmentation. No night-waking habit might develop.

Parents should not project their own emotions or misinterpret these naturally occurring arousals with vocalizations as signifying loneliness, fear of the dark, or fear of abandonment. This might be especially difficult for a mother with depression or anxiety issues (see Chapters 3 and 5), and if so, professional help for the mother might be needed.

If your baby wakes at night and behaves as if she is hungry, feed her. If your baby appears to want to play at night, stop going to her. At night, the question is "Does my baby *need* me or *want* me?"

As mentioned, a second waking for feeding may occur around 4:00 or 5:00 a.m. Some children do not get up at this time, but those children who do awaken are wet, soiled, hungry, or thirsty, and a prompt response is appropriate. While you attend to your baby's needs, maintain silence and darkness so your child will return to sleep. A common mistake is to quietly play with your child, preventing the return to sleep. But the return to sleep around 4:00 or 5:00 a.m. is important, so that with a later wake-up time, at 6:00–7:00 a.m., your child will be able to comfortably stay up in the morning until the time of the first nap. Actually, many children do not need to be fed twice at night; they simply get up at 2:00 or 3:00 a.m. or not at all. A common mistake is to feed around midnight, at 2:00 a.m., and again around 4:00 or 5:00 a.m. If you feed your baby around midnight, please do not respond again at the 2:00 a.m. time; your baby is not hungry then. The general guideline after 4 months of age is to feed your baby overnight when hungry, but no more than two times.

BEDTIME BATTLES, DIFFICULTY FALLING ASLEEP

Past 6 weeks of age, biologically driven bedtimes tend to become earlier. If you are unable or unwilling to allow these early bedtimes, your child will become overtired, develop a second wind at bedtime, and have difficulty falling asleep drowsy but awake. He will protest at bedtime and fight falling asleep. Problems commonly occur (1) in the post-colic child who is dependent on the family bed and breast-feeding to sleep but now needs to sleep much earlier at night than the parents, (2) when parents use day care with a long commute time to bring the child home, causing a late bedtime, or (3) when dual-career families (see Chapter 11) have long commute times from work. In the first situation, the solution involves allowing your child to learn self-soothing. In the next two situations, solutions involve using others to help prepare the baby or child for bed (bathing, dressing for sleep, and feeding dinner) and, as early as possible, the parents beginning a *brief* bedtime routine. Although you will see your child less at night, you will have lovely morning time. To really enjoy the mornings, some parents will have to go to sleep earlier themselves! Other parents may be able to alter their work schedule to come home early on some days or do some of their work at home in the evenings after their child has gone to sleep. In one dual-career family, one parent was able to go to work extra early in order to come home earlier. Obviously, not all parents can come up with a complete solution, but a bedtime that is a little too late is preferable to one that is way too late. If a sleep debt accumulates during the week from a bedtime that is a little too late, try to focus on protecting naps and early bedtimes on weekends.

If circumstances cause your baby to go to bed too late, do the best you can, but try for the earliest bedtime possible.

One mother with an executive position said: "The reality of my job was that I would usually get home around 9:00 p.m. and try to put my child to bed around that time. Now I understand that she is looking drowsy around 7:00 p.m. I was able then to rearrange my schedule so that I could be at home to put my child to sleep around 8:00 p.m. She's sleeping so much better. It's not perfect, but it's my new reality."

NIGHT WAKINGS (SIGNALING), DIFFICULTY STAYING ASLEEP

Night waking normally occurs in all children; the real problem is failure to develop the ability to return to sleep unassisted after the awakening. All sleep problems eventually lead to night waking. The specific treatments depend on the child's age and are discussed in the appropriate age chapter.

In this age range, 4 to 12 months, night wakings are typically the complete arousals from sleep associated with disturbed sleep in post-colic babies and are discussed in Chapter 7. Other causes include severe eczema, chronic snoring associated with partial airway obstruction during sleep, general disorganization of sleep with chronic fatigue, or parental reinforcement of naturally occurring wakings.

Two separate groups of infants after 4 months of age seem especially prone to night waking. The first, larger group—about 20 percent of infants—includes those infants who had colic when they were younger. Not only do these infants awaken more often, but their total sleep time is less. Although boys and girls in this group awaken the same number of times, parents are more likely to state that it is their sons who have a night-waking problem. In fact, boys are handled in a more irregular way than girls when they awaken at night. This was shown in studies using video footage taken in dim light in the children's own bedrooms at home. Even when the colic either has or had been successfully treated with a drug (which is no longer used for colic due to safety concerns) during the first few months, by 4 months of age the children still were reported frequently awakening at night.

One possibility is that biological disturbances in infants can cause an overaroused, too wakeful, hyperalert, irregular state full of fussing and/or crying, especially in the late afternoon or early evening. In the past, the crying part of colic was thought to be the major problem, but as discussed in Chapter 7, fussiness is now considered to be a more common behavior. In any case, though evening crying generally diminishes at about 2 to 4 months, the wakeful, not-sleeping state may continue and thus is more serious and harmful in the long run.

This is because parents, defeated in the short term by colic, prematurely give up the effort to teach self-soothing. They do not realize that after 2 to 4 months of age, regular and consistent attention to bedtimes and nap times really does help their older infant sleep better. The parents' failure to develop and maintain healthy sleep patterns in these older post-colic babies then leads to prolonged fussiness driven by chronic fatigue.

Another possibility is that maternal anxiety leads to fragmented infant night sleep caused by unnecessary feedings at night over the first few months. The fragmented night sleep causes the infant to become overtired, and he fusses and cries more than well-rested infants. Even when biologic factors settle down after 2 to 4 months, the persistent maternal nighttime behavior mediates night waking in her baby. Of course, this is not an either-or scenario: both the child's nature and maternal nurturing practices influence sleep.

The second group of children with frequent night wakings after 4 months includes the approximately 10 percent who snore or breathe through their mouths during sleep (see Chapter 11). This difficulty in breathing during sleep might be due to allergies or large adenoids or tonsils. These infants awaken as frequently as do those with post-colic night waking, but their parents do not label this night waking as a problem. Probably the parents had not worried about night waking, because the infants had not suffered from colic. Those infants who snored also had shorter sleep durations than other infants. As in many sleep disturbances, when one element of healthy sleep is disrupted, other elements are disturbed. Please alert your child's health care provider if your child commonly snores or mouth-breathes during sleep.

Another cause of night waking in this age group is abnormal sleep schedules. Going to bed too late and getting up too late seems to set the stage for frequent night waking. This is especially common among mothers who like to sleep in late in the morning, and so keep their child up too late at night or do not rouse their child early enough in the morning. Sleeping out of phase with biological rhythms produces an overtired and hyperaroused child who has difficulty falling asleep and staying asleep. One child I cared for took two to two and a half hours of soothing, rocking, or holding before she would go to sleep, and then would usually awaken three to four times each night, sometimes as often as ten times. This prolonged period to put a child to sleep is called "increased latency to sleep." It's also called a waste of parents' time, and because the off/on twilight sleep for the child during the rocking, walking, and hugging is light sleep, it represents lost good-quality, restorative deep sleep. Correcting the sleep schedule quickly eliminated the night wakings and long latency to sleep, highlighting the importance of *when* sleep occurs and not just *how long* the sleep period lasts.

Fatigue causes increased arousal. Therefore, the more tired your child, the harder it is for him to fall asleep, stay asleep, or both.

One consequence of increased arousal at bedtime is that *disturbed sleep* produces more wakeful, irritable, and active behaviors during the day. Also, these children often have increased physical activity when asleep. Although all babies can have movements involving the entire body or localized movements or twitches involving only one limb, these are brief motions lasting only a second or less. But chronically fatigued babies who are overly aroused move around more in a restless, squirmy, crawly fashion when sleeping. It seems that their motor is always running at a higher speed, awake or asleep. I will explain how you can reduce your child's idle speed by making sure he gets the sleep he needs.

What is *disturbed sleep*?

Abnormal sleep schedules (going to bed too late, sleeping in too late in the morning, napping at the wrong times)

Brief sleep durations (not enough sleep overall)
Sleep fragmentation (waking up too often)
Nap deprivation (no naps or brief naps)
Prolonged latency to sleep (taking a long time to fall asleep)
Too active sleep (lots of tossing and turning)
Difficulty breathing during sleep

Disturbed sleep or night waking is *not* caused by:

Too much sugar in the diet
Hypoglycemia at night
Zinc deficiency
Pinworms
Gastroesophageal reflux

Teething, contrary to popular belief, does not cause night waking. If you ask parents what happens when teething occurs, the answer is everything! All illnesses, fevers, and ear infections that happen to occur around the time a tooth erupts are blamed on teething. Throughout medical history, doctors used the diagnosis "teething problems" as a smoke screen to hide their ignorance. In fact, at the turn of the twentieth century, 5 percent of deaths in children in England were misattributed to teething.

A proper study, by Dr. Arvi Tasanen, of problems caused by eruption of teeth was performed in Finland in 1968. Based on daily visits and the testing of 233 children between the ages of 4 and 30 months, he concluded that teething does not cause fevers, elevated white blood cell counts, or inflammation. Most important, teething did not cause night waking. Despite this study being published more than forty-five years ago, many parents and professionals still believe in this myth. Two separate studies by Dr. Melissa Wake and Dr. Michael Macknin in 2000 also found no association between infant teething and sleep, wakefulness, or sleep disturbances. Night waking between the ages of 6 and 18 months is more likely due to nap deprivation, fragmented night sleep, or abnormal sleep schedules—not teething.

> **Allowing your child to hold a bottle of milk or juice while falling asleep, or resting the bottle on a pillow when putting your baby to bed, will cause "baby-bottle cavities." Protect your child's teeth. Hold your baby in your arms when you give a bottle.**

Growing pains also do not cause night waking. One study examined 2,178 children between 6 and 19 years of age and found that 16 percent complained of severe pain localized deep in the arms or legs. Usually the pain was deep in the thighs, behind the knees, or in the calves. The pain usually occurred late in the afternoon or in the evenings. But when the growth rates of these affected children were compared to children without pain, there was no difference. In other words, growing pains do not occur during periods of rapid growth! Blaming night waking on growing pains is a handy excuse. But the rubbing, massaging, hot-water bottles, or other forms of parent soothing at night are really serving the emotional needs of the parent and/or child, not reducing organic pain.

Night waking may be caused by:

Fever
Painful ear infections
Atopic dermatitis (eczema; see Chapter 11)

If you think your child is ill, call the doctor. If your child has a diaper rash or eczema that is moderate or severe, consider using thick layers of zinc oxide paste in the diaper region so that no rash will develop when you do not go to your baby at night to change diapers. Ordinary mineral oil will make removal of the paste easier in the morning.

> **Do not attempt to correct unhealthy sleep habits unless you see a clear period ahead of several days when you will be in control.**

Don't trust most relatives or babysitters to do as good a job as you can to correct unhealthy sleep habits. Also, if your child's sleep improves during a training period but suddenly he becomes worse, appears ill, or seems to be in pain, let your pediatrician examine him for the possibility of an ear or throat infection.

COMMON NIGHT-SLEEP ISSUES

Brief Sleep Durations

If your child is on an apparently normal sleep schedule and napping well, you might presume she is getting enough sleep because she doesn't look tired, and thus you might decide that no adjustments regarding sleep will be needed. But then, around 10, 11, or 12 months, your child starts waking at night. What's happening?

Many times, physical and mental activity increases around 9 months. Your child is now moving around more, exploring more, becoming more active and independent. Also, there may have been a third nap that disappeared around 9 months, and afterward your child began to slowly acquire a sleep debt. The problem will often disappear when the bedtime is shifted to an earlier hour. Most families find that if they gradually shift the bedtime earlier in twenty-minute increments, they reach a time when night wakings melt away. Usually this change is easy for the baby, but sometimes it is hard for the parent who returns home late from work to accept that he or she will miss out on playtime with the baby due to the earlier bedtime. Just remember that small changes in sleep patterns often make big differences in sleep quality. Even a small change, as little as an additional *nineteen minutes* of sleep at the front end of the night, can cause a big change in your child's behavior during the day (see Chapter 1 and page 207 in Chapter 4).

Having More than One Child Creates Bedtime Problems

Experienced mothers often try to help their babies learn self-soothing from the day they come home from the hospital (see Chapter 3) in order to create more time to be with their first child. Still, there may be conflicts between the social needs of your older child and the nap or early bedtime needs of your baby. When there are such conflicts, try to strike a balance. For example, perhaps Mom or Dad has to go to an older child's soccer practice on one day, interfering with the baby's optimal nap time, while on another day the older child might be late to some event because it's important for the baby to finish his nap.

Also, an older child, about age 3 years, might not nap and will need to go to sleep fairly early, especially if he has had a very active day. His younger sister, about age 6 months, might be taking three naps and be able to stay up later. If the mother is by herself, she cannot ignore her baby and fully attend to her 3-year-old's earlier bedtime routine. Perhaps the solution is to eliminate the third nap for the baby so she goes down earlier, before her older brother, while the 3-year-old is playing by himself. Sometimes when the older child protests that he has to go to bed earlier than the baby, the solution is to tell the older child that because the baby naps, she can stay up later, and if he wants to nap like the baby, then he, too, can stay up later.

Fraternal twins who have different sleeping schedules, causing different bedtimes, are challenging to parents. Sometimes there is no solution except to put them down at about the same time; if there is any crying associated with falling asleep, then temporarily separate them. More information on twins can be found in Chapter 11 and in my book *Healthy Sleep Habits, Happy Twins*.

Unable to Fall Asleep

Young babies or children may have difficulty falling asleep except when they are in bed with their parents or in their arms. Most of these are children who had colic (see Chapter 5) or whose parents had used the family bed from the beginning. The "no-cry," "maybe-cry," and "let-cry" sleep solutions that may be helpful for these children are discussed in Chapter 4.

Will Not Sleep Anywhere Else

Maybe your baby sleeps well in your home but does not sleep well at Grandma's. Try to play the same music only at sleep times at both homes. Buy something soft and safe for your baby to feel or clutch, and use it only at sleep times at both homes. Spray some fragrance or perfume around the crib or bed only at sleep times at both homes. Try to use the same sleep schedules and nap time and bedtime routines at both homes.

Only One Bedroom

When your baby becomes more curious and aware of the sounds and movements of people around him, and you are using a crib, it might be time to move your baby to his own room. But what do you do if you don't have an additional bedroom? Some families have their baby sleep at night in their bedroom, then use a sofa bed to convert their living room into the parents' bedroom at night. In this way, the baby can go to bed early in a dark and quiet room, and the parents know that their nighttime sounds will not wake him.

> **Sleeping well is a 24/7 process. It's not just about how we get our children to go to bed at night without crying.**
>
> **Solving sleep problems may be a very tough prescription and demands a consistent approach.**
>
> **There may be increased crying in the beginning, but the upside is that crying around sleep will ultimately be eliminated altogether.**

If your child has a sleep problem that requires multiple changes but you are only able to make some of the changes, go ahead and do the best you can. Try to identify the major sleep issue and focus your attention on a solution that you feel comfortable with (see Chapter 4). Be consistent and patient. Anytime you make a change, allow at least four to five days before making another change, in order to see whether you have helped your child. Keeping a sleep log (see Chapter 4) is helpful to see objectively whether the change you made is helping, because you might be under such stress that you fail to see a little improvement in the beginning. For example, there may be protest crying at night that is unbearable for you, but the sleep log shows that for the very first time, your child took a substantially longer nap.

Day Sleep

Please review the sections "Consistency in Soothing Styles for Naps" and "Different Decisions for Different Babies" in Chapter 7.

DAY-SLEEP DURATION BY AGE

In my nap survey of children born between 1984 and 1986, starting at 6 months of age, I divided them into five nap duration groups (see below; each group represented about 20 percent of the children). I found that children typically remained in their initial nap duration group until 21–24 months. In other words, for babies whose average nap duration was 3 hours at 6 months of age, by 9 months it was 2.9 hours and by 12 months it was 2.8 hours; most did not move to a different nap duration group with much shorter or longer naps. Stated another way, children with long naps at 6 months of age continue to take long naps until 21–24 months, and the same is true for children with short or intermediate nap durations. So while there is a large variation in nap duration among children, there is also a stable tendency for nap durations for an individual child. This individual stability of nap durations probably reflects a *genetic* influence over sleep. Also, for the vast majority of infants, nap durations were restricted to narrower time frames (shown below) as the children got older, despite variations in caretaking and social activities. This suggests that *biologic* processes affect naps. Nevertheless, considering the actual minimum and maximum duration of naps, the wide total range of nap durations (shown below) suggests that *parents* do play an important role.

AVERAGE DAY-SLEEP DURATION

Initial Nap Duration Group (Hours)	6 months	9 months	12 months
1–2.5	2.3	2.7	2.5
3	3.0	2.9	2.8
3.5	3.5	3.1	3.1
4	4.0	3.2	3.2
More than 4	4.8	3.6	3.3

Most children nap within a narrow range:

At 6 months: for 80 percent of children, the range is between
    2.5 and 4.0 hours; 5 percent nap less than 2.5 hours and
    15 percent more than 4.0 hours.
At 9 months: for 93 percent of children, the range is between
    2.0 and 4.0 hours.
At 12 months: for 94 percent of children, the range is be-
    tween 2.0 and 4.0 hours.

Some children nap far outside the narrow range that occurs for
most children:

Minimum	1.0	1.0	1.5
Maximum	6.0	5.5	5.5

Average nap durations apply to groups only, of course, not individual children:

Average	3.5	3.1	3.0

As previously mentioned, post-colic children might be overrepre-
sented in the 20 percent of children in the shortest nap duration
group (1–2.5 hours), but the good news is that this is the only group
that did not show a decrease in nap duration between 6 and

9 months; in fact, their average nap duration *increased* from 2.3 to 2.7 hours, suggesting a slower maturation of day-sleep rhythms. This increase of *twenty-four minutes* may seem small, but we know that small changes in sleep can have a huge impact (see Chapter 1 and page 207 in Chapter 4). Although studies on large groups of children show no consistent relationship between the duration of daytime sleep and nighttime sleep, I think it is likely that most of the children who sleep near the minimum number of hours for naps have problems with night sleep and/or naps. This may also be true for some of the children who sleep near the maximum number of hours for naps, although I have encountered some very well-rested children, later determined to be highly intelligent, who had, at these young ages, very long naps.

You may have a well-rested child who does well with short naps, even though his fraternal twin wants long naps or your older child took long naps. Now that you appreciate how wide the nap duration range is, you can see how important it is to not compare your child's naps with other children's naps, because all children are a little different. No matter what the nap duration is for your child, all of these numbers are less important than your observation of whether or not your child is well rested.

NUMBER OF NAPS PER DAY BY AGE

In my nap survey of children born between 1984 and 1986, I asked how many naps were taken per day.

NAPS PER DAY BY AGE

Age (months)	Percentage of Children Taking 1, 2, or 3 Naps per Day		
	1/day	2/day	3/day
6	0%	84%	16%
9	4%	91%	5%
12	17%	82%	1%

By 9 months of age, the vast majority (91 percent) of children are taking two naps. As previously stated, these numbers are less important than how your child looks, but if your child is under 9 months of age and is taking only one nap or your child is over 9 months of age and taking three naps, his sleep schedule may be off and in need of adjustment.

DAY-SLEEP DURATION TRENDS OVER TIME

In addition to the previously discussed trend of bedtimes becoming later, causing less night sleep, data are available from studies by Dr. Price and me that show a trend for less day sleep over time. The cause of this shift is unknown.

AVERAGE DAY-SLEEP DURATION

1979–80	2004
3.2 hours (4–11 months)	3.0 hours (4–6 months)
	2.8 hours (7–9 months)
	2.6 hours (10–12 months)

COMMON DAY-SLEEP ISSUES

Nap Deprivation

When parents have invested the effort to create an age-appropriate sleep schedule and their child is well rested, occasional disruptions due to illness, trips, parties, or holiday visits cause only minor disruptions of sleep. The well-rested child requires only a brief recovery period—for example, a single reset—before getting back on track. But when parents allow poor-quality sleep patterns to emerge and persist, then significant sleep deficits accumulate gradually. Now even minor disturbances might create long-lasting havoc.

In this age range, nap deprivation seems to be a major culprit in ruining healthy sleep patterns. It's only natural that you want to get out more and do more things with your child, who is now full of

new social charms, cheerful, and crawling or maybe even walking . . . why not hang out together and enjoy the good weather at
the park or beach? Children at this age are fearless, full of grace and
self-confidence, and very explorative. Hanging out with parents and
siblings is simply a lot of fun for everyone. The main message is to
enjoy socializing out of the house but not so frequently that your
child is often shortchanged on day sleep.

Willfulness (self-agency) might lead your child to protest naps
because he would rather play than sleep. If you often allow him to
skip his nap, then he will become fatigued. The natural adaptive
response to fatigue is to fight it with stimulating hormones, which
allow him to maintain more wakefulness. However, this heightened
state of alertness or arousal creates an inability to easily fall asleep
or stay asleep for subsequent naps and night sleep. Not only does a
vicious circle of sleep problems begin, but your child may also develop emotional ups and downs or a reduced attention span as a
by-product.

If naps slip and slide too much, a trend of increasing fatigue
will clearly develop. First, the child becomes a little more crabby,
irritable, or fussy, maybe only in the late afternoon or early evening.
You might think it's normal for children this age to be easily frustrated or sometimes bored. Then he starts to get up at night for
the first time ever, "for no reason." Later, maybe following a cold or
a daylong visit with his grandparents, he starts fighting going to
sleep at night, and you wonder why night sleep is suddenly a problem.

When you reestablish healthy, regular nap routines, the witching
hour, bedtime battles, and night awakenings disappear. I have seen
this over and over again. That's why I think nap deprivation and not
a particular "stage" is the culprit behind disturbed night sleep.

**Sleep deprivation may appear as boredom. If your child's motor
is idling and she's not going anywhere, maybe she's short on
sleep.**

Some parents, unsure of when their child naturally shifts to need-ing only one nap, try to get by with one nap before their child is ready. If this occurs, late afternoons full of activities can help smooth over rocky moments of heightened emotionality or grumpi-ness. Anyway, Mom or Dad returns from work shortly thereafter, so there is a loving play period early in the evening.

However, the fatigue from nap deprivation eventually leads to increased levels of arousal and alertness, and this causes difficulties in falling asleep, staying asleep, or both. These changes in the direc-tion of disturbed sleep and behavioral changes during the day may be very gradual, so initially it may appear that a single nap is all right. The effects of persistent sleep deficits are cumulative, though, and eventually your fatigued child starts to behave differently.

Sometimes, the changes in behavior can be striking. For example, two children in my practice, 5 and 6 months of age, had severe bob-bing, turning, and jerking of the head and facial wincing or grimac-ing. The parents of both children were physicians and were worried about neurological problems. So both children were hospitalized and evaluated for seizures or epilepsy, but all the test results were normal. Nap deprivation turned out to be the problem, as I had al-ways suspected, and both children recovered completely when they were better rested, though the movements transiently returned for each child during a temporary period of overtiredness.

Here is one parent's account of how shortening the interval of wakefulness helped her child sleep better during the day.

In November, our third daughter, Rebecca, was born. At that time I prided myself on how well I schlepped our new baby everywhere and how wonderfully she slept in and out of the car seat all day.

Our days were filled with errands and car pools; Rebecca would be nursing and napping on and off all day. What a cooperative baby, I used to think. But I was so exhausted by evening that I found the only way to survive was to sleep with her, waking up every hour or so to shift her so that she could nurse on the other side. I knew then that having her in bed with me wasn't such a terrific idea, but it was the only way for me to get any rest.

When Rebecca turned 5 months old, I placed her in her crib instead of going to sleep with her at my breast. As I anticipated, every few hours she began to cry, expecting me to be by her side. I would quickly run into her room and rock and nurse her back to sleep ... until the next time she woke up.

And so our next pattern began. She would wake up every few hours, and I would faithfully run in and get her back to sleep. I was certain she would grow out of this bad habit ... our other two had.

A few months passed. By now Rebecca was weaned to a bottle and I was sure things would change for the better. That didn't happen. In fact, things got worse. There were many nights when Rebecca would get up every hour on the hour. I tried letting her cry, fifteen minutes at a time, but it was much easier to just go in and give her a bottle.

When Rebecca was 1 year old, this pattern of frequent waking continued. It was difficult leaving her with a babysitter on the occasional evening we went out. I knew that within an hour or so of our leaving she would be up crying for me. I actually felt sick leaving her.

When Rebecca was almost 13 months old we went to see Dr. Weissbluth. When we left his office I felt prepared for battle—armed with all the mental ammunition I needed to change Rebecca's nightly wakings. We started the program of shorter intervals of wakefulness the next day.

In a week's time, the change in Rebecca was phenomenal! She was always a happy baby, but when she began to sleep better, she became even more relaxed, more affectionate, and more fun to be with.

The change in her sleeping pattern has had an effect on everyone in the family. I don't yell and lose my patience with my older children quite as much, for I am better rested and I feel so much better physically and emotionally.

This has been one of the most rewarding and positive experiences that we have shared as parents. We are so proud of Rebecca and also pat ourselves on the backs for a job well done.

Shhh! Rebecca's sleeping!

As this mother wrote, "She was always a happy baby, but when she began to sleep better, she became *even more relaxed, more affectionate, and more fun to be with.*" Parents are usually skeptical that their charming and sweet baby can become even more so with healthier sleep. But it's true!

The treatment strategy to go back to two naps involves (1) shortening the interval of wakefulness *before* the first nap and reestablishing the midday nap by making sure the wakeful period after the midmorning nap is not too long, (2) making sure the midday nap does not start too late in the afternoon, in order to protect a reasonable evening bedtime, and (3) consistency in the nap time ritual. Don't disrupt your efforts by allowing your child to stay up too late before bedtime. If you do, he is likely to become overtired and overaroused, and will experience disturbed night sleep, which in turn means he will start the day short on sleep.

It's not uncommon for a child to sleep well at night but not nap well, especially in the afternoon. At night it is dark, everyone is more tired, and parents want to be regular with bedtimes because they want to enjoy each other's company or just go to sleep themselves. During the day, it is light, everyone is more alert, and parents are more irregular because they want to run errands or enjoy recreational activities.

So during a training period, it's easiest to establish good night sleep than naps, and easier to establish regular midmorning naps than midday naps. Don't expect improvement to occur equally at all times. Still, it's best to implement a twenty-four-hour sleep retraining program, because if you focus only on one feature, such as bedtime, and ignore naps, you will be less likely to succeed.

In general, I recommend a twenty-four-hour sleep package to help restore healthy sleep habits. Here is an example of an exception. A single mother has limited resources for soothing and is completely exhausted. The child does not sleep well day or night. The mother wants to continue breast-feeding, but now she wants to transition the baby from her bed to a crib. The first step might only be a temporarily ultra-early bedtime in the mother's bed to help the child get more sleep. Everything else stays the same. The advice is to do whatever is necessary to maximize sleep and minimize crying during the day. After the child is a little better rested, the second step might be to make the transition to the crib. This might involve crying, but because both child and mother are better rested, the crying may be very little and the mother is more able to cope. The third step is to work on naps. This will now be easier because everyone is better rested. If, instead, this mother had an enormous support system to help her soothe the baby, she might try to do everything at the same time. Her child might become better rested faster, and the greater stress in making all these changes abruptly would be shared by people other than the mother.

Some families have found it difficult to establish naps because their bedrooms are too bright or noisy during the day. One family I know was fortunate enough to have a large walk-in closet, which they furnished like a little bedroom and which was used only for naps. Other families have problems because they live in a one-bedroom apartment and it is difficult for anyone to sleep well when a child shares a bedroom with the parents. These parents sometimes relocate to the living room and turn the bedroom over to the child so that the entire family can stay well rested. If you do not want to have a family bed, expect it to become difficult for your child to sleep well in your room. Plan ahead, before the family becomes overtired.

As long as your child retains the expectation that she can convince you to play during nap time, she won't nap well. If she thinks she can outlast you, she won't give up her protesting.

Fixing Nap Schedules

When the bedtime hour and sleep periods are not in synchrony with other biological rhythms, we don't get the full restorative benefit of sleep. Please refer to Figures 5 and 6 (page 41) for age-appropriate times when children fall asleep or awaken.

At any age, abnormal sleep schedules can lead to night wakings and night terrors in older children. The schedule often gets shifted to a too-late bedtime hour because Mom or Dad (or both), returning late from work, wants to play with their baby. Or parents deliberately keep their baby up late in a misguided attempt to encourage a later awakening in the morning. Or perhaps they discovered that if they kept their baby up late, their child would eventually crash due to exhaustion, and in this way they avoided stressful bedtime battles. Or there may be parent issues (see Chapter 3) causing a late bedtime.

The strategy for bringing sleep schedules back to normal is based on developing an age-appropriate wake-up at 6:00 or 7:00 a.m.; a midmorning nap around 9:00 a.m.; a midday nap, usually around 12:00 to 1:00 p.m., but always starting before 3:00 p.m.; an early bedtime, 6:00 to 8:00 p.m.; and consolidated night sleep. This package of advice ensures good sleep quality, and it is quality, not just quantity, that really matters.

MAJOR POINT

The major fear that inhibits parents from establishing an earlier bedtime is that this will cause their child to get up earlier to start the day. In fact, the opposite will occur. An earlier bedtime will allow your child to sleep later, just as a too-late bedtime will eventually cause a too-early wake-up time. Remember, sleep begets sleep. This is not logical, but it *is* biological.

Q: *Why do you recommend 6:00 to 8:00 p.m. as an appropriate bedtime?*

A: Survey data from my earlier research showed that the vast majority of children between the ages of 4 and 12 months went to sleep between 7:00 and 9:00 p.m., and so I used to recommend those hours. However, as I have helped families correct sleep problems over the past thirty-five years, it has become clearer that children who go to bed earlier tend to not develop sleep problems in the first place. In addition, children in this age range who did have sleep problems almost always benefited from an earlier bedtime. I think we have simply grown accustomed to having overtired children in the evening hours, and because it is so common, we have assumed that fussiness or irritability near the end of the day is normal. Imagine what a "normal" bedtime was before candles, kerosene lamps, electric lights, radio, television, videos, commuting, smartphones, or dual-income families traveling from work to day care to home.

A reasonably early bedtime means that your child wakes up well rested and is better able to nap. So think of an early bedtime and consolidated night sleep as prerequisites for good naps. Naps can be established or reestablished by the nap drill and controlling the wake-up time (see Chapter 4), and by focusing on consistency in soothing style for naps (see Chapter 7).

It's up to *you* to enforce an age-appropriate nap and bedtime schedule. Your child initially may not cooperate by falling asleep immediately. Don't give up.

Studies have shown that when sleep disturbances are associated with abnormal sleep schedules, control of the wake-up time may be sufficient to establish a healthy twenty-four-hour sleep rhythm. In other words, *you* set the clock in the morning!

Nap patterns are as varied as children themselves, family sizes, and parental lifestyles. One 5-month-old always awoke briefly at 6:00 a.m. and then promptly returned to sleep until 10:00 a.m. A long midday nap occurred from noon to 3:00 p.m. and a brief nap from 5:00 to 5:45 p.m. Between 7:30 and 8:00 p.m. the child went to sleep for the night, until about 6:00 the following morning. This child was well rested, and the midday nap coincided with his older brother's single nap. For the time being, this pattern met both children's sleep needs. By 6 or 7 months, this child developed the more common pattern of a midmorning nap and a midday nap.

However, other children whose naps are not in sync with biologic rhythms begin to accumulate a sleep deficit that grows, often slowly, over time. Eventually, daytime mood or behavior problems develop, as do sleep disturbances at night.

Please review "Choose a Sleep Solution" in Chapter 4.

A temporary disturbance or mild variation in sleep schedules, nap patterns, amount of sleep, or early awakenings may not be worth changing. But if chronic or severe problems cause your child to become tired, then try to help your baby become more rested. Watch your child's behavior, not some inflexible schedule.

SLEEP RECOMMENDATIONS

Recall Lisa Matricciani's point from her 2013 review of the literature that published recommendations for children's sleep are not based on empirical evidence, and that "*sleep timing* [the time when sleep occurs] may be even more important than *sleep duration*."

The take-home message is that what is common regarding bedtimes and naps among your relatives, friends, and neighbors might not be what is right for your child. See Chapters 1 and 9 for more information on sleep recommendations.

Commonly occurring sleep patterns among your relatives, friends, and neighbors might not fit your child. Ignore what they

recommend and what you read about bedtimes, naps, and total sleep needs and instead *watch your child*. Don't be surprised if your child needs an earlier bedtime and/or takes longer naps than other children.

When your child sleeps might be more important than *how long* your child sleeps.

MONTHS 4–8

Midday nap from 12:00 to 2:00 p.m.; and a variable late afternoon nap around 3:00–5:00 p.m. develops.

As months 3 and 4 blend into months 5 to 8, your child's behavior slowly changes toward increased sociability, which permits more playfulness and gamelike interactions between you and your infant. Your child may roll over, sit, imitate your voice with babbling, or respond quickly to your quiet sounds. This increased social interaction certainly makes having a baby more fun.

Infants really do enjoy their parents' company; they thrive in response to your laughter and smiles. However, your baby is not like an empty vessel you can fill with love, warmth, hugs, kisses, and soothing until it is full, thus leading to satisfaction, blissful contentment, or undemanding repose. The more you entertain her, the more she will want to be amused. So it is natural and reasonable to expect your baby to protest when you stop playing with her. In fact, the more you play with your child, the more she will come to expect that this is the natural order of things. Nothing is wrong with this, except that there are times when you have to dress your baby or leave her to amuse herself for a while, and she will probably resist the partial restraint needed for dressing or the curtailment of fun and games. When this happens, please remember that leaving your baby alone protesting for more fun with you while you get dressed is not the same thing as abandonment! Similarly, leaving your baby alone protesting for more fun when she needs to sleep is not neglect. You have become sensitive to your child's need to sleep, and she is now old enough for you to recognize and respect her internal timing mechanism for naps. Our goal is to synchronize caretaking activities with your child's needs to be fed, to be kept warm, to be played with, and to sleep.

After 4 months of age, an infant's sleep becomes more like an adult's. Younger infants enter sleep with a period of REM sleep, but around 4 months, like adults, they begin to enter sleep with a non-REM sleep period. Sleep cycling, from deep to light non-REM sleep with interruptions of REM sleep, also matures into adultlike patterns around 4 months of age.

As discussed previously, the five elements of healthy sleep are (1) sleep duration (night and day), (2) naps, (3) sleep consolidation, (4) sleep schedule, and (5) sleep regularity. Now let's look at Figure 7. This circle graph is a navigational aid for parents to help them understand sleep/wake rhythms. Although I designed this graph, I did not create it any more than a mapmaker creates the shape or location of an island. As your child gets older, the times when he will become sleepy become more predictable. Another way of saying this is that the biological sleep/wake rhythms mature. This allows you to change your strategy for keeping your child well rested. Previously, the focus was on *brief intervals of wakefulness* to avoid the overtired state; now you can begin to use *clock time* as an aid to help your child sleep well. Some parents call this sleeping "by the clock," or BTC. Stated simply, you are using your child's natural sleep rhythms to help him fall asleep.

Data for the circular graph below were derived from my research in the late 1970s on children living in northern Indiana and Illinois. The ranges for the wake-up time are about 6:00–8:00 a.m.; the first nap takes place about 9:00–10:00 a.m., and the second nap about 12:00–2:00 p.m. The range for the bedtime includes 8:00 p.m., but this time is too late for children who have brief naps and/or no third nap.

You want your child to sleep well by synchronizing parent-set

Figure 7: Healthy Sleep Schedule for Infants 4 to 8 Months Old

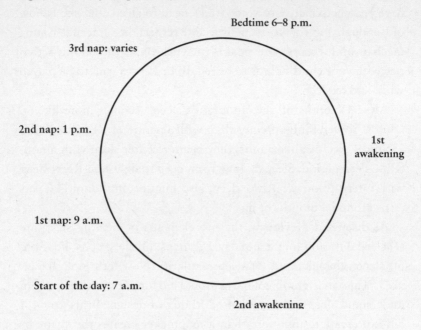

naps and bedtimes with the sleep schedule set by your child's developing internal timing mechanism. Let's start in the morning and go around the clock.

Wake-up Time in the Morning

Some babies tend to wake up early, 5:00 or 6:00 a.m., and return to sleep after a brief feeding or diaper change. This is a true continuation of night sleep and not a nap. Other babies wake up later and start the day then. Most children will awaken to start the day about 7:00 a.m., but there is a wide range (between 6:00 and 8:00). In general, it is not a good idea to go to your child to start the day before 6:00 a.m., even if he is crying, because if you do, he will begin to force himself to wake up earlier and earlier in order to enjoy your company. The natural wake-up time seems to be an independent, neurological alarm clock in these young infants that is somewhat independent of the part of the brain that puts them to sleep or keeps them asleep. In fact, despite what is commonly believed, you usually *cannot* change the wake-up time by keeping your baby up later, feeding solids before bedtime, or awakening your baby for a feeding before you go to sleep. The last seems insensitive, anyway. How would you feel if someone woke you from a deep sleep and started to feed you when you weren't hungry?

When your child is well rested and has no disturbed sleep, an early wake-up hour may be inconvenient but not necessarily changeable. If your child is near his first birthday, you might consider some of the items discussed in the next chapter on older children.

When the Wake-up Time Is Too Early

Make sure that the bedroom is dark and quiet in the morning. Window-darkening shades and a white-noise machine or noise from a humidifier will help reduce the startling effect of street noises. Keep a sleep log to help find the best bedtime.

The most common cause for waking up too early before 4 months of age is extreme fussiness/colic (see Chapter 5); after 4 months, it is a too-late bedtime.

If you suspect the bedtime is too late but are not sure because your child does not appear dramatically overtired, slowly move the bedtime earlier. Try twenty minutes earlier for four nights to see whether your child will fall asleep at the earlier time and sleep in later. Do everything you currently are doing at bedtime, but simply start the bedtime routine earlier. If this seems to help a little, repeat the process, making the bedtime an additional twenty minutes earlier for four more nights. You can repeat this process until it is clear that you have reached a too-early bedtime because your child no longer easily and promptly falls asleep. Now you might want to return to the last step and let your child stay up an additional twenty minutes. This gradual shift in bedtime may produce no protest crying.

If you are more confident that the bedtime is too late because your child appears tired much earlier, then move the bedtime much earlier right away; a slightly earlier bedtime might not help and only frustrate you. The abrupt shift may or may not produce protest crying. Review the "no-cry," "maybe-cry," and "let-cry" sleep solutions in Chapter 4. It will probably be necessary to ignore your child until 6:00–7:00 a.m. For younger children, the option of bringing them to your bed for soothing may produce extra Z's in the morning, but after 6 months this is more likely to be stimulating than soothing.

Sometimes, after 4 months, a child is already going to bed very early, around 5:30 or 6:00 p.m., and this causes the entire schedule to shift: too early a wake-up time causes too-early or poorly timed naps and a very tired child in the late afternoon who goes to sleep easily very early in the evening (see "The 5:30 Bedtime Rut" in Chapter 4). For young children, it may help to simultaneously move their bedtime a little later, maybe twenty to thirty minutes every four nights, and ignore them until about 6:00 a.m. If you move the bedtime abruptly too late, your child might become so overtired that instead of the wake-up time becoming later, she simply wakes up more overtired.

> **Finding the bedtime that is just right for your child might require some back-and-forth adjustments; make one change and then wait four days to see whether it helps. And *be patient*.**

Morning Time Awake

Morning wakeful time will last about two hours for 4- to 5-month-olds or about three hours for 8-month-olds. Some easy babies or babies born early may be able to stay up for only one hour at 4 months of age. In that case, plan a wind-down or nap time routine of up to thirty minutes. You decide what you want to do: bath, bottle, breast-feeding, lullaby, massage—but limit it, because spending hours holding your baby produces only a light or twilight sleep state, which is poor-quality sleep. Begin this routine as drowsy signs emerge (see Chapter 3) or just before they are expected, about half an hour or less *before* the end of your baby's wakeful period, not after it's over. At the end of your predetermined nap time routine, whether your baby is asleep or awake, lie down with her (see co-sleeping and SIDS warning in Chapter 1) or put her in her crib. As one mother commented to me, "I cannot tell you what a liberating experience it was to be able to put my baby down in her crib before she fell asleep in my arms." Your baby may now cry a little, a lot, or not at all.

The temperamentally easy child cries very little, and the routine is repeated for a midday nap. The temperamentally more difficult child, who may have also been an extremely fussy/colicky infant, might now cry a lot. The preemie also may cry a lot, and if so, the following approach might be delayed until 4 months after the expected date of delivery.

Nap #1: Midmorning

There are "windows" of clock time for naps. When your child is awake, watch your baby *and the clock* to determine the time when it is easiest for your child to take an age-appropriate nap. The nap windows of "sleep propensity" open and close, and they represent times during which it is easiest to fall asleep and stay asleep.

This midmorning nap develops first, usually between 12 and 16 weeks of age, counting from the due date. It occurs about 9:00 a.m. and may last an hour or two. Sometimes you can stretch your child's morning wakeful period by a few minutes each day to get to this time, or you might wake him up at 7:00 a.m. in order for him to be able to take this nap. This violation of the rule "Never wake a sleeping baby" is to help maintain an age-appropriate sleep schedule for the benefit of the baby. The rule mainly applies to waking babies for our social convenience, but to their detriment. Try to anticipate your child's best nap time. If he takes this nap too early or too late, then it may be difficult for him to take the second nap on time.

Consider a sleep period to be a restorative nap if it is about an hour or longer. Forty to forty-five minutes is sometimes enough, but most babies in this age range sleep at least a solid hour. Sleep periods shorter than thirty minutes should not count as good-quality naps.

If you are using method A for naps (see Chapter 7) or have a temperamentally easy baby, after putting your baby down for this nap leave him completely alone for no more than one hour to allow him to (1) learn to fall asleep unassisted and (2) return to sleep unassisted until he has slept about an hour in an uninterrupted fashion. Easy babies may cry very little or not at all; the temperamentally more difficult child may cry a lot. Remember, you are responding sensitively to his need to sleep by not providing too much attention. You are decisive in establishing a routine because you are upholding his right to sleep. Be calm and firm and consistent, because *consistency helps your baby learn rapidly.*

He will pick up on your calm, firm attitude and will learn quickly not to expect the pleasure of your company at nap time. You are not abandoning your child in his moment of need; you are giving him all the attention he needs when he is awake. Now he needs to be alone to sleep. Please review, if needed, the prevention of nap problems (Chapter 3) and treatment for them (Chapter 4), and why consistency in soothing for naps may be helpful (Chapter 7).

Q: *How long do I let my baby cry?*
A: No more than one hour.

Q: *What do I do if the nap is short? When I put my child down to sleep, she cries a long time, but for less than an hour, and then falls asleep, but she doesn't sleep very long. Do I let her cry again? Sometimes she doesn't cry when I put her down for a nap, but she still doesn't sleep very long. Do I let her cry after the brief nap to see if she will sleep longer?*
A: If the nap is substantially less than thirty minutes, you might

try to leave her alone for an additional thirty to sixty minutes, even if she cries, to see whether she will return to sleep unassisted. If the nap is substantially more than thirty minutes, it is less likely that she will return to sleep unassisted, so you might want to leave her alone for an additional thirty minutes or go to her immediately and not let her cry anymore. In general, the shorter the nap and the less restorative it appears, the longer you should leave her alone to see if she will return to sleep unassisted. Alternatively, you might want to try to lengthen the nap by rushing to your child at the first sound of awakening from a brief nap (less than an hour) and attempting to soothe her back to sleep for a continuation of the nap. However, especially over 6 months of age, this might be counterproductive and simply stimulate your child to fight sleep more for the pleasure of your company.

Q: *After one hour of crying, what do I do?*
A: Go to your baby and soothe her. Now you have two choices. Your baby might remain wakeful, and you might decide that this was so stressful for you or her that you want to go outside for a walk, relax, and try again the next day to get a midmorning nap. Or after all this crying your baby might be falling asleep in your arms when you pick her up; if you feel that she will now be able to fall asleep, put her back down to see if she will nap. But do not let her cry any more if this new attempt fails.

Q: *What's wrong if I quickly check my baby when she first cries, and I give her a pacifier or roll her back over? She always immediately stops crying and returns to sleep.*
A: Checking on your baby like this when she should be napping may not interfere with naps or night sleep in some infants between 4 and 6 months. But please be careful, because eventually all babies learn to turn these brief visits into prolonged playtimes. This learning process may develop more slowly if it is the

father who does the checking and provides minimal intervention.

Q: *My child had extreme fussiness/colic. Now she is about 5 months old. How do I get her on a 9:00 a.m. and 1:00 p.m. nap schedule?*
A: Make sure she is sleeping well at night. Control the wake-up time; try to start the day around 6:00 to 7:00 a.m. by not going to her before 6:00 a.m. or by waking her up at 7:00 a.m. if she is still sleeping. Try intense but brief stimulation outdoors. Expose her to wind, rustling leaves, moving clouds, street noises, voices, barking dogs, sand in the playground, motion in the jogger or soft sling on your chest, swings, splashing in a swimming pool, and so forth. Try to stretch her wakeful period to about 9:00 a.m., but be mindful not to allow her to become so frantically over-tired that she will not be able to subsequently sleep well. She will get a little geared up, and initially she might get close to but not make it to 9:00 a.m. Tone it down a little as you get close to 9:00 a.m. Plan for a much longer and relaxing soothing-to-sleep routine before her midmorning nap, because she will be a little overtired. Consider including a bath for relaxation, not for hygiene. Bathing might be stimulating, but more often it is calm fun for babies. Around 9:00 a.m., lie down to sleep with her (see co-sleeping and SIDS warning in Chapter 1) or put her down to sleep. If she has a decent nap of close to one hour, repeat the same steps for her 1:00 p.m. nap. If she does not nap in the morning, get out of the house and try to not let her sleep until about 11:00 a.m. Try the same soothing-to-sleep routine around 11:00 a.m. This means no car rides at 10:00 a.m.

Parents of post-colic babies or babies with a more difficult temperament might want to begin to practice method A (see Chapter 7) at this time. Many of these parents have been using method B (your baby always begins naps in deep sleep with your help). Ideally, you have been very consistent with method B up until now, because the better rested your baby is when you make the transition from method B to method A, the easier it will be.

WARNING

It may be very difficult to establish regular naps at 4 to 5 months of age in some babies because their biological nap rhythms are maturing very slowly. Some babies don't evolve into a schedule of regular long naps until 5 or 6 months of age, especially if they had extreme fussiness/colic when younger or if their parents were inconsistent or irregular about naps during the first 4 months.

Focus on the Midmorning Nap

For the difficult-temperament or post-colic baby, establishing the midmorning nap may be the toughest parenting maneuver that you have attempted so far. By focusing on the midmorning nap we try to help a post-colic baby learn self-soothing skills. It's best to begin establishing an age-appropriate nap schedule with the midmorning nap because it is the first one to develop; it is the nap that should be the easiest to obtain, because your baby is most rested from the night sleep, and parents usually can be more consistent in the early morning, when scheduling conflicts are less likely to develop compared to the afternoon. After your child's day starts, look at the clock. *Within one hour of waking,* you will want to clean him, feed him, and then begin to soothe him using method A. If there is bright morning light during this hour, open up all your shades, because exposure to morning light might help establish sleep rhythms. If there is no bright natural light, make the room as bright as you can with room lights. Darken the room as you begin your soothing to sleep. After several minutes of soothing, which may include feeding, put your baby down to sleep. Remember, the soothing also occurs within the one-hour period of wakefulness. This ultra-short period of wakefulness is designed to prevent the overtired state from developing. Another reason it is important to establish the midmorning nap by keeping the interval of wakefulness very short is that the midmorning nap might represent a continuation of night sleep. The midmorning nap contains more REM sleep than the midday nap, and large amounts of REM sleep are a characteristic feature of a baby's night sleep. Eventually, this midmorning nap will be gradually and slowly delayed until about 9:00 a.m.

Q: *What if my child wants to go to sleep but is unable to do so?*
A: Here is a report from a mother who observed that her child was "so sleep deprived he could not go to sleep. . . . Though he seemed to want to go to sleep, he appeared unable to get there."

I'll never forget the night and early morning at about 3 months of age when Eric was so sleep deprived he could not go to sleep. I tried everything—nursing, rocking, walking, bouncing, and singing. Eventually he did fall asleep while I pushed him around the house in the stroller listening to his favorite CD, only to wake up the second I tried to move him into his crib. The hours stretched on and Eric became more and more tired, overstimulated, and agitated. He began trying to pick the flowers off my pajamas. Though he seemed to want to go to sleep, he appeared unable to get there. I felt I didn't have any choice but to put him in his crib, awake and crying. After about twenty minutes of crying, he fell asleep.

He did best with his first midmorning nap, crying only one or two minutes, if at all, before going to sleep. The evenings remained the most difficult. The longest crying episode was twenty-one minutes. My husband and I would sit in the den holding hands, listening to the baby monitor, and engaging in self-doubt: "Does he need us? Are we bad parents for letting him cry?" We kept reminding ourselves that Eric was learning a valuable skill that would serve him (and us!) well for life. After about three days, we felt he had achieved suc-

cess. He has been a terrific sleeper ever since. Now, at age 11 months, he sleeps from 7:00 p.m. to 7:00 a.m. and naps twice for an hour or two. Everyone who meets him says he is happy, joyful, and alert.

This story describes the hyperaroused state caused by lack of sleep that interferes with sleeping well. It becomes a vicious circle. To prevent or correct this problem, consider rereading the parent reports about successfully helping babies with extreme fussiness/colic at ages as young as 8 weeks in Chapter 4 and babies with common fussiness/crying at ages as young as 3–4 weeks in Chapters 3 and 5.

If there is crying when you put your child down for a nap and you cannot leave your child for one hour, ignore the crying for between five and twenty minutes. You be the judge of how much crying you think is appropriate, but watch the clock, because three minutes of hard crying might feel to you like three hours. The reason you might not let your difficult-temperament or post-colic baby cry for an hour, as you might with an easy-temperament baby, is that they have increased difficulty falling asleep unassisted. Parents of these babies are usually extra stressed as well. I would, however, like to point out that some babies scream their brains out for two minutes, moan and whimper for three minutes, and then go to sleep for a great nap! You might lose the chance for a long nap if you do not let your child blow off steam for a minute or two. As before, when you feel there has been enough crying, rescue your child and try again the next day—or maybe put him back down if you think he will now go to sleep. For the remainder of the day, try to keep each interval of wakefulness to no more than two hours, or do whatever works to maximize sleeping and minimize crying.

An alternative to putting children in their crib for naps is to sleep with them in your bed (see co-sleeping and SIDS warning, Chapter 1). This may work well for first-time mothers who do not have other children to care for. However, as your child becomes older, she becomes more aware of her environment while awake, drowsy, and asleep. So you might have to use a co-sleeper next to your bed to ensure that your child is not stimulated by your body movements, coughing, or snoring.

Midmorning Nap Problems

Morning Nap Is Absent, Too Short, Too Long, or at the Wrong Time

The midmorning nap develops at 3 to 4 months of age in 80 percent of all children and a few months later in the 20 percent of children who had colic.

Sometimes the midmorning nap does not develop because the bedtime is way too late and your baby sleeps in too late in the morning to take a nap around 9:00 a.m., or he wakes up too early to make it until nine o'clock.

Sometimes the midmorning nap is short because that is all the sleep your child needs at that time—that is, your child is a short napper. As discussed earlier, about 20 percent of children between 6 and 21 months always have short naps in the morning and afternoon, no matter what parents do. These children may be well-rested. In contrast, midmorning naps for other children between 6 and 9 months of age may be short, and the child may take many such short naps—or, as one mother called them, "snaps"—throughout the day. These children often appear tired even though the bedtime is early. However, as long as the bedtime is early, by 9 to 12 months most of these children are taking fewer and longer naps and no longer appear tired. I think that most of these short or irregular nappers are those who had colic when younger, and their biologic nap rhythms need a longer time to mature, so their naps are actually longer at 9 months than at 6 months.

The most common cause of an absent or a too-short midmorning nap may be an interval of wakefulness that is too long between the wake-up time and the beginning of the nap. For the child under 4 months of age, sometimes starting the midmorning nap after only one hour of wakefulness allows the child to be soothed back to sleep before she becomes overtired. In an older child, starting the nap at the wrong time, either too early or too late, may either shorten the nap or make it less restorative; then it messes up the rest of the day. Use the midmorning nap rhythm as an aid to help your child sleep. If needed, stretch the interval of wakefulness, using approximately 9:00 a.m. as your target time. You might only get to 8:30 or 8:45 a.m. because your child is becoming overtired. It's a balancing act: you want to start the nap when the biological nap time begins, but you also want to avoid the overtired state. You are willing to allow the child to become a little overtired but not to become so wigged out that he has great difficulty falling asleep (see "Competing Goals" in Chapter 4).

Sometimes an older brother or sister has a scheduled activity that interferes with the midmorning nap. Some options are to try to get relatives or a neighbor to watch your younger child at home while you drive your older child to the activity, or try to carpool to reduce the number of days per week your younger child misses out on a good midmorning nap. Often the younger child might fall asleep in the car seat during the drive; then the parent can allow the child to continue to nap in the car seat, either in the parked car or when the car seat is placed in the crib. Transferring your child to the crib usually awakens her and ends the nap. It looks awkward to us, but many young children appear to sleep well in the cozy car seat.

Sometimes the wake-up time is too late because the bedtime is too late and your child cannot fall asleep at 9:00 or 10:00 a.m. for a nap. Controlling the wake-up time (see Chapter 4) simply means waking your child around 7:00 a.m. in order to get a good-quality nap to begin around 9:00 a.m. To avoid an overtired child, the bedtime will also have to be moved earlier. Parents may not like this solution, perhaps because they like to play with their child late at night or they like to sleep later in the morning.

If the midmorning nap is too long or too late in the morning, it may interfere with your child's ability to fall asleep easily around

12:00 to 2:00 p.m. for the second nap, and the result is an overtired child by late afternoon. The reason the midmorning nap is too long or too late is usually because the bedtime is too late. Limiting the midmorning nap to one to two hours by waking your child is necessary because it is important to protect the second nap. But many parents reject this suggestion because sleep is so precious! So it becomes essential to move the bedtime earlier, which will cause your child to awaken in the morning better rested, and this will then automatically shorten the midmorning nap.

NAP HINTS

Before the midmorning or midday nap, go outside to briefly but intensely stimulate your child with physical activity at the park or in the sandbox; expose your child to light, wind, clouds, voices, music, traffic sounds; go for rides in the jogger or stroller. Then tone it down as you get near nap time. Now spend an extra-long time soothing; if your child finds baths soothing, include one in the nap time routine. Make the room dark and quiet.

Midmorning Time Awake

Expect your baby to be ready for another nap after two to three hours of wakefulness, depending on the length of the midmorning nap and whether your child is closer to 4 months or 12 months. In general, avoid long excursions, which might lead to mini-snoozes in the car or park. Although I've been emphasizing sleep rhythms, remember that there are also wake rhythms—times during the day when the body clock automatically switches to a wakeful mode, just as it switches to sleep mode at night and at nap times. Wakefulness turns on as sleep turns off. The development of wakefulness is an active process; it is not just the turning off of sleep. During a wakeful mode, it is hard to fall asleep or stay asleep. Very tired children will sleep during the wakeful mode, but sleep quality during a wakeful mode—the ability of the sleep period to restore alertness and a sense of well-being—is lower compared to the same amount of sleep occurring during a sleep mode; that is, the sleep is less restorative. The result is similar to jet lag syndrome. It is equally important to sleep during the biologic sleep mode and not sleep during the wakeful mode. If your child did not take a midmorning nap, do not allow him to take a snooze in the car or stroller at a time when he should be awake, because if your baby naps when he should be awake, it will throw the remaining sleep/wake schedule for the day off kilter.

For adults, there is a dramatic wakeful mode associated with a period of physical relaxation between about 6:00 and 9:00 p.m. Even if you are drowsy or sleep deprived, it is hard to fall asleep during this time. This distinct zone of decreased sleepiness or increased arousal during the early evening hours has been called the "forbidden zone" for sleep. This wakeful period has been recognized by the television industry, which calls it "prime time." This is the time when most adults do not and cannot sleep. Recent research also shows that there is also a "forbidden zone" for sleep in infants (see page 304).

MAJOR POINT
It is as important to not let children sleep when they are in a biological wakeful mode as it is to help them sleep when they are in a biological sleep mode.

Usually if a nap doesn't occur, it is best to keep your baby awake and go to the next sleep period, whether it is another nap or nighttime sleep. Probably this next sleep period will take place a little earlier because of the missed nap. Try to strike a balance between not letting your child become extremely overtired by keeping him up, and at the same time preserving or protecting the age-appropriate sleep pattern.

Nap #2: Midday, Early Afternoon

The second nap usually occurs between noon and 2:00 p.m., most commonly around 1:00 p.m., but in any case it should usually begin before 3:00 p.m. in order to not interfere with an early bedtime. The nap should last about an hour or two. Please remember, this is an *outline* of a reasonable, age-appropriate, healthy sleep pattern, *not a set of rigid rules*. In order to describe sleep patterns, we have to use clock time and the number of hours of sleep, but it is more important to watch your baby than to watch the clock. There is nothing absolute about napping at 1:00 p.m. or any other time in this sleep schedule. You'll have to make some adjustments to fit your own lifestyle and family arrangements. There will be special occasions when your child does not get the sleep he needs. But he will recover from these exceptions faster if you have a regular pattern on most days. The problem with some families is that they never establish a regular pattern, so the child is always somewhat overtired, and exceptional days of missed naps create more extreme overtired behavior. The return to baseline in these children, which is slightly overtired behavior, is slow and stressful for families.

The midday nap commonly continues until the third birthday, but after age 3 it begins to drop out.

Midday Nap Problems

Nap Is Absent, Too Short, Too Long, or at the Wrong Time

The most common problem with this second nap is that the interval of wakefulness following the first nap is too long. Maybe you lost track of time or traffic delayed your return home. Being up too long causes your baby to become overtired, and he has difficulty either falling asleep or staying asleep. If you are using method A (see Chapter 7), please leave your baby completely alone for one hour after soothing to see if he will fall asleep.

If the duration of crying and sleeping associated with the midday nap puts you way past 2:00 or 3:00 p.m., forget this nap and try to get your child to nap in the late afternoon if your child is substantially younger than 9 months and has usually been taking a third, midday nap. If there is no midday nap and no third midday nap, prepare for a rocky afternoon and a long soothing period as you put your child to sleep super early that night, around 5:30 p.m. Even though your child might appear very sleepy at 4:00–5:00 p.m., going to sleep this early is likely to backfire with a too-early wake-up the next day.

Bad timing is a common cause of problems associated with the midday nap. If it is too early, way before noon, because of a too-short midmorning nap, the midday nap will not be as restorative and your child might be overtired by late afternoon. One mother said her son was a "French fry" by the end of the day because he was crispy. Under 9 months of age, this might lead to a late or long third nap that causes the bedtime to become too late. If the midday nap starts too late, way after 2:00 p.m., or if it lasts past 3:00 p.m., it may interfere with an early bedtime.

Sometimes the midday nap conflicts with scheduled activities, such as preschool for the child or scheduled activities for older brothers and sisters. Try to minimize these conflicts regarding the older children by using babysitters or car pools, or by skipping some (but not all) of the classes for your infant. An earlier bedtime might be essential when the midday nap is shortened or skipped.

Center-based day care may be associated with poor-quality naps because of bad timing for soothing to sleep, not enough help for long soothing, too much light or noise from the environment, or crying from other children. Sometimes there are no alternatives available to the family in their choice of day care, and although it is especially hard on these families, an earlier bedtime will help these children.

If the midmorning or midday nap is sometimes way too short or skipped, try to keep the child up and go to the next scheduled

sleep time, but move it a little earlier. Protect the sleep schedule.

Nap #3: Late Afternoon

About 16 percent of children are still taking a third nap at 6 months; the frequency of this nap drops to 5 percent at 9 months and to 1 percent at 12 months. Therefore, after 6 months of age, more than 84 percent of children have no third nap, and their longest wakeful period occurs in the afternoon. This is the time to go on longer excursions, errands, or shopping trips. Scheduled events such as baby exercise classes and outings to the park may be fun during this longer wakeful period. In contrast, the morning wakeful period between the two major naps might not be very long.

If the late afternoon nap does occur, the time when it starts may vary between 3:00 and 4:00 p.m. Also, the duration of this nap may vary, but it is usually very brief, maybe thirty to forty minutes. Some children take it daily and others take it occasionally. The presence of a third nap after 6 to 9 months is often associated with a bedtime that is too late, which in turn causes issues with the two major naps and may contribute to the bedtime battles that eventually emerge around 9 to 12 months of age, when there is increasing self-agency. If so, eliminate the third nap in order to accomplish an earlier bedtime. The earlier bedtime then abolishes the tiredness that had made the third nap appear necessary. Early bedtimes are especially difficult in families where both parents work outside the home (see Chapter 11), but the benefits for the entire family outweigh the difficulties (see Chapter 2). Try to overcome these difficulties as best you can.

Late Afternoon Nap Problems

Sometimes, around 9 to 12 months of age, a child falls asleep around 4:30 to 5:30 p.m. and awakes around 7:30 or 8:00 p.m., then is kept up playing with parents for a few hours until 10:00 p.m., and finally goes back to sleep but may not sleep well at night. The parents think the child is taking a third nap at 4:30 to 5:30 p.m. But in reality the child needs a very early bedtime, maybe around 6:00 p.m., and no playing between 7:30 and 10:00 p.m. Eventually, the lost evening sleep during the wakeful evening play period produces a cumulative sleep debt.

REAL LIFE
Special events often result in skipped or shortened naps for children. Do not become a slave to your child's nap schedule. But the more you protect the sleep routine for regular days, the less disruptive those special days will be.

Q: *How long should my child nap?*
A: Ask yourself this question: does your child appear tired during the day? If your baby is tired in the late afternoon or early in the evening, this *might* indicate insufficient naps. A possible solution is simply to put your child to bed earlier at night. Keeping a baby up too late produces fatigue and sleep deprivation, and will ultimately lead the child to resist falling asleep or to wake at night. This may be a problem, especially when a working parent or parents arrive home late, feeling guilty about being away from the family so long.

To Sum Up: Months 4 to 8
In this age range, most babies accept naps without protest and fall asleep at night without difficulty. These easy babies may still awaken once or twice in the middle of the night. I consider this behavior normal, natural, and not something that needs to be changed—as long as it's for a brief feeding and not prolonged playtime.

Choose the one or two times when you'll go to feed your baby and change diapers, and don't go at any other time. Please review the earlier discussion on arousals (see Chapter 1) if you are puzzled as to why babies sometimes get up or make sounds frequently throughout the night. If you have an intercom or baby monitor that allows you to hear all the quiet cries or sounds that occur during the arousals, turn it off. All you are accomplishing by listening to your child's awakenings is messing up your own sleep. A mother's sleeping brain is so sensitive to her baby's crying that any loud, urgent call will awaken her. You do not need an amplification system to ruin your sleep over every little quiet sound your baby makes!

Most mothers will partially synchronize feedings to sleep patterns so that their child is fed around the time he gets up in the morning, around the time of (either before or after) the two naps, around bedtime, and one or twice at night under 9 months of age. In other words, bottle-feedings or breast-feedings now occur four times during the day. Frequent sips, snacks, or little feedings throughout the day are not necessary for nutrition, but the overtired child might appear to be "hungry" like this because sucking is soothing.

Gradually your child will begin to associate certain behaviors on your part, certain times of the day, his crib, and his sensation of tiredness with the process of falling asleep for naps. If you started early to teach your child self-soothing (see Chapter 3), falling asleep for naps usually involves no crying. If your child had extreme fussiness/colic or did not learn self-soothing early, learning to fall asleep for naps might involve "maybe-cry" or "let-cry" sleep solutions (see Chapter 4).

Stranger wariness or stranger anxiety may be present in some babies by about 6 to 9 months of age, and with this new behavior, some mothers note some separation anxiety—that is, the child shows distress when the mother leaves. I do not think this type of separation anxiety directly makes it more difficult for a child to fall asleep unassisted. I have observed that babies with separation anxiety learn to sleep well as rapidly as any other babies when their mothers leave them alone at sleep times. The problem is that some mothers also suffer from the thought of separation and will not leave their children alone enough at sleep times to allow healthy sleep habits to develop. Self-agency, described above, also develops around 6 months of age and may lead to major bedtime battles or signaling at night if your child is short on sleep.

A major problem in implementing an age-appropriate sleep schedule for naps and early bedtimes is that it is *inconvenient*. Many parents resent the fact that their babies are now less portable. It is inconvenient for parents to change their lifestyle to be at home twice a day on most days so that their baby can nap. But when parents initially suffer through the process of establishing a good sleep schedule and their child is well rested, occasional irregularities and special occasions that disrupt sleep usually produce only minor and transient disturbed sleep. The recovery time is brief, and the child responds to a prompt reestablishment of the routine.

Bluntly put, when parents are unwilling to alter their lifestyle so that regular naps are never well maintained or the bedtime is usually a little too late, the child always pays a price. The child's mood and learning suffer, and recovery time following outings or illness is much longer. These parents often unsuccessfully try many "helpful hints" to help their child sleep better. I'm not sure any or all of these hints can ever substitute for maintaining regular sleep schedules. Parents in my practice who have utilized regular sleep schedules have rarely, if ever, found these hints to be useful after 4 months of age.

Bureau of "helpful" hints of dubious value to soothe your baby to sleep:

Lambskins

Heartbeat sounds

Womb sounds

Elevating head of crib

Maintaining motion sleep in swings

Changing formulas or eliminating iron supplement

Changing diet of nursing mother

Feeding solids only at bedtime

You are harming your child when you allow unhealthy sleep patterns to evolve or persist—sleep deprivation is as unhealthy as feeding your child a nutritionally deficient diet.

Babies seem to respond quickly at this age to a somewhat scheduled, structured approach to sleep. If you can learn to detach yourself from your baby's protests and not respond reflexively by rushing in to her at the slightest whimper, she will learn to fall asleep by herself. As one mother said of her child, "She now goes down like warm butter on toast!"

COMMON DAY-SLEEP ISSUES IN MONTH 9

Needs Two Naps but Can Get Only One

The bedtime might be too late and/or the wake-up time too early, causing your child to be very tired in the morning. This morning sleepiness causes him to take a mega-nap in the morning that interferes with his ability to take a midday nap. As a result, he is not well rested in the late afternoon or early evening. Or scheduled morning activities might conflict with a nap around 9:00 to 10:00 a.m., resulting in a very late midmorning nap around 10:30 or 11:00 a.m. Even if this is a brief nap, it may recharge your child's battery and interfere with a long midday nap.

The solution for needing two naps but only getting one is a bedtime that is twenty or thirty minutes earlier. More sleep at the front end allows young children, who need two naps, to wake up better rested, which means they are better able to take two naps. In older children who appear to need two naps but are really old enough for just one, more night sleep with an earlier bedtime erases the apparent need for two naps.

Needs to Nap but Refuses to Nap

When I studied naps in children, about 10 percent of children gave up naps early because of some stressful event that *disorganized home routines,* such as the death of a parent, divorce, moving to a new home, or the birth of twin siblings. Simply having a new sibling did not cause a change in napping. Also, there were three children who stopped napping for about a year during a period of marital discord or problems with caretakers. After resolution of the conflicts, all three children resumed napping and continued to nap for years. Additionally, there were many other children whose families experienced deaths (including SIDS), divorces, or moves but without associated napping problems. It appears that when parents and caretakers maintain nap routines despite potentially disruptive stressful events, most children continue to nap.

Holidays, trips, illnesses, or other changes in routine might cause your child to give up napping and be very tired during the day. Another common cause of no napping occurs when the child drops the midmorning nap but the parents do not make the bedtime a little earlier. Over many weeks or months, your child develops "cumulative sleepiness" until he hits a wall and becomes way overtired. In this state, it is difficult for him to nap because his body is geared up to fight the fatigue. When you try to reestablish the nap, he just plays in his crib, cries, or does a combination of both.

Try a temporarily super-early bedtime to help him wake up better rested. In other words, for four or five nights, put him to sleep when he is drowsy at 5:00 or 5:30 p.m. This might backfire and cause him to wake up too early. If this happens, for those four or five mornings ignore him until 6:00 a.m. Often the temporary super-early bedtime will help erase his sleep debt so he is more able to relax and take a nap. To help reestablish the nap habit, you might want to have intense morning stimulation and an extra-long and soothing nap time ritual. Leaving him alone in his crib for no more than one hour, even if he cries, often will allow the nap to occur because he is tired and not receiving any stimulation from his parents (see "Nap Drill" in Chapter 4). Or you might have to lie down with him in your bed to help induce sleep. If this is successful, then you would very slowly and gradually transition him back to his crib.

Once the nap has been reestablished, the bedtime can be made a little later. Children who slip in and out of good sleeping patterns are usually going to bed slightly too late every day. They don't have major problems, but they are always on the edge of becoming overtired and they easily and quickly become very overtired whenever there is a disruption of sleep routines.

Here is a report of how a temporarily super-early bedtime helped create long and regular naps and a change in personality:

When our pastor asked us if our 8-month-old son, Henrik, was a "serious, sullen" boy, I knew we had a problem. Just one month before, my friend had sent us a note saying how Henrik was the happiest baby she'd ever seen. She could elicit a belly laugh from him with just a sideways glance. Now, our pastor, an experienced grandfather, was pulling out all the stops—goofy faces and exaggerated sneezing— and Henrik wouldn't crack a smile. But it wasn't because he was suddenly sullen or serious; he was exhausted.

What I had hoped was just a napless phase that he'd outgrow was catching up to him and choking his vibrant personality. We needed help. While Henrik was sleeping better at night, his daytime naps were becoming history. Over the past two months, his decent, if erratic, nap schedule had faded into two brief naps and then disappeared altogether.

Getting my son to fall asleep was never an issue; nursing or rocking soothed him easily. The problem was getting him to stay asleep once I set him down. As soon as I'd set him in his crib, his back would arch and he'd be choked up before he touched the mattress. "Nap time" had come to mean Henrik crying in his crib until my nerves couldn't take it anymore, or him sleeping soundly on me.

I knew he needed to learn to soothe himself to sleep, but crying it out just didn't seem to work. The longer I'd let him cry, the more he would work himself up. I knew sleeping on me wasn't a good solution, but when I'd see the dark circles under his eyes and hear his voice husky from crying—and especially when he got his first cold—I just couldn't let him cry anymore. He needed sleep. So I'd get comfortable with him on the sofa and hope a good movie was on cable.

We set off for our consultation with Dr. Weissbluth. After studying our son's erratic sleep patterns, he recommended an earlier bedtime and regular wake-up times for my son. Dr. Weissbluth explained that Henrik was going to bed too late and wasn't getting enough sleep at night. (Henrik usually fell asleep between 8:00 and 9:00 p.m. and woke up around 7:00 a.m.) This lack of sleep and a consistent schedule—as odd as it may seem—is what was keeping him from being able to cry himself to sleep during the day. He was too over-tired to sleep! Dr. Weissbluth suggested a 7:00 p.m. bedtime and a 7:00 a.m. wake-up for the long-term goal, but said that we'd probably be looking at a 5:30 p.m. bedtime until Henrik's napping got better.

Once Henrik was up in the morning, we were to stimulate him through walks, outings, and vigorous play. After that, a soothing period would precede his attempt at a 9:00 a.m. nap. I was to continue putting Henrik to sleep in my normal way (nursing and rocking) and then set him down in his crib. I was then to leave him alone for one hour either to sleep, cry, or a combination of the two.

Then, after his midmorning nap, we were to repeat the process for his attempt at a 1:00 p.m. nap (or earlier if no midmorning nap was taken). And then we'd go about our afternoon until it was time for the evening soothing. He asked us to chart our sleep data so we could clearly see Henrik's progress.

When we got home, we played and played, and then I soothed Henrik to sleep. When I set him down for his after-noon nap, he cried. I said a quick prayer, told him I loved him, walked out, and closed the door on my wailing son.

As I walked down the stairs, I breathed in slowly, reminded

myself that I was doing this for my son's well-being, and hit the pause button on my emotions. I spent fifty-nine minutes emailing friends with one ear to the monitor to see if and when he'd stop crying. "Didn't work today," I was telling myself on the way back up the stairs. But by the time I got to his door, I realized he was quiet. He fell asleep after fifty-nine and a half minutes of crying. If I had gone up one minute sooner, I would've cheated him out of this accomplishment. We were on our way.

The midday nap was the first to get back on track. It took about a week for him to be able to go down at all without crying, and he was still only sleeping for a half hour at a time. But he was sleeping—and on a schedule! I used to think that because Henrik was an erratic sleeper, a sleep schedule wouldn't work for him. Now I know that Henrik was an erratic sleeper because he lacked that schedule. While the idea of a schedule sounds limiting, establishing a schedule was the most freeing thing for our family. We are now able to make accurate plans instead of having to wait around and guess when our son would be ready to go.

The midmorning nap was more of a challenge. For two weeks he cried through his entire midmorning nap. It was difficult to put him down each day knowing he would cry, but his success in the afternoons, along with the giant hug I'd receive when I came to get my teary son, gave me the strength to keep going. Then one day he cried himself to sleep after just twenty minutes, and from then on he would stay sleeping after we put him down. It took two weeks for Henrik to get back to two naps a day, but he did it.

Despite Henrik's sleeping for only thirty to forty-five minutes at a time, Dr. Weissbluth told us we should get him as soon as he woke up. He suggested we keep the 5:30 bedtime, which would naturally help lengthen his naps. Our days are now virtually tear-free.

My son is thriving on his new schedule. He's back to his giggly, healthy, and well-rested self. Instead of being the sullen boy in church, he's now the chipper angel who sings out loud with joy—with or without the rest of the congregation.

As mentioned earlier, self-agency becomes more apparent at 9 months of age. Strong-willed, willful, independent-minded, stubborn, headstrong, uncooperative. Sound familiar? These are the words parents often use to describe their toddlers. You may observe that your young child is simply less cooperative. A psychologist might use the term *noncompliance* to describe this lack of cooperation, but the psychologist would also point out that these behaviors go hand in hand with the normal, healthy evolution of the child's autonomy or sense of independence. All infants can now express what they do and do not want, what they like or do not like, with greater energy and persistence than previously. Parents discover that their child is not as easily distracted as before. Get used to it, because self-agency only becomes stronger with time! But don't forget that your child is also exhibiting positive qualities of drive and determination, qualities that, along with self-sufficiency, will stand her in good stead as she grows.

Usually, experts tell us, the times when you should expect the most difficulties, or "oppositional behaviors," are at transitions: for example, stopping play for dressing, mealtimes, and bedtimes. Since this is the beginning of the "stage" of autonomy (and noncompliance), some experts claim that it is natural for this independence/stubbornness to cause either resistance in going to sleep or night waking. I think this "stage" theory is an incorrect interpretation of fighting sleep, but self-agency and separation anxiety do develop around this age and are often used by parents to justify not helping their child sleep; they tell themselves, incorrectly, that all children have trouble sleeping during these stages.

Children in this age range also often develop behaviors described as social hesitation, shyness, or fear of strangers. A child also might cry or appear distressed when his mother leaves him alone in one room while she goes to another room or when she leaves the child with a babysitter. Psychologists call this behavior stranger wariness, stranger anxiety, or separation anxiety. So if a child develops increased resistance in going to sleep at night at this stage, some experts might say that separation anxiety, or fear of being away from the mother, is the cause. I think this is an incorrect interpretation also.

In my general pediatric practice, I have seen many children with intense self-agency and dramatic separation anxiety who have absolutely no problems with sleeping. Additionally, the vast majority of children with sleeping issues do not have big problems with self-agency or separation anxiety. When some children with significant challenges regarding self-agency or separation anxiety plus sleep problems see child psychiatrists or child psychologists, these professionals tend to misattribute the sleep problems to self-agency or separation anxiety. In part, as previously discussed, this is because there is little attention given to sleep during their professional training. But my experience and research show that the direction of effects is often likely the opposite: when overtired children become better rested, they then become more cooperative and less fearful.

Nap #3 Disappears

As mentioned above, the major sleep change that occurs before or around 9 months is the disappearance of the third nap. If the late afternoon nap persists, it often causes the bedtime to become too late. Also, children do not need to be fed at night after 9 months; children who are bottle-fed during the night are likely to develop a night-waking or night-feeding habit. If your baby goes right back to sleep after a feeding, then do not necessarily stop the feedings. But if he decides to play with you and does not easily and quickly return to sleep after the feeding, then stop going to him at night. Again, if you are breast-feeding in the family bed (see co-sleeping and SIDS warning, Chapter 1), no night-waking habit might develop. Additional changes in sleep routines are coming soon; the midmorning nap is going to disappear.

COMMON DAY-SLEEP ISSUES IN MONTHS 10 TO 12

Nap #1 Begins to Disappear

Beginning around 9 months of age, a small number of babies (4 percent) are now taking only one midday nap. This increases to 17 percent by the first birthday. The vast majority of children between 6 and 12 months are taking two naps. When your child drifts toward a single nap, which is always the midday nap, often the bedtime has to be twenty or thirty minutes earlier because children in this age range tend to get more tired near the end of the day. Sometimes it is the midday nap that starts to disappear because the midmorning nap is too long. In this case, move the bedtime much earlier; you can also wake your child after an hour or an hour and a half into the midmorning nap in order to protect the midday nap.

You may think your baby needs only one nap now, but most babies in this age range still need two naps. One clue that two naps are still needed is that some parents notice that their babysitter can have their child take two good naps, but they themselves can only get her to take one, if that. The child is obviously more rested after the sitter leaves, and the parents wonder how the sitter does it. Well, children are very discriminating at this age. They know that the sitter, following parents' instructions, has a no-nonsense approach and will put them to sleep on a fairly regular schedule. But they figure that with Mom or Dad, enough protesting may gain them more playtime together. After all, sometimes it works. And so long as your child retains the expectation that you will come to her and take her out of her boring, quiet room, she will fight naps.

Summary and Action Plan for Exhausted Parents

Now that your baby is older, the times when your baby will become sleepy are more predictable. Another way of saying this is that your baby's biological sleep/wake rhythms are more mature. This allows you to change your strategy to keep your child well rested. Previously the focus was on *brief intervals of wakefulness* to avoid the overtired state; now you can begin to use *clock time* more as an aid to help your child sleep well.

REMEMBER
Timing is important, but watch your baby more than the clock.

Let's start in the morning and go around the clock.

Starting the day: Most children will awake to start the day about 7:00 a.m., but there is a wide range (between 6:00 and 8:00).

First nap: The first nap occurs about 9:00 a.m. and may last about an hour or two. Sometimes you will stretch your child to get to this time, or you may wake your child at 7:00 a.m. in order for your child to be able to take this nap. Previously you focused on maintaining short intervals of wakefulness, but now you try to anticipate your child's predictable best nap time. If your child takes this first nap too early or too late, then it is difficult for him to take the second nap on time. The midmorning nap begins to disappear between 9 and 12 months, but 84 percent of children at 12 months are still taking this nap.

Second nap: The second nap occurs around 1:00 p.m. and may last about an hour or two. The most common problem at this nap time is too long an interval of wakefulness after the first nap. This causes your child to become overtired.

The window for this second nap is between noon and 2:00 p.m., but you may notice that your child's own window, during which it is easiest for her to fall asleep, is much narrower. The midday nap commonly continues for about 3 to 4 years.

Third nap: The third nap may or may not occur. If it does occur, it may vary between 3:00 and 4:00 p.m. Also, the duration of this nap may vary, but it is usually a very brief nap. Usually this nap disappears by about 9 months.

Bedtime: Because of the variability of the third nap, the bedtime may also vary. Most children are asleep between 6:00 and 8:00 p.m. The most common problem at bedtime is keeping your child up too late. If your child is put to sleep after his sleep wave has crested, he will have more difficulty falling asleep and staying asleep. If you keep your child up past the time when he is drowsy, for example, because you return home from work and want to play with your child, then you are depriving your child of sleep. Please try to avoid making your child overtired in this way, just as you would never deliberately make your child go hungry by withholding food.

First night waking: This may occur four to six hours after your child's last feeding. Some children do not get up at this time. Feeding your child differently or giving cereal will not help your child sleep better. There is a shifting from deep sleep to light sleep throughout the night. Partial awakenings or light sleep stages called arousals occur every one to two hours when your child is asleep, and sometimes your child will make quiet, nondistressed sounds or loudly call out or cry during these arousals. Loud crying during these arousals usually signifies an overtired child. If your baby is not sleeping with you in your bed, going to your child at the time of these partial awakenings will eventually lead to a night-waking or night-feeding habit, causing fragmented sleep. This is because the social stimulation that occurs when you pick up your baby, hold your baby, and feed your baby will eventually cause your baby to force himself to a more alert state during these arousals. Consequently, he will learn to expect to be fed or to enjoy the pleasure of playtime with his parents at every arousal. However, if you are sleeping with your baby and breast-feeding, you might promptly nurse at all of these arousals while your baby is still in a somewhat deep sleep state, and then no night-waking habit might develop. The most common problem regarding these naturally occurring arousals is to project psychological problems onto our children, such as saying that they must be lonely or afraid. *Just because the parents may be experiencing these emotions does not mean the child shares them!* However, four to six hours after the last feeding, many children are actually hungry, and you should promptly respond by feeding.

Second night waking: This may occur around 4:00 or 5:00 a.m. Some children do not get up at this time. Most children who do awaken at this time are wet, soiled, or hungry, and a prompt response is appropriate. Maintain silence and darkness, because your child should return to sleep. A common mistake is to play with your child and prevent the return to sleep. The return to sleep is important so that your child will wake up well rested and be able to comfortably stay up to the time of his first nap. Although this pattern of getting up once in the middle of the night and/or in the early morning is common, some children will simply get up once around 2:00 or 3:00 a.m. or not get up at all. Some night wakings for feeding are very common during the first 8 to 9 months.

Sleeping through the night: This may be defined in different ways, but if the bedtime is too late or if unnecessary feedings or attending to your child cause fragmented sleep, then your child will continue to wake up at night.

There are trends over time for the bedtime hour to become later and for children to sleep less during the night and, for some children, to sleep less during the day. Pay attention to your own child's mood and behavior to determine what's best for your child. Ignore advice from others or what you read. There is enormous variation at specific ages for bedtimes and sleep durations for night sleep and day sleep. Don't compare your child's sleep to other children's sleep.

There are three dramatic turning points in sleep maturation for young children:

1. At 6 weeks of age, night sleep becomes organized.
2. At 4 months of age, day sleep is developing and night sleep is becoming adultlike in terms of sleep cycles.
3. At 9 months of age, the third nap is eliminated, naps may be longer for post-colic babies, and there is no need to feed babies at night.

These turning points are so highly predictable and independent of parenting practices that we know they reflect maturation of the brain. Anticipating these changes and allowing them to occur naturally will set the stage for preventing all common sleep disturbances.

It cannot be emphasized enough that the major sleep problems in babies from 4 to 12 months old develop and persist because parents

- Reinforce bad sleep habits by unnecessarily feeding or attending to their baby at night
- Interfere with an important learning process in their child, namely, learning how to soothe themselves to sleep unassisted
- Do not respect the child's biologic nap and bedtime rhythms

The failure of children to fall asleep and stay asleep by themselves is the direct result of parents' behavior. Don't underestimate your child's competence and ability to learn healthy and unhealthy sleep habits during these early months!

CHAPTER 9

Healthy Sleep Habits in Early Childhood: Age 1 to 7

Total Sleep Duration Trends over Time

A study by Dr. Ivo Iglowstein showed that total sleep durations decreased from 1974 to 1979 and from there to 1986. For example, "at two years of age, the decrease between 1974 and 1986 was from an average 14.2 hours to 13.5 hours for total sleep duration." Also, a review by Lisa Matricciani found that "over the last 103 years, there has been consistent rapid declines in the sleep duration of children and adolescents."

This trend was confirmed by studies by Dr. Anna Price and me for middle-class or middle-socioeconomic-status (SES) families:

AVERAGE TOTAL SLEEP DURATION

Age (Years)	1979–80	2004–8
1	13.8 hours	13.4 hours (2004)
2	12.8 hours	—
3	12.4 hours	11.7 hours (2006)
4	11.9	—
5	11.4	11.1 (2008)

As noted previously (see page 207 in Chapter 4), cumulatively small differences in sleep—for example, among the 5-year-olds, a decrease from 11.4 to 11.1 hours (*19 minutes*)—may have major consequences.

This same trend was noted for higher-SES families by Dr. Josephine Foster in the early part of the twentieth century and by Dr. Avi Sadeh at the beginning of the twenty-first century:

AVERAGE TOTAL SLEEP DURATION

Age	1927	2006
12–17 months	13.6 hours	12.8 hours
18–23 months	13.4 hours	12.5 hours
2–3 years	12.8 hours	11.9 hours
	(24–29 months)	(24–36 months)

Night Sleep

SLEEPING THROUGH THE NIGHT

What does the phrase "sleeping through the night" mean? This is discussed in detail in Chapter 8. In my experience, all children who are napping well and have early bedtimes are sleeping uninterrupted through the night by *9 months or earlier.*

> **Don't hide behind excuses; there will always be one handy! Some families use extreme fussiness/colic (birth to 6 months), teething (6 to 12 months), separation anxiety (12 to 24 months), "terrible twos" (24 to 36 months), and fears (36 to 48 months), one after another, to "explain" why their child wakes up at night and has trouble returning to sleep by himself.**

BEDTIME HOUR TRENDS OVER TIME

I want to illustrate the enormous variability in children's sleeping, both in the past and currently. The age of your child is most important; older children stay up later and sleep less. But at every specific age, there is a wide range for the bedtime hour and for the duration of night sleep, day sleep, and total sleep. I present the average numbers to help you understand the main points. But, for clarity, I have deliberately excluded the very wide ranges that accompany each average number in order to present a rough guideline to show how *most* children were sleeping in the past. This guideline may or may not inform you how your child should sleep today. It may be reassuring that your child's early bedtime was commonplace in the past, when parenting may have been less complicated. Skip all the number stuff if you wish; what counts is your child's mood and behavior—so watch your child!

As discussed in Chapter 8, it is only recently, over the long history of parenting, that children have been able to stay up late at night. Data collected by Drs. Iglowstein, Price, and me (1979–80) show that the bedtime hour has shifted over the years to a later clock time. The cause of this shift is not known.

BEDTIME HOUR (P.M.) BY YEAR

Age	1974	1979	1979–80	1986	2004–8
1 year	7:08	7:41	8:00	8:16	8:00 (2004)
					(10–12 months)
2 years	7:08	—	8:30	7:46	—
3 years	7:35	7:53	8:15	8:07	8:15 (2006)
5 years	7:46	7:56	8:10	8:11	8:15 (2008)

After about 1980, the trend toward a later bedtime plateaued among young children around 1 year and younger, perhaps because increasingly later bedtimes would eventually be significantly disruptive to the child and the family. But the trend for ever later bedtimes for 3- and 5-year olds continued through 2006 to 2008. Although the wake-up times were a little later in children 1, 3, and 5 years old (three, seventeen, and four minutes, respectively), these later wake-up times failed to fully compensate for the later bedtimes, resulting in less night sleep than in the past. When the bedtime is always too late, then you should expect behavioral, emotional, and academic problems, even if your child gets up a little later or takes longer naps. *When* your child sleeps at night is as important as *how long* your child sleeps, and longer naps are not a substitute for less night sleep (see Chapter 1).

A possible contributing factor to the trend of later bedtimes over time might be that, over the same time frame of Dr. Iglowstein's survey (1974 through 1986), other data show that between 1975 and 1985 the percentage of women in the labor force who had children under age 18 dramatically increased, by 14.7 percent. Afterward, this began to taper off: between 1985 and 1995, the increase was only 7.6 percent, and between 1995 and 2005, the increase was only 0.8 percent. More mothers in the workforce might be associated with more center-based day care (also associated with shorter naps) and later bedtimes so that parents could enjoy the company of their children after work. In support of this suggestion, families using child care in centers as their primary child care arrangement more than doubled (13 percent to 28 percent) between 1977 and 1990. By 1995, the increases in the percentage of children ages 3–6 enrolled in center-based care began to taper off.

In addition to later bedtimes (1974–1986), many more mothers entering the workforce (1975–1985), and increased use of center-based day care (1977–1990), another trend occurred: the number of first births among women ages 35–39 started to increase in the mid-1970s and rose sixfold from 1973 to 2006. Sleep issues in children appear to be more common among older parents (see Chapter 5).

The trend of having televisions in the bedroom, causing later bedtimes, began in the later 1980s, after Dr. Iglowstein's survey, but this trend has dramatically increased among children with the addition of newer screen-based technology. Television and other electronic screen-based devices in the bedroom have recently become even more popular. These intrusive objects cause later bedtimes, which, as we have seen, are associated with less sleep and sleep problems (see Chapter 10).

BEDTIME

For younger children, time cues can be used as stimulus control to enforce the bedtime hour. Use a digital clock and a matching picture or photo and say, "Oh, look, it's seven o'clock [say 'seven, zero, zero']—time for your bath." After the bath, hugs, stories, and kisses, say, "It's now seven-thirty [say 'seven, three, zero']—time to go to sleep." Or use a timer to control the duration of the soothing bedtime routine. Then turn out the lights and close the door. No returning or peeking. Your child learns that after a certain hour, no one will come to play with him, so he falls asleep and stays asleep until the morning. He learns to amuse himself with crib toys or other toys in his room until the wake-up time. For older children, Sleep Rules with silent return to sleep work well. Chapters 3 and 4 give more information regarding how to establish parent-set bedtimes and maintain them without bedtime battles.

BEDTIME BATTLES AND NIGHT WAKING (SIGNALING)

In one study of children between 1 and 2 years of age, about 20 percent woke up at night five or more times a week, while in another study of 3-year-old children, 26 percent experienced night waking at least three times a week. If your child behaves this way, consider this behavior to be worth changing. Unfortunately, you simply cannot assume that difficulty returning to sleep unassisted will magically go away. Returning to sleep unassisted is a learned skill; you should expect problems to persist in your child until she learns how to soothe herself back to sleep without your help.

Also in the study of 1- and 2-year-old children, those children who woke up frequently were much more likely to have an injury such as a broken bone or a cut requiring medical attention than those who slept through; while only 17 percent of good sleepers had injuries, 40 percent of the night wakers were injured! The reason is that fragmented night sleep causes daytime drowsiness and inattentiveness and, maybe, impulsiveness that can lead to injury (see Chapter 11).

Surveys have shown that the majority of children between the ages of 1 and 5 years have a bedtime routine less than thirty minutes long, go to sleep with the lights off, and fall asleep within about thirty minutes after lights out. Night waking occurs in the older children in this group once a week; only a few awaken more than once a night. If your child's pattern between the ages of 1 and 5 is substantially worse (longer latency to sleep or more night wakings), consider the possibility that your child is among the 20 percent of children in this group with disturbed sleep. If so, you might also notice later the excessive daytime sleepiness that has been observed in about 5 to 10 percent of children between the ages of 5 and 14 years.

If your child has had a long history of resistance to falling asleep or of night waking, then reread Chapter 4 and work on establishing a healthy sleep pattern in general.

Q: *Does this mean that after my baby falls asleep I can never peek in and never go in to soothe or comfort him?*

A: No. Only during the period when you are establishing a new sleep pattern is it important to avoid reinforcement. After your child is sleeping better and becomes well rested, there is nothing wrong with going in to check on him at night.

Q: *I took his older brothers out of their bedroom so his crying wouldn't disturb them. When can they go back into their old bedroom?*

A: Allow several days or a couple of weeks to pass before making changes. The more rested the baby becomes, the more flexible and adaptable he will be. Changes then will be less disruptive.

Q: *My 2½-year-old son understands what I'm saying; why can't I discuss these problems with him?*

A: You want to avoid discussions or lectures at the time the problem is taking place because your reasoning at that time calls attention to the problem and thus reinforces it. It's like shining a flashlight on a problem. Instead, choose some low-key casual playtime to gently voice your concerns regarding his lack of cooperation. Now he is more likely to be in a better mood to reflect on what you are saying. But when there *is* some cooperation, make sure to praise the *specific behavior:* "Thank you for staying in bed" or "Thank you for trying to sleep." Praising your child ("Thank you for being a good boy") but not the behavior fails to tell him exactly what it is that you want him to do again.

If there has been long-standing ambivalence or inconsistency regarding putting your child to bed at night, then naturally occurring separation anxiety will only aggravate or magnify bedtime problems. The same is true for the naturally occurring fears of darkness, death, or monsters that children often express around age 4. In order to deal with separation anxiety or fears at night, we must understand that all children experience them, and that they can learn not to be overwhelmed by them at the bedtime hour with the help of the consistent, calm resolve of their parents. The routine of a set pattern in a bedtime ritual reassures the child that there is an orderly sequence: sleep will come, night will end, the sun will shine again, and parents will still be there smiling.

COMMON NIGHT-SLEEP ISSUES

When your child starts to walk, babble, and show more personality, you will naturally begin to treat him less as an infant and more like a person. Please try to avoid the trap of endlessly explaining, nego-tiating, or threatening when it comes to sleep times. Save your breath; let your behavior do the talking.

Teaching self-soothing during the first year may or may not have been easy, but the benefits become clearer as your child grows older. Here is how one parent described her journey:

My friends and family look at me in disbelief when I tell them my 14-month-old daughter goes to bed around six-thirty on her own (without a bottle or rocking or crying) and sleeps soundly until seven the next morning. The training exercise of putting the baby to bed drowsy but awake so they can learn self-soothing is the key. The crib, her bedroom, naps, and bedtime are a place and time of relaxation and enjoyment for our daughter and for us! No crying, no anxiety. I will admit it wasn't always easy and there were trials and tribulations ... but once you get over whatever humps are your challenges, it's relatively smooth sailing. My experience this past year can be described as follows: 0–3 months is unnerving and exhausting, especially for the first-time parent; 3–6 months is anxious, wondering if you are doing the right thing; 6–9 months is more rewarding as you start to see your efforts really paying off; 9–12 months brings a sense of satisfaction and accomplishment; and 12 months and over makes all the training worth it.

Your child's developing personality and awareness of himself as an individual means that his second and third years will be a time of testing, noncooperation, resistance, and striving for independence. Your child has stronger self-agency. Sleep problems in 12- to 36-month-olds are related to this normally evolving stubbornness or willfulness in children, who now want to do their own thing. For example, they may want to get out of their crib or bed at night, not take naps, get up too early to play, and, of course, resist falling asleep and wake up at night. This last problem might have started during the first year and may now continue during the second year as an ingrained habit.

> **Don't confuse these issues:**
> • **Needs versus wants**
> • **A sad cry versus a protest cry**
> • **Being abandoned versus being alone**

Fears

Nightmares, monsters, fear of separation, fear of darkness, fear of death, fear of abandonment . . . don't fears cause disturbed sleep at this age? Many experts tell us that night fears are common among children between 2 and 4 years old. Thunderstorms, shadows, barking dogs, loud trucks, and many other events over which we have no control can frighten our children.

If your child has been a good sleeper up to now, you should expect any disturbed sleep triggered by these events to be short-lived. Reassurance, frequent curtain calls, open doors, or a longer bedtime routine will help your child get over his fears. Night-lights might help, but a closet light or even a conventional night-light might keep a sensitive baby from sleeping well. Instead, try a .03 watt guide light that produces a faint yellow glow; this will usually provide sufficient illumination. A new teddy bear, to serve as a protector, might help fight off fears. A parent might walk around the room and capture the "monsters" and put them into a bag or box and then remove them from the room. Guardian angels, charms, or dream catchers may help make your child feel more secure.

My recommendation is to spend extra time soothing your child to sleep or go to him once for reassurance, but use a kitchen timer to control the duration of the extra soothing time. The timer is set to the number of minutes you want to spend with your child, and is then placed under a pillow or cushion to muffle the noise. Tell your child that when the buzzer or bell sounds, you will kiss him and leave. The child learns to associate the sound of the timer with your departure and learns that this signals the end of your hugging, massage, or lullabies. This is called "stimulus control" (see Chapter 4). Just as you know the play is really over when the final curtain call ends, or just as you know to slow down when the green light turns to yellow, your child learns to associate the sound with the end of your soothing effort. Because crying will not bring you back, the crying ends.

An older child might be given a bell to summon his mother or father with the understanding that he can use it only once, or a pass that allows him to leave his room once at night (see Chapter 4). Knowing that he can have some attention at night gives the child confidence, and he will sleep better. The goal is to provide extra attention at night without it becoming open-ended or a ploy to fight sleep. If you are uncertain whether your child is fearful or willful, it may be useful to meet with a child psychologist. Also, if your child now appears during the day to be extremely frightened, withdrawn in new surroundings, shy, or fearful, then it is very difficult for parents to give less attention at night, even if the goal is to enhance consolidated sleep. If this is the case with your toddler, a child psychologist can give you good advice on where to draw the line between supporting the child and encouraging him to learn to overcome his fears.

Some child care experts believe severe sleep disturbances are commonly caused by night fears, because they tend to see mostly children with long-standing sleep issues and fears. These children with serious sleep problems and fears who did not sleep well at younger ages then have their current situation misinterpreted as caused by an age-appropriate concern or "stage."

Q: *My 15-month-old child shows separation anxiety during the day, and at night she wants me to hold her and sit with her on the sofa until she falls asleep. How can I leave her alone at bedtime, when she is most anxious?*

A: Separation anxiety, stubbornness, or simply exhibiting a preference for parents' company over a dark, boring room might separately or in combination cause your child to behave this way. Please understand that it is normal for children to feel some anxiety, and learning to deal with anxiety and not be overwhelmed by it is a healthy learning process. Let's not use separation anxiety as an excuse for our own problems in dealing with a child's natural disinclination to cooperate at bedtime. On the other hand, anxiety issues can occur in your children, and if you suspect that this might be the case with your child, discuss this with your child's primary care provider.

If your child has not been a good sleeper up to now, increasing cumulative sleepiness might contribute to increasing fearfulness. It's time to review Chapters 1–3, because sleep problems do not go away on their own. Some parents misattribute their child's sleep problems first to gastroesophageal reflux, then to teething, then to separation anxiety, and lastly to fears, but not to their own behaviors.

Getting Out of the Crib or Bed

It's quite natural for social and curious 2- and 3-year-olds to repeatedly climb out of the crib or bed to check out the interesting things they think their parents are up to. Or maybe they just want to watch the late late movie or have a bite to eat! This is the jack-in-the-box syndrome. Of course, what these children like to do best is to come visit with their parents and get into their bed. This not only disrupts their parents' sleep but also harms the child. For a young child who does not understand consequences, consider a crib tent (see Chapter 4) to protect sleep and prevent the development of sleep problems. You may have to use duct tape to keep the child from getting to the zipper. Parents are often reluctant to use a crib tent because they imagine their child will feel like a caged animal in a zoo, restricted, or abandoned. Of course, there might be some protest crying for a few days. However, many children quickly come to enjoy the comfort zone, treating it like a teepee or fort; they do not appear sad or angry.

Some parents do not want to use a crib tent but feel more comfortable putting up a gate or latch lock on the door. If you stand at the door preventing your child from leaving the room, your child will fight sleep all the more because he is getting attention from you. If parents want to put a lock on the door, I ask that they have the child watch them put the lock on. One parent felt that the additional step of bringing her 3-year-old child to the store where she purchased the lock for the door helped convince him that she was serious. The child is told that if he leaves the room, he will be put back in and the door will be locked. Almost all the time, the child picks up on the parents' serious demeanor and does not even attempt to leave the room in the first place. If, however, the child tests the rules and leaves the room, and the parents place him back into the room and lock the door, although there may be loud and long protest crying, it is usually only for one night, because the child is now highly motivated to prevent the door from being locked in the future.

Sleep Rules and silent return to sleep are used for the older child, about 2½, who will not stay in bed and understands consequences. Here, too, some parents know that they cannot be consistent at night with silent return to sleep, so they want to put a latch lock on the door. These treatments and others are discussed in Chapter 4.

A Regular Bed and the Arrival of a New Baby

One rearrangement is moving your child to a big-kid bed. There is no special age when you should make this change. As long as the crib is large enough, you should not feel that your child must be placed in a regular bed by a certain age. Many parents make the switch around the second or third birthday. Let your child ask for a big bed. One mother described feeling that she had made the move too soon; she thought the big bed must have seemed "oceanic" compared to the crib, because her son always slept curled up in one corner of the bed—that is, when he slept. He slept much better when returned to his crib. Before she made the move back to the crib, his mother wondered whether this would cause a "regression" in her child. It did not. But it did result in a better-rested family.

If the move to a regular bed is needed because of a new baby brother or sister, consider making the move when your newborn is about 4 months old. By then, your newborn has regular sleeping habits. Before your baby reaches this age, there is a constant shifting of household routines due to your infant's naturally irregular sleep pattern. This may cause confusion or insecurity in your older child because he does not know when Mom or Dad will be available, or why he has to wait when he wants to go outside and has gotten used to doing just that. When your newborn is 4 months old and her sleep pattern is stable, events in the house are much more predictable. Your older child now becomes adjusted to the new family arrangements. Your baby goes to the crib and the older child graduates with pride to the big bed for big kids. He does not feel displaced. Before your newborn is actually moved from the bassinet to the crib, feel free to leave the crib up and empty for a while with the understanding that if your older child gets out of bed once, then it's back to the crib.

Moving to a big bed too early—for example, in anticipation of the birth of a new baby—often invites a problem: the commotion and excitement surrounding the arrival of your new baby may create confusion or insecurity in your older child, who may call out or cry at night. The more difficult situation is when your older child starts to get up every night to visit his parents.

If the move to a regular bed prompts frequent nocturnal visits, curtain calls, calls for help going to the bathroom, or calls for a drink of water, think before you act. A habit may slowly develop in which your child learns to expect you to spend more time with her, putting her to sleep or returning her to sleep. Imagine what would occur if a babysitter gave your 2-year-old candy every day instead of a real lunch. Once you discovered this, you would immediately stop the candy for meals. Your child might protest and cry, but would you give in and let her have the candy? No. If you are spending too much time at night with your child when she should be sleeping, consider what you are doing to be giving "social candy"—not needed and not healthy for the child. Be firm in your resolve to ignore the expected protest from your child when you change your behavior.

Day Sleep

DAY-SLEEP DURATION BY AGE

Here are data from my nap study (for children born between 1984 and 1986) regarding the percentage of children taking naps and the total duration of naps. The nap durations are greater than in other reports, presumably because I followed these children since birth and gave the parents advice about sleeping at every visit. So my data might represent optimal naps.

NAP STUDY, 1984–86

Age (months)	Percentage of Children Taking Naps	Average Duration, Total Hours per Day	% in Range: Total Hours	Minimum-Maximum Hours
12	100%	3.0	94%: 2.0–4.0	1.5–5.5
15	100%	2.7	91%: 1.5–3.5	1.0–5.5
18	100%	2.5	98%: 1.5–3.5	1.0–4.0
21	100%	2.4	97%: 1.5–3.5	1.0–4.0
24	100%	2.3	99%: 1.5–3.5	1.0–4.0
36	92%	2.1	80%: 1.5–2.5	1.0–3.5
48	57%	1.9	80%: 1.5–2.5	0.5–5.0
60	27%	1.7	89%: 1.0–2.0	1.0–3.0
72	12%	1.6	90%: 1.0–2.0	0.5–2.5

At every age, the vast majority of children have nap durations within a narrow time frame, but the actual range of nap durations among all children is very wide because a few children have extremely short or long naps. Between 2 and 6 years, the most common duration of day sleep is about two hours for those children still taking naps. All children are taking naps every day until age 3 years. But naps start to disappear around that age: 8 percent of 3-year-old children are not napping, and among those who continue to nap, they nap, on average, six days per week. In Japan, it is customary to have naps in nursery school, and in one study of 441 children 3 to 6 years of age, the naps caused the children to go to sleep later at night.

Looking at these numbers may reassure you that your child's naps are appropriate for his age, but due to the variability at every age, it is more important to look at your child's mood and behavior than at these numbers.

Individual Stability of Naps

In my nap survey, I divided 6-month-old children into five nap duration groups (see Chapter 8). Children typically remained in their initial nap duration group until 21–24 months; this individual stability of nap durations probably reflects a *genetic* influence over sleep. In other words, the group of babies whose average nap duration was 3 hours at 6 months of age had nap durations of 2.9 hours by 9 months, 2.8 hours by 12 months, 2.6 hours by 15 months, 2.5 hours by 18 months, and 2.4 hours by 21 months. The babies did not move to a track of much shorter or longer naps. Stated another way, children with long naps at 6 months of age continue to take long naps until 21–24 months; the same is true for children with short or intermediate nap durations. Also, infants' nap durations, for the vast majority of children, remained within a narrow range despite variations in caretaking and social activities, suggesting that *biologic* processes affect naps. Nevertheless, considering the actual wide range of nap durations among all the children as a group (shown above) and the fact that many children move away from their initial nap duration group after 21–24 months, it does seem likely that *parents* play an important role regarding naps as well.

Although studies on large groups of children show no consistent relationship between the duration of daytime sleep and nighttime sleep, I think it is likely that most of the children who sleep near the minimum number of hours for naps have problems with night sleep, naps, or both. This may also be true for some of the children who sleep near the maximum number of hours for naps, although I have encountered some very well-rested children, subsequently determined to be very intelligent, who had very long naps at these young ages.

But very long naps might develop as a result of a bedtime that is too late even though night-sleep duration seems normal; in this case, despite the long naps, the child is impaired. Long naps are not a substitute for a bedtime that is too late (see Chapter 1). This is similar to the situation described by Dr. Seog Ju Kim in Chapter 10 for older teens who stayed up late on weeknights to study and then slept in for catch-up sleep on weekends: the later the bedtime on weeknights, the greater the weekend catch-up sleep a student achieved. But Dr. Kim found that "increased weekend catch-up sleep as an indicator of insufficient weekday sleep . . . is associated with poor performance on objective attention tasks." So weekend catch-up sleep does not substitute for or fully compensate for late weekday bedtimes.

NUMBER OF NAPS PER DAY BY AGE

Here are some data from my nap study for children born between 1984 and 1986 regarding the disappearance of naps:

CHILDREN TAKING 1 OR 2 NAPS PER DAY

Age (months)	1 Nap	2 Naps
12	17%	82%
15	56%	44%
18	77%	23%
21	88%	12%
24	95%	5%
36	100%*	0%

* 100% of those still napping take only one nap, but 8% are not napping

As you can see, the majority of children switch to a single nap between 15 and 21 months of age; Dr. Iglowstein observed the transition age to be 18 months. If your child is substantially less than 1 year old and taking one nap, or more than 2 years old and taking two naps, there might be an unappreciated sleep problem.

DAY-SLEEP DURATION TRENDS OVER TIME

In addition to the trend over time for bedtimes to become later, causing less night sleep, data are available from studies by Dr. Price and me (1979–80) that show a partial trend over time for less day sleep. The cause of this shift is unknown.

NAP TRENDS, 1979-80 TO 2004

Age	Average Day-Sleep Duration	
	1979–80	2004
	3.2 hours (4–11 months)	3.0 hours (4–6 months)
		2.8 hours (7–9 months)
		2.6 hours (10–12 months)
1 year	2.3 hours (12–17 months)	2.5 hours (13–15 months)
3 years	1.4 hours (30–41 months)	1.2 hours (29–33 months)
		1.0 hours (34–39 months)

TRENDS OVER TIME: PERCENTAGE OF CHILDREN TAKING NAPS AND NUMBER OF NAPS PER WEEK

Comparing my data with Dr. Foster's study from 1927, it appears that in the past, between the ages of 4 and 6 years, a higher percentage of children took naps, but they had fewer naps per week.

NAP TRENDS, 1927 AND 1984–86

Age (years)	Percentage of Children Who Nap		Number of Naps per Week	
	1927	1984–86	1927	1984–86
1	100%	100%	Daily	Daily
2	100%	100%	Daily	Daily
3	90%	92%	5	6
4	75%	57%	3.5	5
5	49%	27%	1.7	4
6	20%	12%	0.5	3

Dr. Foster wrote in 1927, "Up to the age of five (the usual age for entering kindergarten) more than half of the children [nap]. The drop from 68 percent at 4½–5 years to 30 percent at 5–5½ years" reflects entry into school. This 38 percent decrease is similar to the decrease noted in 1984–86 of 35 percent between 3 years (92 percent) and 4 years (57 percent), but it is occurring a year earlier! Perhaps this earlier decrease reflects a trend toward earlier involvement in preschool, day care, or scheduled activities. In other words, more scheduled activities during the day now, compared to 1927, might interfere with naps. But also, later bedtimes today might be driving more naps per week in those children who are given the opportunity to nap. Whatever the cause or causes for these trends, it is clear that parents influence nap behavior and, over time, parenting practices change.

But for the moment let's ignore my nap study (1984–86), because it might represent optimal napping. Other studies, by Drs. Foster, Iglowstein, and Lavigne, still report a trend toward fewer naps per week, and fewer children napping.

NAP TRENDS: NAPS PER WEEK

Age (Years)	Number of Naps per Week	
	1927	1990s
1	7	—
2	7	5
3	5	3

NAP TRENDS: PERCENTAGE OF CHILDREN NAPPING

Age (Years)	Percentage Taking Naps	
	1927	1974–93
1	100%	100%
2	100%	87%
3	90%	50%

Comparing these data on the number of naps per week and the previously discussed data on duration of naps to my nap study and the experience of caring for many children over forty years leads me to the conclusion that many children today are being denied the opportunity to take a nap, and to take a long nap when they do nap. The developing famine in sleep may be a direct contributor to the spreading epidemic of obesity and attention deficit hyperactivity disorder.

However, as previously discussed, taking long naps or more frequent naps might also be an attempt to partially compensate for a bedtime that is too late. In Dr. John Lavigne's study of children 2 to 5 years old, the lowest-SES group of children went to sleep later, awakened later, and took longer and more frequent naps compared to children in all other SES groups. Total sleep duration was similar to the other SES groups, but the children with later bedtimes had more externalizing problems. Also, as mentioned previously, Dr. Seog Ju Kim showed that when older children's bedtimes are too late during the school week, there is more catch-up sleep on weekends, and those children with the largest amount of weekend catch-up sleep have the poorest performance on objective attention tasks (see Chapter 10).

So sleeping later in the morning, taking more naps or longer naps, or trying to catch up on sleep on the weekend does not fully compensate for the harm done by a bedtime that is too late.

If the bedtime is often too late, sleeping later in the morning and sleeping more during the day does not fully compensate. *When* **you sleep is as important as** *how long* **you sleep.**

COMMON DAY SLEEP PROBLEMS

Specific prevention and treatment strategies for common day-sleep problems are discussed in Chapters 3 and 4.

Routines and Schedules

Although most 2- to 3-year-old children in my survey went to sleep between 7:00 and 9:00 p.m. and awoke between 6:30 and 8:00 a.m., I think that an earlier bedtime is better. A single nap between one and three hours occurs in over 90 percent of children. Try to be *reasonably* regular about nap time and bedtime, and be consistent in your bedtime rituals. There are no absolute, rigid, or firm rules, because every day is somewhat different. Reasonable regularity and consistency imply reasonable flexibility.

How about scheduled, organized activities that take place when your child needs to take her midday nap? If your child is unable to take her midday nap two or three times each week and you are able to get an extra-early bedtime on those days, then there may be no problem, as long as your child is sleeping well in general. But if your child is not sleeping well, for whatever reason, frequently losing a few naps can be quite problematic. Also keep in mind that children are likely to pick up minor illnesses from each other in group settings, and these minor illnesses may disrupt your child's sleep and push her into an overtired state. In general, be cautious regarding preschool classes during the flu season. Have fun with your child, but occasionally take what my wife called a "declared holiday." Missing a swim class, gym class, or any other preschool event now and then because your child is tired and needs to nap, or leaving a class soon after you arrive because some other children look sick, will not jeopardize your child's college plans!

Be aware that your lifestyle helps or hinders your child's sleep patterns, and remember that there will be changes due to growth and rearrangements in relationships within the family such as the arrival of a new baby.

Refusal to Take a Nap

Playtime in the park or shopping together is so much fun; who wants to take a nap? Ask yourself whether not napping is *your child's* problem or *your* problem. Some parents simply find it too inconvenient to hang around the house to enable their child to get his needed daytime sleep. But reflect on how inconvenient it is to drag a tired child around while shopping. Please review Chapters 1 and 2 if you feel that naps are not that important.

Refusal to take a nap often occurs after a special event, such as a holiday, party, or vacation. There was so much excitement the day before; your child doesn't want to miss anything again! Sometimes the refusal to nap develops because of unappreciated chronic fatigue due to an abnormal sleep schedule, brief night-sleep duration, or sleep fragmentation. If these problems are present, work on them as you work on day sleep. Refusal to take a nap might take place "all of a sudden" after a slow buildup of cumulative sleepiness, such as might occur from a bedtime that is only slightly too late during long summer days. Another common cause of cumulative sleepiness occurs when the child drops the midmorning nap but the parents do not make the bedtime a little earlier. For whatever reason, if your child develops cumulative sleepiness, he becomes way overtired and "suddenly" hits a wall. In this state, it is difficult for him to nap because his body is geared up to fight the fatigue.

If your child is substantially under 3 years old and you want to help him nap, try a temporarily super-early bedtime so that he wakes up better rested. For four or five nights, put him to sleep when he is drowsy at 5:00 or 5:30 p.m. That might set things right. However, be aware that it might also backfire and cause him to wake up too early. If this happens, for those four or five mornings, ignore him until 6:00 a.m. Often the early bedtime will help erase his sleep debt, so he is more able to relax and take a nap. Also, to help reestablish the nap habit, you might want to have intense morning stimulation and an extra-long and extra-soothing nap time ritual. Leaving him alone in his crib for no more than one hour, even if he cries, often will allow the nap to occur because he is tired and not receiving any stimulation from his parents. Or you might have to lie down with him in your bed to help induce sleep. If successful, then you would very slowly and gradually transition him back to his crib. Once the nap has been reestablished, the bedtime can be made a little later. Children who slip in and out of good sleeping patterns are usually those who are always going to bed slightly too late. They don't usually have major problems, but they are always on the edge of becoming overtired and they easily and quickly become very overtired whenever there is a disruption of sleep routines. Getting naps back on track is also discussed in Chapters 4 and 8.

If your child is close to or past his third birthday, trying to reestablish the nap may not make sense because some children are now naturally outgrowing naps, but trying to establish an earlier bedtime might help your child sleep better anyway.

Keep a sleep chart, log, or diary; pick a time interval that you think is right, and put your child down in the crib at that time. *You* are controlling the nap time. Spend as much time as you want—ten, twenty, or thirty minutes—hugging, kissing, rocking, and nursing to soothe your child. Then down is down—leave him alone for one full hour.

If your child has been quite well rested up to now, the crying may be brief. But if your child has a history of chronic fatigue, prepare yourself for a full hour of crying. Here's one mother's account of how her 14-month-old daughter responded.

My daughter was 14 months old, ate poorly, resisted naps, woke two or three times in the night, needed to be rocked to sleep, and was tired all the time. My husband and I were exhausted, angry, resentful, and blaming each other for the situation we were in.

We were ambivalent, scared, concerned, and skeptical about letting our daughter cry, as the treatment plan recommended. We thought she would feel unloved and worthless if no one responded to her.

After only one episode of crying, she learned how to lie down and fall asleep on her own! It was very difficult listening to her crying, but when she woke in the morning smiling and kissing us good morning, we were reassured that she loved us. Now she naps regularly, sleeps through the night, eats better, plays better, and is able to play in her crib before going off to sleep on her own.

The more rested your child is, the quicker you'll see improvement. A very tired child might require several days of training before he relearns how to nap.

Your goal is to establish an age-appropriate nap routine so your child associates being left alone in a certain place and a familiar soothing routine with feelings of being tired and taking a nap. No more playtime, no more games, just sleep. If your child is young, then every day at about 9:00 a.m. and 1:00 p.m. parents should put their child down to nap; older children may be put down only at midday. I call this "nap structuring"; we are trying to use natural sleep rhythms to help your child sleep best. After one hour, if there is no nap, then we go to the next sleep period, but a little earlier.

Parents who would rather hold their child in a rocking chair or let her catnap in the stroller are robbing their child of healthy sleep. This lighter, briefer, less regular sleep is less restorative—it's not as effective in returning your child's energy and attentiveness to its best levels. Remember, sleep is also measured in *quality*, not just *quantity*.

Q: *My problem is not that my child refuses to nap or resists naps, but that her nap schedule is very irregular. What's wrong?*

A: If your child is well rested, it may be that you are in fact very sensitive to her need to sleep and are placing her in an environment conducive to sleep when she needs it. Differences in daily activities produce differences in wakeful intervals and differences in the duration and timing of naps. Perhaps you have unrealistic expectations regarding the regularity of naps according to clock times. If your child is very tired, however, she might be crashing at irregular times when she is totally exhausted. A common problem here is a bedtime that is slightly too late. Early bedtimes appear to regularize and lengthen naps.

Q: *My problem is that my baby takes such long naps that we don't have much time to play together. Are long naps a problem?*

A: There may be a problem if your child snores or mouth-breathes when asleep (see Chapter 11). These are symptoms of respiratory allergies or large adenoids or tonsils and should be discussed with your child's physician. Another possible problem is that the bedtime is too late and the long naps are attempts to compensate for the lost sleep. In the long run, this compensation will fail because the too-late bedtime causes cumulative sleep deficits. Or maybe your child needs long naps; long sleep durations are associated with higher intelligence levels, so protect his long naps! Don't worry: you will have more playtime together in the future when your child's naps naturally become shorter.

Getting Up Too Early

Getting up too early is another major problem in toddlers. The first question to ask is, how early is too early? If your child gets up at 5:00 or 6:00 a.m. and is well rested, perhaps this pattern is not changeable. You may try encouraging her to sleep later by making the room darker with opaque shades. Getting everyone together in a family bed at that hour may also allow all of you to get some more snooze time. Often families give their baby a bottle at this early hour, after which she returns to sleep for a variable period of time.

While bottles given early in the morning may help your child return to sleep, be aware that if your baby is allowed to fall asleep with a bottle of milk, formula, or juice in her mouth, the result is decayed teeth. This will not occur if the bottle contains only water. Unfortunately, some parents go to their child at 4:00 or 5:00 a.m. with a bottle of milk and then let the baby feed herself.

Treatment for the well-rested child who has a habit of taking an early morning bottle is to first switch to juice, and then gradually, over about a week, dilute the juice more and more until it is only water. Once your child is drinking only water, place a water bottle at either end of the crib, point them out to her at bedtime, and stop going in.

One mother used to allow her child to watch a video every morning as soon as she woke up. This allowed the mother to have some free time to take care of herself. But her child started waking up earlier and earlier in order to enjoy the video. Stopping the routine of watching videos in the morning was part of the solution.

If your child wakes up too early and is not well rested, work hard to establish a healthy sleep pattern. In the morning, don't go to her until the wake-up hour.

REMEMBER

Getting up too early may be caused by going to sleep too late. Earlier bedtimes often prolong night sleep and prevent early wake-ups. Sleep begets sleep.

For a 3-year-old child, you can try a variation of controlling the wake-up hour using *stimulus control* (see Chapter 4). We previously used a digital clock as a signaling device to indicate bedtime. Now we are going to use a digital clock to signal the wake-up time. Place a digital clock in her room and set the alarm for 6:00 or 7:00 a.m., which may be *after* the expected spontaneous wake-up time. Draw a picture of the clock face showing 6:00 or 7:00—the time that corresponds to when the alarm will go off. Or you might use a clock radio set to turn on at the designated time with quiet classical music or a color-changing bunny light programmed to change color at the desired clock time.

Do not respond to her cries before this wake-up time. Then, at the wake-up time *you* have picked, you bounce into her room, exclaim how the clock matches the picture or the music is on or the color has changed, and exclaim, "Oh, see, it's time to start the day!" Shower her with affection, open the curtains, turn on the lights, bring her into your bed, or give a bath. Be dramatic, wide-eyed, and happy to see her. The child learns that the day's activities start at this time. The pattern on the digital clock, the quiet music, or the color change in the light acts as a cue, just as a green traffic light tells you to start moving. Before the wake-up time, the child has her water bottles but no parental attention.

Sleep Recommendations

Lisa Matricciani's 2013 review of the literature concluded that published recommendations for children's sleep are not based on empirical evidence (see Chapter 1). She points out that differences exist among individuals to cope with less sleep: "Interestingly, children from different parts of the world have radically different habitual sleep durations. At any given age, children from Asia sleep 60–120 minutes less each day than children from Europe, and 40–60 minutes less each day than children from the United States. Either there are genetic differences in sleep needs, or sleep needs can be modified by sociocultural context, or Asian children are catastrophically sleep deprived."

She adds that "*sleep timing* [the time when sleep occurs] may be even more important than sleep duration." In a separate 2013 paper titled "Sleep duration or bedtime?" the authors studied 2,200 children 9–16 years old and concluded that "*late bedtimes and late wake up times* are associated with poorer diet quality *independent of sleep duration*" (emphasis added).

Months 12 to 15

NIGHT SLEEP

Dr. Jacqueline Henderson reported that among a group of 12-month-old children whose average bedtime was 8:30 p.m., many were not sleeping through the night (see Chapter 8). Based on my research and experience, I think that 8:30 p.m. is too late a bedtime for many, if not most, 12-month-old children.

The percentage of children who were not sleeping uninterrupted between midnight and 5:00 a.m. was 13 percent, and 14 percent were not sleeping uninterrupted for 8 hours minimum between sleep onset and time awake in the morning, while 27 percent were not sleeping uninterrupted from at least 10:00 p.m. to 6:00 a.m. I suspect that the factors that caused these children to be unable to sleep uninterrupted at night at 12 months are primarily associated with a failure to learn self-soothing well during the first year of life; the bedtime may also have been too late. The main reasons for not learning self-soothing are post-colic sleep problems and the parent issues described in Chapter 3. Because these may be difficult challenges for some parents, if your child is not sleeping through the night at 12 months, I urge you to consider just a simple change that might make a huge difference; that is, move the bedtime a little earlier as described in Chapter 4.

NAP #1 (MIDMORNING) BEGINS TO DISAPPEAR

At 12 months of age, 82 percent of children have two naps and 17 percent take only a single midday nap. But by 15 months of age, 44 percent of children are taking two naps and 56 percent take a single midday nap. This is a dramatic change occurring over a short time period. The majority of children make the shift from two naps to one nap between 15 and 21 months.

This transition, however, may not be smooth. You might have a few rough months when one nap is not enough but two are impossible. Here are some ideas for making the transition easier.

Move the Bedtime Earlier

The midmorning nap is always the first nap to naturally disappear. If the bedtime is moved a little earlier, most parents will notice that their child's midmorning nap becomes briefer or turns into a quiet playtime without sleep. Most of these children do not appear to become very tired in the morning, because more sleep at night eventually erases the need for a midmorning nap.

Other children take longer and longer midmorning naps and then appear to actively resist or be unable to take the second midday nap. Often, because this second nap was short anyway, many parents forget it. The result is a child who is overtired late in the afternoon or early evening and who quickly becomes way overtired by bedtime. Instead of, or in addition to, an earlier bedtime, you might want to shorten the midmorning nap by waking your child after about one or one and a half hours so she will be more tired around the midday nap time. But truthfully, very few mothers like the idea of waking their sleeping child to help set a better schedule; sleep is so precious! However, if you do try this, also try to get out of the house immediately following this parent-shortened midmorning nap to provide fun-filled intense stimulation to manage sleep inertia; but tone it down as you get to the middle of the day. Provide extra-long and relaxing soothing to sleep for the midday nap. Maybe also consider moving the midday nap to a slightly later hour so your child is a bit more tired. But what if your child continues to take a midmorning nap and none of the above causes her to take a midday nap? Here's another plan.

Move Back the Midmorning Nap and Skip the Midday Nap

At the usual time of the midmorning nap, delay its onset by ten or twenty minutes. This might require more intense and prolonged soothing to sleep. Anticipate that the late afternoons might be a bit rocky for a while. Slowly, over many days or weeks, continue to delay the midmorning nap until it is occurring near the middle of the day. During this transition, the bedtime might have to be temporarily ultra-early because your child gets pooped every afternoon. After the shift of the midmorning nap to the midday is accomplished, the bedtime might now be moved a little later. However, this new little-later bedtime (associated with a single, midday nap) should be earlier than the original bedtime that was based on having two naps every day. The earlier bedtime means that a working parent coming home late might not see their child then. If that is the case, that parent can get up extra early to have a longer morning playtime with their child before going off to work.

BE FLEXIBLE

Another solution to getting through the transition from two naps to one nap is to declare some days as two-nap days and other days as one-nap days, depending on when the baby awakens, how long the midmorning nap lasts, scheduled group activities, or the time you want your baby to go to sleep at night. Flow with your child and arrange naps and bedtimes to coincide with his need to sleep as best you can. Be sensitive to the growing need for earlier bedtimes. Eventually, the midmorning nap disappears.

Sleep problems around 1 year of age might involve first attempting to establish two naps with the understanding that it might not succeed; if so, after several days regroup and try a plan that involves a single nap. Here is one mother's account of how an early bedtime did *not* help her child become better rested and able to take two naps, but subsequently it did help when the single nap was delayed until midday.

Sophie has always been inconsistent when it comes to napping. Some days she would sleep for half an hour, others she wouldn't sleep at all. And if I was lucky, she would take an occasional hour nap. I decided it was time to get help before the situation became worse.

Sophie was 13 months old when I met with Dr. Weissbluth. She was sleeping for thirty minutes in the morning; her midday naps were unpredictable. At night, getting her to sleep was even more frustrating. Sophie had always been a great nighttime sleeper. Then, all of a sudden [cumulative sleepiness], she was waking up several times throughout the night. Not only was her mental state unbearable, but physically she did not look well. As for me, I was becoming mommy the monster. There were days when I thought I was going to lose it. I blamed myself for her sleeping disorder, even though I was doing everything right—putting her to bed early, keeping a consistent nap time, and putting her down in her crib for her naps instead of allowing her to sleep on the go.

After looking over Sophie's sleep log, Dr. Weissbluth gave me several options: try an earlier bedtime (5:00 p.m.), lots of stimulation when awake, and soothing her longer at night. The goal was to allow her to catch up on her sleep.

My husband and I put the plan to work. He supported the decision of an earlier bedtime, even though his time with her was already limited. Unfortunately, Sophie's sleeping did not improve. She continued to take one nap for thirty or forty-five minutes and then skip her midday nap. She and I were both exhausted, and my frustration level was sky high at this point.

During our follow-up conversation, Dr. Weissbluth asked if I would consider dropping her midmorning nap. He recommended the continuation of an earlier bedtime (5:00 p.m.), which, surprisingly, she welcomed. Although I was hesitant to drop her midmorning nap, I was determined to get my happy child back.

So, I put plan B to work. For the first several days, Sophie could barely keep her eyes open past 10:30 a.m. I was able to keep her up until 11:00 a.m. and then 11:30 a.m. for the next several days. She continued to take thirty-minute naps. I called Dr. Weissbluth and he reminded me that she was still trying to catch up on sleep, that it would take several days for her to feel rested. After day four, she was staying awake until 12:30 and sleeping for an hour. And she was sleeping through the night—no more nighttime waking. By the end of the week, she was starting her nap at 12:30 and waking up at 2:00 p.m. And Sophie and mommy were happy.

Obviously, any combination of parents' scheduling for their convenience and the baby's need to sleep can shape nap patterns as long as the biologic nap rhythms are respected (see Chapter 1). If you love naps for yourself, you may protect your child's nap schedule differently from the parent who does not customarily take naps.

HELPFUL HINT

Some children appear to hate their bedroom in the afternoon and scream as you approach it. One mother solved this by doing

all the pre-nap soothing in the living room and then quickly went into her child's room.

Q: *How long should my child nap?*

A: Does your child appear well rested? You be the judge. All of us have good days and bad days, but if you notice a progression toward more fussiness, brattiness, or tantrums, your child may need longer naps.

Months 15 to 21

NAP #1 (MIDMORNING NAP) BEGINS TO DISAPPEAR

The midmorning nap is on its way out. At 18 months, 77 percent of children take a single midday nap; by 21 months, 88 percent of children sleep only in the midday. Sometimes the child is taking only the midmorning nap and the plan discussed above does not work because the general recommendation of an early bedtime backfires. You try an early bedtime, and all you get is an earlier wake-up time, which makes your child more tired in the morning and makes him need the midmorning nap all the more (see "The 5:30 p.m. Bedtime Rut" in Chapter 4). Under these circumstances, you might temporarily put your child to bed a little later at night with the hope that he will sleep in later. It may take several days or a few weeks to build up enough sleep pressure to cause the later wake-up time. Be careful to avoid a second wind (see Chapter 1), because if you put him to bed much too late he will have difficulty falling asleep and staying asleep. So this will require some patience and trial and error. Still, wake him, if he is asleep, at 7:00 a.m. and then proceed with one of the plans previously described to get a midday nap.

Q: *What do I do if my child is healthy but cries at night, and the crying stops as soon as I pick him up?*

A: Ask yourself if there is anything you can do to regularize the total sleep pattern, such as timing naps better or making the bedtime earlier. Was there anything that recently disrupted his schedule to cause him to become overtired? Does he snore or mouth-breathe during sleep, or might he be starting to become ill? Look at the big picture, not just the night crying. In general, you will not want to attend to the night crying, because you want to encourage consolidated sleep. If you go to your child, you will cause fragmented sleep, which is poor-quality sleep. If your head says that not going to your child is the right thing to do, but your heart won't let you do it, try some of the following suggestions. One mother tied a ribbon around her ankle and her husband's ankle so that she did not shift into autopilot mode at night and go to her child when he cried. Another mother waited for her husband to go away on business for a few days so she could ignore the crying without having her husband undercut the plan. Sleep temporarily farther away from your child; use earplugs, earphones, pillows over the head; take a shower. Do what is best for your child, but don't torture yourself.

Months 21 to 36

The midday nap usually lasts until about 3 years of age and then gradually disappears. If the midday nap disappears too soon, your child may become overtired in the late afternoon and have difficulty falling asleep at night. Either reestablishing the midday nap (if your child is substantially under age 3) or moving the bedtime earlier (if your child is substantially over age 3) should help. If the midday nap persists in much older children, the bedtime might progressively get later and later, causing bedtime battles to develop. Eliminating the midday nap will permit an earlier bedtime and help erase bedtime battles.

SINGLE MIDDAY NAP BEGINS TO DISAPPEAR

The majority (80 percent) of children between the ages of 2 and 3 years have a nap length in a narrower band between one and a half to two and a half hours. The most common nap duration between the ages of 2 and 6 years is two hours. The stability of the two-hour nap over different ages is another argument for a strong biological influence over sleep, but it does not necessarily mean that your child needs a two-hour nap. Some children need less and some need more daytime sleep.

Q: *When do I transition my child from a crib to a bed?*
A: As he approaches his third birthday, let your child ask for a big bed. If you move him too soon, he may not stay in his bed because he is curious and wants to see what's going on elsewhere in the house.

Years 3 to 7

The list of new concerns for older children is long: school start times, organized weekend and afterschool activities, and enrichment classes or lessons (music, dance, math, or religious). Health habits may appear to be less important to parents than the development of children's academic, social, athletic, or artistic skills. But the contribution of healthy sleep habits to a child's well-being does not diminish with age.

Some of the subjects to review for the prevention and treatment of sleep problems in this age range, discussed in Chapters 3 and 4, are: bedtime routines, early bedtimes, parent-set bedtimes, parent issues, no television in the bedroom, sleep log, Sleep Rules and silent return to sleep, control the wake-up time, day correction of bedtime problems, fading, pass system, and choose a sleep solution.

Here are some simple ways to help your child settle down for day or night sleep. Consider them to be a sleeping routine for preschool children. Choose those items that work best for your child and do them at all sleep times.

Slowdown activity
Close physical contact
Gentle massage or mild stretching
   Cuddle up with the child in a chair
   Nestle or snuggle in her bed
Quiet voices
   Share a fun event
   Tell a story, talk about your family
   Read a book
   Sing or hum a song
   Chat about the day
   Say good night to everyone and everything in the room
   Play a favorite tape, maybe grandparents singing or saying
      good night, sounds of nature
Comfortable room
   Photos of family and pets
   Favorite stuffed animals or dolls
   Night-light or flashlight
   Dream catcher or guardian angel for protection

Please don't think that it is all right to have a late bedtime just because there is a late wake-up time and a long nap. In a study of 1,105 Japanese 3-year-olds, it was observed that half fell asleep at 10:00 p.m. or later. For all children, the later they went to sleep, the later they woke up in the morning and the longer they napped. However, the later bedtime was associated with less total sleep compared to those with an earlier bedtime. The later wake-up time and longer nap did not compensate for the later bedtime.

My research and experience suggests that among *well-rested* young children with early bedtimes, in general, there is no strong association between the duration of night sleep and day sleep. After a special occasion that causes a late bedtime, they might sleep in later or have a longer nap the next day only. In contrast, *overtired* children usually have chronically late bedtimes, and the later the bedtime, the later the wake-up time and the longer the naps. But they may still be short on total sleep, and, even when not, the late bedtime causes problems in the child.

Let's look at the issues that may occur in this age range and some of the strategies we can use to deal with them.

NIGHT SLEEP

Three-year-olds may no longer have tantrum behaviors, but they may call parents back many times and clearly express their feelings of love for their parents or fears of the dark. How to reassure your older child without reinforcing undesirable behavior?

In an English study of children about 3 years of age, a *fade* procedure (as described in Chapter 4) was particularly effective: 84 percent of the children who displayed difficulty in going to bed, night waking, or both, improved. Not surprisingly, the two factors that most likely predicted success were both parental: the absence of marital discord and the attendance of both parents at the consultation sessions. (The important role of the father is discussed in detail in Chapter 3.) And although half of the mothers in this study had current psychiatric problems requiring treatment, this did *not* make failure more likely. Another study from England (described in Chapter 4) that used a *fade* procedure included children who took at least an hour to go to bed, who woke at least three times a night or for more than twenty minutes at a time, or who went into their parents' bed. Among those families who completed four or five treatment sessions, 90 percent showed improvement. "Once some success was obtained, the *morale and confidence of the parents rose* and they were reinforced in their determination to persist by the more peaceful nights."

I have seen this over and over again; when you see even partial improvement, you gain confidence and no longer feel guilty or rejecting when you are firm with your child.

Your 4-year-old might be helped to sleep better if you make a schedule and post it in his room: time for bath, time for sleep routine, lights off, and so on. Regularity helps, but the times might include a range, because not all days are the same. Try to engage or enlist cooperation with your child by doing something together such as singing, reading out loud, or doing artwork as part of a bedtime routine.

It appears that sharing your plans with your older child is more likely to lead to cooperation. In office consultations, it often seems that the child is listening to the treatment plan discussed, because parents often report back that their child slept better that very night!

Regular Bedtimes

Q: *How important are regular bedtimes?*
A: In general, the bedtime should reflect your child's needs. With decreasing naps and increasing physical activity, your child's night-sleep needs may increase. Therefore, the bedtime often needs to be a little earlier, and not later simply because he is older. To maintain orderly home routines such as meals and baths, you might want to keep the bedtime within a narrow range.

Dr. John Bates's study of 204 children 4 to 5 years old examined in great detail the home environment, behavior at preschool, and sleeping patterns. The researchers noted that the *more variable bedtime,* as well as the lateness of bedtime, predicted poor adjustment in preschool, even after considering the roles of family stress and family management/discipline practices. This study provides evidence that sleep problems directly cause behavioral problems in children at preschool. Other research suggests that when older children are overtired, they learn to no longer bother their parents, but instead they bother their teachers.

Regularizing the sleep/wake schedule has also been shown to reduce daytime sleepiness and promote long-lasting improvements in alertness. It appears that regularity itself improves the ability of sleep to reverse daytime drowsiness. But some children are so excited at the end of the day, they have trouble unwinding whether they are overtired or not. Hot lavender bubble baths may help make the transition to sleep easier.

Some previously well-rested children who slip into a night-waking mode need only gentle reminders to return to sleep. As related in Chapter 4, my wife used to teach the "dolphin game" to one of our sons. She would read a story about how the dolphin swims deep in the water but sometimes has to come up for air before returning to a deep underwater sleep. Then she told our son to pretend that he was a dolphin at night and that it was perfectly all right to come up from sleep, but that he had to go back by himself. It worked.

Some previously very overtired children are so unmanageable at night that the family resources are stretched to the limit. In such cases the idea of more extreme measures such as extinction, using gates, or locking the door may come up (see Chapter 4). But before trying these measures, some parents try to avoid bedtime issues altogether by keeping their child up very late, until he crashes, in the hope that he will sleep in later in the morning and be all right during the day. Unfortunately, this only makes matters worse.

Q: *Why can't I just keep my child up later at night to see if he will sleep in later in the morning?*

A: If your child has been well rested up to now, then slowly try a slightly later bedtime. If you move it too late, he might just become more overtired and have difficulty falling asleep and staying asleep in the morning. If your child has always been a problem sleeper and overtired, a later bedtime will only make matters worse, because sleeping later in the morning or taking a longer nap usually does not make up for the lost sleep from a later bedtime. It just throws the rest of your child's sleep schedule out of whack.

Most children between 3 and 6 years of age, according to my survey, still go to sleep between 7:00 and 9:00 p.m. and awaken between 6:30 and 8:00 a.m. As previously discussed, I think that these bedtimes, derived from survey studies, are too late for many children. Going to bed too late may cause bedtime battles, night waking, or early morning wake-ups, or it may mess up the nap schedule. One mother described her son as turning into a "crank monster" at 4:00 p.m. every day because he was going to bed too late, waking up tired, and taking a midmorning nap, which prevented a midday nap and so caused cumulative sleepiness by late afternoon. Another mother described her child's new early bedtime as "a rescue maneuver to get back the old good pattern he fell out of."

THE SLEEP-TEMPERAMENT CONNECTION

I studied a group of sixty children at about 4 months old and again at 3 years old. At both ages, children with easy-to-manage temperaments slept longer than children with difficult-to-manage temperaments. Easier children were more regular, approaching, adaptable, mild, and positive in mood than the more difficult children. Which came first, the temperament traits or the sleep?

I don't think sleep habits, temperament, and fussing or crying are independent; rather, I believe they are all interrelated. However, we name and measure items such as sleep duration, temperament traits, or fussiness in the same way we might describe different features of a rose: its color, its smell, or its texture. But the rose is still a rose and a baby is still a baby; even though we give names to different features, none of them could exist without the whole.

It seems to me that after about 4 months of age, parenting practices such as loving attention during wakeful periods and encouraging good-quality sleep during sleep times can modulate or influence those features we call temperament (see Chapter 7). At age 3 years, among those children who had been easy-temperament infants at 4 months, some remained easy and were sleeping a total of 12.4 hours, while some became more difficult and slept less, 11.8 hours. So to help keep easy infants easy when they arrive at toddlerhood, protect their sleep.

What about those difficult infants? Some of them remained difficult at age 3 years and slept only 11.4 hours, but others became easy and slept 12.0 hours. I think part of the reason why some difficult infants mellowed into easy 3-year-olds is that they were handled in a more structured and regular fashion, learning more social rules and becoming better rested. The power of sleep to modulate temperament is reflected, at age 3 years, in the rank order of hours of total sleep durations: 12.4, 12.0, 11.8, and 11.4, respectively.

TEMPERAMENT AND SLEEP DURATION

Temperament at 4 months	Temperament at 3 years	Total Sleep Duration at 3 years (hours)
Easy	Remained Easy	12.4
Difficult	Became Easy	12.0
Easy	Became Difficult	11.8
Difficult	Remained Difficult	11.4

Adaptability, the ease with which children adjust to new circumstances, was the only temperament trait that showed individual stability over the three-year study. Remember, temperament traits are not like fingerprints, which are completely biologically based, unchanging over time, or unique identifiers. Temperament traits are more like hair. Our hair has a biological basis, but it changes over time; texture, length, curliness, and color can change naturally or at our will. How we care for our hair affects its health and appearance.

And how we care for our children, including how we care for their sleep, influences temperament. Helping your fussy baby sleep better will make him less of a fussy child when older. Between 4 months and 3 years, there was *no individual stability* regarding the durations of total sleep, night sleep, or naps, which means this time is the window of opportunity for parents to teach healthy sleep habits.

You shouldn't be surprised if your colicky 3-month-old has a difficult temperament at 4 months, but that doesn't predict anything for the future, not even for 5 months. A fussy nature may persist when colic and parental mismanagement together cause enduring post-colic sleep deprivation, or it may vanish when the child develops healthier sleep habits. You cannot change the fundamental personality of your child, but you can modulate it.

As previously mentioned, among the children I studied were three between the ages of 2 and 3 who stopped napping during a period of marital discord or problems with caretakers. When they stopped napping, they underwent what looked like a personality transplant! Fatigue masked their sweet temperaments. But after resolution of the conflicts, all three resumed napping and continued to nap for years. The resumption of napping restored their original or "natural" temperament.

Reestablishing naps was discussed earlier, but it is worth restating that in this study the kinds of stressful events that tend to disorganize home routines—the death of a parent, divorce, a move to a new home, the birth of twin siblings, or the death of a sibling—did not cause any napping problems in 90 percent of the children. It appears that when parents and caretakers maintain nap routines, children continue to nap despite disruptive and stressful events.

After the publications of my original discovery on the association between sleep patterns and temperament—in infants in 1981 and in toddlers in 1984—many other studies in preschool children have confirmed and extended my findings. In adults, sleep loss has been shown to affect mood more than cognitive or motor performance; we all get a bit testy or cranky when we are tired, but we can still learn and perform reasonably well. For children it may be a different story, because the developing brain may be more sensitive to sleep loss than the mature brain. Evidence to support this suggestion comes from animal studies, which have shown that less light was needed to affect the sleeping and behavior of young animals. In other words, the developing brain may suffer more, and in more ways, than the adult brain from the harmful effects of insufficient sleep.

Q: *Is it ever too late to see benefits from better sleep quality?*
A: No. It is never too late—nor too early—to help *healthy* children sleep better. In addition, some neurologically impaired children can be helped to have fewer seizures by becoming better rested. Sadly, other children have neurological diseases or medicine requirements that directly disrupt sleep. And tragically, recent research suggests that children who were severely traumatized by abuse or neglect beginning in infancy might not respond to ordinary sleep training like healthy children.

THE SLEEP-BEHAVIOR CONNECTION

Many research studies have shown more daytime behavioral problems in preschoolers who are poor sleepers. In some studies, "externalizing" problems such as aggression, defiance, noncompliance, oppositional behavior, acting out, and hyperactivity were associated with less sleep. When parents listed the types of daytime behavior problems their children were expressing, it became apparent that the less sleep they had, the longer the list! In other studies, there was an association between sleep and "internalizing" problems such as anxiety or depression. A recent study by Dr. Wendy Troxel showed a direct relationship between sleep problems at 36 months and internalizing problems at 54 months.

So sleep duration is clearly a factor associated with behavior and emotional problems. Still, we do not have absolute scientific proof on whether (1) less sleep directly causes daytime behavior problems, (2) parenting or biological forces cause both the daytime behavior and nighttime sleep problems, or (3) daytime problems cause the nighttime problems. However, as mentioned earlier, research by Dr. John Bates on 202 children 4 to 5 years old shows that sleep does have a direct effect on daytime behavior in children, in support of the first theory. My impression is that parents who are somewhat regular, consistent, and structured—in terms of both meeting the child's need to sleep and helping the child learn social rules—enable the child to have fewer behavior problems. In contrast, circumstances such as a parent who works late and keeps the child up too late in order spend time with her produce an overtired child; then behavioral problems will be more frequent.

Another study of preschool children noted that the poor sleepers who had more behavioral problems did not get up more frequently than good sleepers, but that the poor sleepers were unable to soothe themselves back to sleep unassisted. They always disturbed their parents' sleep with signaling behaviors. I think the ability to return to sleep unassisted to avoid fragmented sleep (and to avoid upsetting parents!) is learned behavior. So consolidated sleep doesn't just mean longer sleep: it helps to avoid behavior problems.

Regular bedtimes also seem to be important, maybe even when the total amount of sleep is not quite enough. There were fewer school adjustment problems in Dr. Bates's study where a regular bedtime was maintained by the parents. Research on 5- and 6-year-old children in Japan and Germany has also shown a connection between short sleeping hours and *obesity* (see Chapter 11). In the Japanese study, the later the bedtime, the greater the risk for obesity. In both studies, the shorter the duration of sleep, the more likely the children were obese. The researchers controlled for many of the variables, such as parental obesity, physical inactivity, long hours watching TV, and so forth. Maybe these overtired children felt stressed and dealt with it by eating. We know that American society is becoming more overweight; maybe our modern lifestyle is causing us to become more overtired, and this sleep loss is directly causing more obesity. In addition to prevention of obesity, many other benefits from healthy sleep are discussed in Chapter 2.

One study of 499 children showed that sleep problems at age 4 years predicted behavioral and emotional problems, such as depression and anxiety, when the same children were age 15. So although your older overtired child may not bother you as much as he did when he was younger, that does not mean that the sleep problem has gone away. Sleep issues in young children may be somewhat hidden, only to resurface later, much like too little calcium in our diet causes weak bones when we are older.

PREVENT AND SOLVE SLEEP PROBLEMS

Chapters 3 and 4 cover the prevention and treatment of sleep problems in the preschool-age range. The emphasis is on reasonably early bedtimes and no screen-based media in the bedroom.

Difficulty Falling Asleep

In one survey of about one thousand children, where the average age was between 7 and 8 years, about 30 percent resisted going to bed at least three nights per week. This was the most common sleep complaint of the parents. About 10 percent of the children had difficulty falling asleep once they were in their beds. Many took up to an hour to fall asleep on more than three nights per week. Some children both resisted going to bed and had *difficulty falling asleep,* and these children had a host of other problems: fears, anxiety, night wakings, need for reassurance, closeness of parents, complaints of fatigue, and a *history of not being able to successfully self-soothe.* Please review Chapters 3 and 4 regarding how to help your child learn self-soothing.

Another study emphasized the distinction between bedtime resistance (bedtime battles) and *difficulty falling asleep.* If your child resists bedtime and does *not* have difficulty falling asleep, then treatments such as an earlier or more regular bedtime, Sleep Rules, and other solutions described in Chapter 4 are likely to help. But if your child has no bedtime resistance and instead has *difficulty falling asleep*, has never slept well, and exhibits chronic mild anxiety-related symptoms, then consulting with a child psychologist or other mental health professional may be needed. This study also confirmed other observations that night wakings in early childhood tend to persist. Persistence of sleep problems is a theme in many reports, and it is only ignorance among some professionals that leads to the advice "Don't worry, he'll outgrow the problem."

Bedtime Becomes Later

Preschool and school-age children appear to be sleeping less today than in the past as the bedtime hour has gradually became later and later. If healthy sleep habits are not maintained, the result is increasingly severe daytime sleepiness.

Recurrent Complaints

Some children complain of aches and pains for which no medical cause can be found: abdominal pains, limb pains, recurrent headaches, and chest pains. Children who suffer from these pains often have significant sleep disturbances. Stressful emotional situations thought to cause these complaints include real or imagined separation of or from parents, fear of expressing anger that might elicit punishment or rejection, social or academic pressures, or fear of failing to live up to parents' expectations.

These are real pains in our children, just as real as the tension headaches adults get when we work too hard or sleep too little. All laboratory tests or studies during these episodes of tension headache will have normal results. All tests will also show normal results in children who have similar somatic complaints if the cause is sleep deprivation. Unless there is a strong clinical sign pointing toward organic disease, performing laboratory tests to rule out obscure diseases should be discouraged, because of the pain of drawing blood, the risks of irradiation, the expense, and, most important, because of the possible result of creating in the child's mind the notion that he is sick. Also, a slightly abnormal test result might lead to more and more tests, all of which, in the end, are likely to show basically normal results.

No Apparent Solution

Parents with older children have more scheduled activities to attend, and they are more likely to have more than one child requiring attention. What happens if the parent is a shift worker, or works in a bakery or restaurant with extremely early or late hours, or travels a lot for her job, or has irregular hours built into the job like some physicians? In these cases, it can be hard to arrange to be present when your children participate in an important scheduled school, music, or sports event. I have met some mothers and fathers who are absolutely dedicated to their children and try very hard to strike a balance between the time requirements of child care and their work outside the home. Usually there is a sharing of responsibilities regarding putting the children to sleep at night. However, what do you do if both parents have work schedules that make it difficult to be home reasonably early at night for bedtimes? To further complicate matters, one parent alone cannot easily manage different bedtimes for two or more children. To make it even more of a problem, what if the parents are blinded by their love for their children and their own subjective blindness to sleep loss (see Chapter 1) and cannot see that the late afternoon tiredness, headaches, or developing academic problems are connected to unrelenting mild sleep deprivation in their child? For some parents, it appears impossible to change their lifestyle or work schedule in order for their children to have a reasonably early bedtime.

When the children were much younger, as infants and preschoolers, morning times were available to enjoy being together as a family, but now mornings are a frantic blur trying to get ready for out-of-the-house activities. So the night is the only quiet and relaxed time the family has together. These factors converge into a too-late bedtime. It may seem that there is no solution to this problem, but in fact it's not that the solution isn't apparent. The problem is that the solution is not easy. But many worthwhile things are not easy. And as parents, we often have to place the welfare of our children above our own desires and comfort. This is such a time. An earlier bedtime, even at the cost of less family time at night, is the solution.

DAY SLEEP

Naps naturally become less common after the third birthday. Some parents stop their child from napping, but as a group, the children whose parents stopped naps did not have different nap patterns from those children who naturally outgrew naps. In other words, naps were not stopped because they were too short or too long. There were three reasons why parents stopped their children from napping. First, among 3- to 6-year-old children, scheduled preschool or school activities conflicted with the nap (60 percent of families). Second, parents of 5-year-olds wanted their child to go to sleep earlier, because their children were fighting going to sleep around 9:00 to 10:00 p.m. (30 percent of families). Finally, stressful events that disorganized home routines caused an additional 10 percent of parents to stop naps.

Summary and Action Plan for Exhausted Parents

1. Sleeping through the night may be defined in different ways, but if the bedtime is too late, if there are unnecessary feedings, or if you attend to your child too often, fragmented sleep will be the result, which in turn will cause your child to wake up at night, even when older. This will lead to earlier wake-up times in the morning, leaving your child in the position of always

playing catch-up when it comes to sleep needs. This a recipe for chronic sleep deprivation, with the network of negative consequences we have seen.

2. There are trends over time for the bedtime hour to become later, for children to sleep less during the night, and for some children to sleep less during the day. Pay attention to your own child's mood and behavior to determine what's best for your child. Ignore advice from others or what you read.

3. There is enormous variation at specific ages for bedtimes and sleep durations for night sleep and day sleep. Don't compare your child's sleep to other children's sleep.

4. Transitions from two naps to one nap may require trial and error, a temporarily earlier bedtime, and patience.

5. Difficulty in falling asleep, as distinct from resistance to bedtime, might require a referral to a mental health professional.

CHAPTER 10

Healthy Sleep Habits in Older Children: Age 7 Through Adolescence

Total Sleep Duration Trends over Time

Dr. Ivo Iglowstein showed that total sleep durations decreased from 1974 to 1979 to 1986 from age 6 months to 16 years. For example, among 5-year-olds, sleep decreased from 11.5 to 11.2 hours, and among 14-year-olds, sleep decreased from 9.0 to 8.5 hours. Comparing Dr. Anna Price (2008 data) with my own data (1979–80) indicates that this trend has continued past 1986.

AVERAGE TOTAL SLEEP DURATION

Age (Years)	1979–80	2008
5	11.4 hours	11.1 hours
9	10.5 hours	10.0 hours

Other studies have shown similar trends. In one study, for 10- to 15-year-olds, school-day sleep duration was seen to have been reduced between 1985 and 2004, due largely to later bedtimes. For example, bedtimes went from 9:47 to 10:12 p.m., while sleep duration dropped from 9.2 hours to 8.7 hours. Also, Dr. Katherine Keyes documented the trend over time for less night sleep among adolescents between 1991 and 2012. A 2012 review by Lisa Matricciani found that "over the last 103 years, there has been consistent rapid declines in the sleep duration of children and adolescents." Small nightly deficiencies in sleep—as little as *19 minutes* (see page 207 in Chapter 4)—may cumulatively have major consequences.

Bedtime Hour Trends over Time

In the history of parenting, it is only recently that children have been able to stay up late at night, as discussed in Chapter 8. But now it is so common that we don't even think about it. Data collected by Drs. Iglowstein, Anna Price, Jennifer Falbe, and me (1979–80) document how the bedtime hour has shifted over time to a later clock time. The cause of this shift is not known.

BEDTIME HOUR (P.M.) BY YEAR

Age	1974	1979	1979–80	1986	2004–8	2012–13
5 years	7:46	7:56	8:10	8:11	8:15 (2008)	—
10 years	8:45	8:50	8:50	8:59	9:00 (9 years)	9:15 (Grade 4)*
14 years	9:43	9:47	9:54	10:02	—	10:12 (Grade 7)*

(* = lower SES)

After about 1980, the trend toward a later bedtime plateaued in children 1 year old and younger, perhaps because an increasingly later bedtime would eventually be significantly disruptive to the child and the family. It is possible that the trend of ever later bedtimes has continued in older children because of increasing viewing of television and other screen-based media in the bedroom. For 5-year-olds, the wake-up times were a little later (four minutes), but the later wake-up times failed to fully compensate for the later bedtimes. The wake-up times for the 10-year-olds did not change over time, and for the 14-year-olds it was eleven minutes earlier! The take-home message is that because of later bedtimes, children are getting *less night sleep* now than in the past

Older surveys of sleep durations by age (but not newer surveys) showed that the gradual decline in total hours of sleep flattened out around age 13 or 14, and it even appeared that some 14- to 16-year-olds actually slept more before the gradual decline with age resumed! There might be an increased biologic need for sleep during a portion of adolescence, but modern life makes it more difficult to satisfy this need.

In the past, it appears that some teens, 14–16 years, needed more sleep to maintain optimal daytime alertness.

TELEVISION AND SCREENS IN THE BEDROOM

The growing popularity of television and other electronic screen-based devices in the bedroom is directly associated with less sleep and sleep problems. Here are some data from different studies to illustrate this trend:

1988: 10 percent of 3- to 10-year-old children have TV in the bedroom.

1999: 26 percent of 4- to 10-year-old children have TV in the bedroom. More TV viewing is associated with less sleep and more sleep problems

2005: 40 percent of 3- to 6-year-old children and 18 percent of children under 2 years old have TV in the bedroom.

2012: 75 percent of fourth and seventh graders (mean age, 10.6 years), sleep with a TV in the bedroom and 54 percent sleep near a small screen (smartphone or iPod Touch). It appears that sleeping near a small screen is worse than having a TV in the bedroom: Children sleeping near a small screen reported 21 minutes less night sleep (18 minutes less for those with a TV in the bedroom), the bedtime was 37 minutes later (31 minutes later for those with a TV in the bedroom), and reported perceived insufficient sleep (not reported for those with a TV in the bedroom).

2013: More television viewing is associated with later bedtime and less sleep in 10- and 11-year-olds. More TV viewing, computer use, smartphone use, and video gaming is associated with less sleep among 11- to 18-year-olds.

2014: 17 percent of 4-year-olds and 23 percent of 7-year-olds have TV in the bedroom.

Television and media viewing may cause the bedtime to be too late, or the content might make it more difficult for the child to fall asleep. Alternatively, among infants and young children, more viewing may be a parental response to their child not sleeping well. As described in Dr. Jenny Radesky's 2014 paper, parents might be *allowing more screen time as a coping strategy:*

Our findings demonstrate that, longitudinally, infants with regulatory problems [excessive fussiness, poor self-soothing, difficulties in falling asleep and staying asleep and modulating their emotional state] do watch more TV and videos later in their toddler years. However, the relationship is probably not unidirectional: child self-regulation abilities and media habits likely influence each other through a transactional process whereby parents might try to soothe fussier infants through screen time, which reduces the amount of enriching parent-infant interactions and other developmental activities, exposes infants to potentially inappropriate content, and contributes to continued regulatory difficulties, which in turn predict greater media exposure, and so on.

Wake-up Hour Trends over Time

A trend toward earlier wake-up times was also observed by Dr. Iglowstein for 14-year-olds between 1974, 1979, and 1986: 6:41, 6:39, and 6:30 a.m., respectively.

Sleep Recommendations

Lisa Matricciani's 2013 review of the literature concluded that published recommendations for children's sleep are not based on empirical evidence (see Chapters 1 and 9). She found that "sleep timing [the time when sleep occurs] may be even more important than sleep duration." In a separate 2013 paper titled "Sleep duration or bedtime?" the authors studied twenty-two hundred 9- to 16-year-old children and concluded that "late bedtimes and late wake up times are associated with poorer diet quality independent of sleep duration."

Commonly occurring sleep patterns among your relatives, friends, and neighbors might not be what is right for your child. Ignore what they recommend and what you read about bedtimes and total sleep needs and instead *watch your child*. Don't be surprised if your child needs an earlier bedtime than other children.

When your child sleeps might be more important than *how long* your child sleeps.

Years 7 to 12

The contribution of healthy sleep habits to a child's well-being does not diminish with age even though parents have many new concerns: school assignments, organized after-school activities, individual lessons, parties, more homework, dating, and riding with teens who are driving cars. Healthy sleep habits may appear to be less important to parents than the development of their children's social, athletic, artistic, or academic skills. But healthy sleep does interact with skill development. Two sleep surveys of about one thousand preadolescents, one from Belgium and the other from Taiwan, show that school achievement difficulties were encountered significantly more often among poor sleepers compared to good sleepers. For those children on a college path, the more academic pressure they felt, the fewer hours they slept.

Young children who have difficulty sleeping become older children with more academic problems. But children who are academically successful risk not getting the sleep they need!

PREVENT AND SOLVE SLEEP PROBLEMS

Chapters 3 and 4 cover the prevention and treatment of sleep problems in the school-age range, with an emphasis on reasonably early bedtimes, no screen-based media in the bedroom, relaxation training, and stimulus control/temporal control. For issues related to difficulty in falling asleep, please see Chapter 9.

Optimal Wakefulness

School-age children are sleeping less and less as the bedtime hour gradually becomes later and later. In my study (1979–80), most 12-year-olds went to sleep around 9:00 p.m.; the range was from about 7:30 to 10:00, and the range for total sleep duration was about nine to twelve hours. These findings are in close agreement with those from a study at Stanford University where researchers found that the prepubertal teenager needs nine and a half to ten hours of sleep in order to maintain *optimal wakefulness* during the day (see Chapter 2). Their finding has been cited often as a recommendation for how much sleep is needed, but the sleep duration needed at any age varies from child to child, and the time when the sleep occurs is important for sleep quality. As mentioned above, instead of paying close attention to published recommendations about bedtime hours and sleep duration, watch your child.

Recurrent Complaints

Many children in this age range complain of aches and pains for which no medical cause can be found: abdominal pains, limb pains, recurrent headaches, and chest pains. Children who suffer from these pains often have significant sleep disturbances (see Chapter 9).

Adolescence

In addition to increased use of screen-based electronic media in the bedroom, there are worrisome new trends in high schools that place more pressure on our teens. Some high schools have scheduled activities that start before the regular school day or allow students to opt out of the lunch period to take an additional class (honors or Advanced Placement courses) or electives (band, choir, or foreign language). Further, some high schools require a twelve-month commitment to sports such as volleyball or football that is incompatible with other regularly scheduled elective activities such as drama or debate. These trends and the decrease in sleep durations from 1974 to 2008 as a result of later bedtimes are a recipe for mental health problems. A report by Dr. Jean Twenge showed that symptoms of depression (trouble sleeping, thinking, and remembering; shortness of breath) among high school students have increased from the

1980s to 2010: "More than twice as many 2010–2012 teens (8%) reported having trouble sleeping on 20 or more days a month compared to 1982–1984 (3%). . . . Apparently, the pressures, lifestyle, and social forces of modern life have led people to experience more psychosomatic issues such as sleeping issues and difficulty concentrating." As will be discussed later, the salient role of insufficient sleep, as a cause of depression in adolescents or a contributing factor, is highlighted in the American Academy of Pediatrics 2014 recommendation for later start times for high schools.

Chronic sleep deficits were observed in 13 percent of teenagers in a Stanford University study that included more than six hundred high school students. These poor sleepers attributed their sleep problems to worry, tension, and personal, family, and social problems. The students appeared to be mildly depressed. Of course, we don't know which came first, disturbed sleep or the mood changes. Perhaps both the mood changes and the sleep disturbance develop from the same endocrine changes that occur naturally during adolescence or which might be a result of the pressure in school to perform well both academically and athletically. But healthy lifestyle habits, including sensible sleep patterns, might prevent or lighten the depression seen in so many adolescents.

How do you know if your teenager has disturbed sleep? Here is how the Stanford University sleep researchers defined chronic and severe sleep disturbances in adolescents:

- Forty-five or more minutes required to fall asleep on three or more nights a week

or

- One or more awakenings a night followed by thirty or more minutes of wakefulness occurring on three or more nights a week

or

- Three or more awakenings a night on three or more nights a week

So if your teenager exhibits any of these sleep patterns, don't dismiss it as a "normal" part of growing up.

In New Zealand, as in California, about 10 percent of teenagers had sleep problems. They appeared anxious, depressed, and inattentive, and they had conduct disorders more often than those without sleep problems. Anxiety and depression were also common symptoms of poorly sleeping teenagers in Italy, where about 17 percent of all teens met research criteria for sleep problems. A separate survey study of 3,136 children between ages 11 and 17 showed that 17 percent were experiencing sleep that wasn't sufficiently restorative, just as in the Italian study.

Solid research, published in 1991, has documented that adolescents' sleep time has decreased one hour over the past twenty years. The evidence is clear, whether it's from Belgium, Taiwan, China, South Africa, New Zealand, or Italy: teenagers are increasingly at risk for becoming overtired. (See "Sleep Recommendations" in Chapters 1 and 9).

In two separate studies of experimental sleep restriction in children 10 to 14 years of age, the researchers limited night sleep either to seven hours for three days or to five hours for a single night. Although rote memory task performance and routine performance were maintained, higher cognitive functions such as verbal creativity and abstract thinking were impaired. This highlights an important point: that our children can and do perform quite well even when mildly sleep deprived—as long as they are not challenged to write or be creative. Mild sleep deprivation is often trivialized or overlooked because more routine memorization tasks and athletic performances are successfully accomplished.

Another experimental sleep restriction study was performed on 11- and 12-year-olds. Comparisons were made between sleeping ten hours on six nights versus six and a half hours on six nights. The sleep restriction caused measured inattentiveness, irritability, noncompliance, and academic problems.

PREVENT AND SOLVE SLEEP PROBLEMS

Chapters 3 and 4 cover the prevention and treatment of sleep problems in the school-age range, and the emphasis is on reasonably early bedtimes, no screen-based media in the bedroom, relaxation training, and stimulus control/temporal control. An analysis of adolescent sleep patterns by Dr. Megan Hagenauer concluded that teens would be well served by falling asleep earlier, a goal that could be "enhanced by the incorporation of greater physical activity into the school day and [the time of falling asleep] could be shifted earlier by parental restrictions on screen time in the evenings and a reduction of evening light exposure."

It may take a long time for public awareness to develop regarding the risks of certain long-standing activities (see Chapter 2). For example, among some teenage football players, a concussion used to be seen as a badge of honor, but now, in some schools, concussion awareness and prevention is becoming a topic in health education classes. In the nineteenth century, French student architects were given assignments requiring them to work furiously overnight to finish the project; and the term used to describe this period of intense, focused, and sustained work is "charrette." Architecture students today still might do a charrette, but most students refer to it as an "all-nighter," and even say with pride, "I pulled an all-nighter." The harm from not sleeping at all overnight has not yet reached a high level of public awareness.

Sleep Spa and Beauty Sleep

Sometimes I have recommended to a teenager who is short on sleep that he or she take a five-day "sleep spa" treatment. No, that doesn't mean having their parents book them into an expensive resort! It simply means dedicating five days to going to sleep earlier than usual. Afterward, I ask the teenagers to reflect on whether the earlier sleep made a difference. Usually they report, rather sheepishly, that it did. Also, for some teenage girls, I point out how important it is for models, musicians, and actresses to have radiant skin and glowing dispositions, and how important beauty sleep is to maintain their appearance. Of course, that is not a suitable incentive for all young girls, but in the battle for sleep, one must pick one's weapons carefully! One mother reported to me after her daughter's sleep spa:

> Overall Sophia is not feeling as tired. She seems much more willing to go to bed earlier now that you advised her rather than me. She is turning in her computer and phone to be charged outside of her bedroom so she isn't tempted or interrupted by texts. Most 15-year-old girls want to look better and have great skin!
>
> I asked Sophia to make a list of how extra sleep helped her feel, and she wrote: "After getting the new routine I feel a lot better. I'm in a way better mood and feel more positive and have a ton more energy. I feel more willing to do things and feel more active and happier in general. I perform better in sports and am able to strategize and process things faster. I enjoy music more. I am ready to do more things throughout the day and feel more social because before I wasn't up to doing much. I wake up earlier in the morning and have more time to do things throughout the day."

Another teenager who went to bed earlier during the summer so she could accompany her father to work in the early morning compared her new lifestyle to that of her two older sisters, who liked to stay up later and sleep in: "By the time they get up, they've killed half the day."

DIFFICULTY FALLING ASLEEP

As your child gets older, it becomes harder to determine what is cause and what is effect regarding disturbed sleep and problems of mood and performance because of the development of mental health problems and increasing pressure to perform academically during adolescence. It is possible that chronically disturbed sleep causes children to grow up experiencing excessive daytime sleepiness, low self-esteem, or mild depression in adolescence. In one study, about 13 percent of teenagers with disturbed sleep were reported to be like this. They usually took longer than forty-five minutes to fall asleep or woke frequently at night. As previously mentioned, about 10 percent of 7- and 8-year-olds took up to an hour to fall asleep, and difficulty falling asleep in younger children was associated with anxiety. Some of these preteens and teenagers may simply have never learned self-soothing skills to fall asleep easily when they were much younger. As adults, they are described as insomniacs. Consider seeking professional help if your child takes a long time to fall asleep.

Many school-age children have difficulty falling asleep because they worry about their grades, test scores, appearance, or sports skills. Anxiety about not doing well academically or athletically might lead to impaired performance. This is called "performance anxiety." Impaired sleeping likewise occurs when there is too much worrying or nagging about not getting enough sleep. Worrying too much about not sleeping well creates anxiety or stress, interfering with the relaxation needed to successfully perform the task, which is to fall asleep. The solution to this vicious circle might be relaxation training. If your child, at any age, appears to need more sleep, and he wants to sleep but cannot easily fall asleep, please consider working with a professional to help your child learn to relax and avoid performance anxiety. Working with a therapist, older children can learn to sleep better through relaxation training techniques as a stand-alone strategy or in combination with stimulus control and temporal control (see Chapter 4). The attempt is to reduce the level of arousal, therefore permitting the sleep process to surface.

SHIFTING SLEEP SCHEDULES

In 1913, Dr. Lewis Terman noted that adolescents shifted toward a later bedtime and later wake-up time. This shift toward delayed sleep patterns occurs in all adolescents, in all countries and cultures. So although electronic screen-based technology use at night among children is new and tends to cause bedtimes to be even later, there appears to be a biologic shift that predates modern times. He also suggested that early start times for school may cause sleep deprivation in these children. Now, more than a hundred years later, there is a trend toward shifting the start time for school later (see Chapter 2 and page 553).

Delayed Sleep Phase Syndrome

In addition to problems associated with falling asleep and staying asleep, there are normal shifts in sleep patterns that begin in preadolescence or adolescence. Do you notice that your teenager is going to bed later and later? A biological process associated with the development of puberty might cause a shift to a later bedtime. Eventually your child might consider herself to be a night person, an owl. This tendency of your teenager to delay going to sleep may be normal, and so, too, may be her need to wake up later. If this is the case, then the late bedtime is not the problem; rather, it's the too-early start of the school day that's causing problems. Alternatively or additionally, what may be occurring is the development of cumulative sleepiness, causing an inability to fall asleep at a socially and biologically appropriate time

In healthy adolescents, the trend toward a later bedtime and later wake-up time is called the delayed sleep phase syndrome: your child has no difficulty falling asleep or staying asleep, but only when sleep onset is delayed, maybe to 1:00, 2:00, or 3:00 a.m. When she tries to go to sleep earlier, she can't. On weekends and vacations, she'll sleep later, so her total sleep time is about normal. But on school days it's always a struggle to get her up for those early classes.

As a consequence of delayed sleep phase syndrome or an unhealthy sleep schedule, schoolwork suffers and your child's mood may swing widely—the long-term result of brief sleep on school days or a chronically abnormal sleep schedule. Some teenagers try to combat the fatigue with internal stimulation (anger or elation) or external stimulation (sports or exercise).

Chronotherapy

Treatment for delayed sleep phase syndrome is called "chronotherapy," or delaying the internal sleep clock. Let's say your child can easily fall asleep at 2:00 a.m. The therapy consists of forcing him to stay up until 5:00 a.m. and then letting him sleep as long as he wishes. (Obviously, we don't do this during the school year!) The next night, his sleep is allowed to start at 8:00 a.m. the following day and at 11:00 a.m. the day after that. In other words, you are allowing sleep to occur about three hours later every cycle. Over the next few days, sleep begins at 2:00 p.m., 5:00, 8:00, and finally 11:00. Sleep onset, the bedtime, has been shifted from 2:00 a.m. to 11:00 p.m. by delaying the sleep period. Now, keeping careful watch over clock time, *always* try to have your child go to sleep at 11:00 p.m. You have shifted the sleep clock around to a more conventional time, and usually this can be maintained by sustaining a regular nighttime sleep schedule. Advancing the internal sleep clock by moving the bedtime a bit earlier on successive nights might also work. Exposure to bright light in the morning and avoidance of light (especially from electronic screens) at night might also be helpful.

Not Enough Time to Sleep in the Morning

Research has shown that most teenagers would probably be much better rested if they were allowed to sleep longer in the morning. Starting school or practice times for sports early in the morning often causes teenagers to have to nap in the afternoon, which interferes with going to bed at a reasonable time or may force them to get up too early in the morning to finish homework. In Israel, starting times in school were examined for children 10 to 12 years of age. One group started at 7:10 a.m. at least two times a week and the other group always started school at 8:00 a.m. The children in the early start time group had less total sleep, suffered more daytime fatigue and sleepiness, and complained more about difficulties in attention and concentration compared to the later start time group.

Dr. Mary Carskadon, a pioneer in adolescent sleep research, points out that earlier start times for school are a fairly recent development, and their impact on sleep deprivation for older children is only now being appreciated. Dr. Carskadon "compares sleep deprivation to walking at the edge of a cliff on a path that gets narrower and narrower until you are balancing on a rail. Sleep usually gives you a healthy buffer zone, but when you're seriously sleep-deprived, if the wind blows, you've got nothing. Take one false step and you're done."

A report by Dr. Julie Boergers on 15- and 16-year-olds showed that when the school start time was delayed from 8:00 a.m. to 8:25 a.m., there was a twenty-nine-minute increase in sleep duration on school nights. The researchers measured significant improvements in daytime sleepiness (including less falling asleep in the classroom, less tardiness, and less napping), mood (less depression), and less caffeine use. While the twenty-nine-minute improvement may seem trivial, small changes, as little as *nineteen minutes,* can cumulatively make a big difference (see Chapters 1 and 4). In fact, in this study the percentage of students getting eight or more hours of sleep on a school night dramatically increased from 18 percent to 44 percent! Judith Owens co-authored that study, and in another report, she described how "students reported going to bed earlier after start times were delayed, resulting in a greater-than-expected increase in average school night sleep duration. . . . [A]necdotal student comments suggest that the perceived benefits of additional sleep motivated students to further modify their sleep-wake behavior to optimize sleep duration. It appears that the later classes start, the more academic performance improves."

These and other studies showing that later bedtimes are associated with lower grade point averages and that short sleep durations are associated with more car and pedestrian accidents (see Chapter 2 for other problems with teenagers) led to a 2014 policy statement from the American Academy of Pediatrics that schools should not start before 8:30 a.m. "Delaying school start times is an effective countermeasure to chronic sleep loss and has a wide range of potential benefits to students with regard to physical and mental health [e.g., lower rates of obesity and depression], safety [e.g., crashes caused by drowsy driving] . . . academic performance, and quality of life." Here is the AAP's list of the impacts of chronic sleep loss in adolescents:

Physical health and safety
    Increased obesity risk
    Metabolic dysfunction (elevated cholesterol and type 2 diabetes)
    Increased risk for hypertension or stroke
    Increased rates of motor vehicle crashes
    Higher rates of caffeine consumption
    Use of stimulant medication by diversion
Mental health and behavior
    Increased risk for anxiety, depression, suicidal ideation
    Poor impulse control and self-regulation; increased risk-taking behaviors
    Emotional dysregulation, decreased positive affect
    Impaired interpretation of social/emotional cues in self and others
    Decreased motivation
    Increased vulnerability to stress
Academic and school performance
    Cognitive deficits

Impairments in executive function (organization, time management, persistence)

Impairments in attention and memory

Deficits in abstract thinking, verbal creativity

Decreased performance efficiency and output

Lower academic achievement

Poor school attendance

Increased dropout rates

Starting school later is an effective countermeasure to chronic sleep loss in adolescents. An early bedtime is an effective countermeasure at any age. A slightly earlier bedtime may cumulatively have a big impact, but children may be blind to their own sleep deprivation, so parents have to enforce bedtimes.

Starting school later will help adolescents get more sleep, but if parents continue to allow the bedtime to be later and later because of screen-based media, then the trend toward more problems associated with sleep deprivation, such as somatic complaints or depression, might continue.

Naps after school usually do not fully compensate either for bedtimes that are too late or for a wake-up time that is too early. For example, in a study of about ten thousand Japanese junior high and high school students, 50 percent napped after school at least once a week. Because the late naps made the bedtime later, the result was less sleep at night. My impression is that when teenagers are almost exhausted after school or around dinnertime, it is better not to nap then; instead, they should eat, do a little homework, go to bed early, and wake up much earlier to complete the unfinished homework. I think doing homework very late at night or way after midnight, after a late afternoon or early evening nap, is much more inefficient because the brain is in sleep mode. It might take two hours to finish an assignment between 1:00 and 3:00 a.m. after an after-school nap, but only one hour to finish the same assignment between 5:00 and

6:00 a.m. with no after-school nap, an earlier bedtime, and several hours of night sleep.

Dr. Michelle Stone studied sleep and physical activity in 856 children between 10 and 12 years separately for school weekdays and weekends and related her findings to *weight status*. Obese children sleep less throughout the week and are less likely to experience weekend catch-up sleep. But although weekend catch-up sleep helps prevent obesity, it also displaces time for physical activity. "It is not enough to have 'catch-up' sleep over the week-end for maintaining a healthy weight," Dr. Stone concluded. "Children who maintain recommended levels of sleep across the [entire] week have the most healthy and consistent levels of physical activity. . . . The findings suggest that it is not enough to have 'catch-up' sleep over the weekend, sleep regularity matters for maintaining healthy levels of activity. . . . Engaging in higher intensity activity throughout the week could enable children to fall asleep quicker and therefore maintain healthy sleep habits." Also, school-age children may experience short sleep duration during the week because they stay up too late at night and use an alarm clock to get up early, but on the weekend, they might get more sleep because, even though they might stay up later, they are able to sleep in much later in the morning (delayed sleep phase syndrome). This chronic cycling between weekday sleep restriction and weekend delayed sleep phase is called "social jet lag." Social jet lag may also occur in some very young children attending day care who might alternate between different sleep schedules on weekdays and weekends. The symptoms (problems in sleep and performance) that occur with travel-induced jet lag are transient, but with social jet lag, they may be chronic. According to Dr. Till Roenneberg, social jet lag may directly cause obesity. Separately, in a recent review by Dr. Alison Miller, in early childhood, "late bedtimes (after 9:00 p.m.) magnified and independently predicted the association between short sleep duration and obesity."

Similarly, regarding academic performance, catch-up sleep on weekends probably does not fully compensate for grueling school schedules. A study of almost three thousand Korean 17-year-olds showed that on weekdays they slept an average of 5 hours 42 minutes; on weekends it was 8 hours 24 minutes, a difference of 2 hours 42 minutes. But the greater the weekend catch-up sleep, the greater the number of errors of omission and commission observed on attention tasks. "Increased weekend catch-up sleep as an indicator of insufficient weekday sleep is associated with poor performance on objective attention tasks," concluded Dr. Kim.

We see excessive tiredness, daytime sleepiness, or decreased daytime alertness in many adolescents—there simply are not enough hours in the day to do everything. The time demands for academics, athletics, and social activities are enormous. Even without worrying about sex, drugs, alcohol, and loud music, parents worry that their teenagers may become burned out from lack of sleep.

> Social pressures and early start times for schools cause reduced sleep times and chronic sleep deficits.

IRREGULAR BEDTIMES

Dr. Carskadon also identified irregular sleep times at night to be a significant problem independent of short sleep duration (see Chapter 1). Her research showed that the more irregular the bedtime hour, the more impairment of grades, the more injuries associated with alcohol or drugs, and the more days missed from school. Previous research among preschool children also focused on the importance of bedtime regularity regarding school adjustment behaviors.

DRUGS AND DIET FOR SLEEP

Prescription drugs and over-the-counter sleeping medicines don't solve sleep problems (see Chapter 4).

Dietary changes that are known to make some people sleepy include high-carbohydrate meals and foods high in the amino acid tryptophan. It is possible that the contents of a nursing mother's diet affect the carbohydrate content of her breast milk, and this may indirectly influence the levels of tryptophan in the baby. In one study of infants, tryptophan caused the babies to begin quiet sleep twenty minutes earlier and active sleep fourteen minutes earlier. But the total amount of sleep time was not affected. So giving tryptophan to infants or other children will probably not make them sleep longer. Furthermore, tryptophan administration in adults has been associated with severe diseases, even though tryptophan is a naturally occurring amino acid. Melatonin is another naturally occurring chemical that has been popularized as a sleep aid. The safety and effectiveness of tryptophan and melatonin have not been established for infants or children.

There are no scientific data on nutrition in children that could be translated into a sleep-promoting diet. Eliminating refined sugar, because of the commonly held belief that this makes children hyperactive, also does not appear to have any effect on sleep patterns.

One report suggested that cow's milk allergy could cause insomnia. But the results of the study could have been caused by a placebo effect, because the parents knew when they were giving a cow's milk challenge and when they were eliminating cow's milk from the diet. Dietary challenges and elimination diets are best performed when both the parents and the researchers, at the time of the challenge, are ignorant of whether the child is or is not receiving the substance in question. Only then can bias or wishful thinking be reduced.

PARENTS' ADVICE

I asked the same parents that I surveyed in Chapter 2 if they continued later to put forth the effort, with age-appropriate modifications, to encourage healthy sleep in their preteen or teenager, or whether they were forced to abandon trying to help their older child sleep well because it was an impossible task. To summarize their responses: helping preteens and teenagers to sleep well continues to be a part of parenting, but there are many challenges, individual variations, and no guarantees. Here are some reports from different parents.

Guidance and Suggestions, but Not Mandates

Battles with teens are many. I have consciously decided not to make sleep one of them. We provide guidance and suggestions, but not mandates.

Ellen is in eleventh grade. For her, we try to encourage sleep without bludgeoning. Alice is now a freshman in college. At this point, when it comes to Alice's sleep, we offer advice when solicited but feel it is no longer our place to comment. Our approach with the girls has always been to treat them, first and foremost, with respect. As they have gotten older, we recognize that when they choose to go to sleep is their decision, but as their parents, we are still in a position to help them see their options.

Sleep patterns and the effectiveness of early childhood sleep discipline depend on the child. I can't help but think the early foundation is helpful. I am confident that up to this point in my children's lives I have laid the foundation for healthy sleep habits, and I'm willing to give them some freedom with respect to their sleep rituals to find out what works best for them.

Work Backward from the Bedtime

Broadly, I would say that the challenges during the preteen and teen years are the pushback, or resistance, from the child, who is developing independence, and the difficulty of saying no to an overscheduled lifestyle that burdens the children and the whole family. I work with our son and daughter to decide on a reasonable bedtime for them. They are actually in their school and have a better understanding of what they need to do and how much time they need to do it. Preteens and teens want to develop independence, so working together to come to an agreement is both instructive and age-appropriate. We sort of back into the bedtime. What I mean is that once the bedtime is agreed upon, we work backward to get everything finished in time in order to respect the bedtime. So set the bedtime. Work back and set the dinnertime. How much time is needed in between? Work back to include all activities and homework. Work back to the time the child arrives home. How much time is required after school for all the activities and work to get done before bedtime? We still maintain a two-step routine. When the children were young there was the time to go for reading and the time to go to sleep. Now we have a time to go get ready, no phone or computer allowed. Whether this means reading independently or together, talking, or getting organized for tomorrow, this is winding-down time. Then there is the time that the light goes out.

Our children are limited in the number of activities they are allowed to do because we feel this is the number one obstacle to reasonable bedtimes. What we know, plain and simple in our family, is that our children function better in every aspect of their young lives when they are rested. They are happier, kinder, work harder, are more focused, and generally our family functions better. The drama and stress of tween and teenage years are inevitable. We can't control those outside influences, but we can influence what we believe helps our children navigate these challenges. Over the years, without question, we believe our children can self-regulate and cope much better when they are rested. The *key for us is to find the right bedtime and prioritize. Our focus has always been to "work backward" from the time we wanted the children to be in bed—with enough downtime to allow for reading. That means planning dinner, homework, projects, and outdoor time to be finished early enough so that the bedtime isn't compromised. What we learned very early on was to stick to a schedule a majority of the time, and when the exceptions happen, the healthy habits are still intact.*

Naps After School: Pro, Con, and Compromise

Up until about age 14 or 15, I tried to enforce what I thought were healthy sleep habits, meaning come home from school or sports, eat dinner, do homework, go to bed at a reasonable hour (by eleven or twelve). But Sam, age 17, was so tired after he got home that sometimes he would fall asleep after dinner, or before dinner. He would wake up at 9:00 p.m. or 9:30 p.m. and stay awake until 1:00 a.m. or later. Then he'd get up at 7:00 a.m. the next day. For a while, I'd wake him up from these evening naps, insisting that he finish his homework and then go to bed at a more reasonable hour. One day, his patience came to an end, and he said it really bothered him that I kept waking him up. He pointed out that he was managing his grades, his activities, his job, and his family chores just fine. He just wanted to do it his way. So I stopped. He continued to be successful at school, in sports, and in his community.

Doing homework following a long nap after school means exercising the brain around the middle of the night, when, theoretically, learning should be less efficient because of circadian rhythms. Additionally, falling asleep after midnight means that the student is likely to be in a sleep-deprived fog at school the next morning. I usually recommend that adolescents not take a nap after school; instead, they should do a little homework, go to bed early, and set the alarm clock early in the morning to finish the homework. I think that studying early in the morning after a good night's sleep should be more efficient.

> When they came home after school, if they were exhausted, I would insist that they take a nap to refresh before starting their homework if at all possible. Usually they fell right asleep and awakened refreshed. This nap was maybe only thirty to forty-five minutes, but it helped.

Sleep-In Days

> The saving grace for both our children was that we strictly adhered to a one-day-per-week, nonnegotiable, no exceptions, sleep-in day. Usually Sunday there were no scheduled events until possibly dinner. We found that the children were able to make up for and compensate for their inadequate sleep during the week. It would not be uncommon for Elizabeth to sleep until noon or 1:00 p.m. Once high school began, in addition to exponentially more homework, sports occurred both before and after school. The sleep-in day became a lifeline.

> We declare a sleep-in "holiday" on the mornings following a late night.

> Sometimes, though, with challenging classes, they had too much homework and they stayed up later. We tried to compromise; we allowed our children to miss practice or go to school late or miss a day of school rather than stay up past midnight. We called it a "mental health day," because it was just too much. If they would have stayed up really late, they

would have ended up not feeling well all the next day anyway.

Sleepovers

Through the years, we felt pressure to skip naps and have sleepovers from our relatives and friends, rather than from our boys. Neither of our boys loved sleepovers; they didn't love staying up late and feeling horrible the following day. One sleepover experience for them was enough to not want to have another. We never had arguments regarding sleepovers.

I would say it gets more difficult each year to maintain healthy sleep habits because of the added demands on the child's time. We only allowed a few sleepovers a year.

The preteen years, when sleepovers and slumber parties became part of the landscape, posed some challenges since they always resulted in loss of sleep and, often, crabbiness the following day. This wasn't really a problem for long as the girls self-corrected. While we did not want to deprive them of the social aspect (we hosted quite a few sleepovers and slumber parties ourselves), we did feel that it would be best if they took more responsibility for their behavior as they got older. We gently reminded them that the grumpiness induced by inadequate sleep is unpleasant for everyone, the perpetrators especially! After a few years, the novelty wore off and the girls realized that they didn't miss out much if they came home and slept in their own beds. I believe that their cognizance of their sleep needs—a direct result of their early sleep "training"—was at the heart of their decision.

Individual Variation

There is individual variation in the need for early bedtimes, duration of night sleep, and the ability to cope with less than optimal sleep. Please don't expect all your children's sleep needs to be the same or similar to those of their classmates.

It was important to recognize that the twins had different sleep patterns. John likes early to bed, early to rise. Elizabeth prefers staying up and sleeping in. Naps for Elizabeth are more important due to her sleep patterns. She also sleeps much later and longer on her sleep-in day, compensating for the fewer hours of sleep during the week.

Performance

We try to hold tight with a 9:00 p.m. weekly bedtime. Trystan (age 13) knows he swims better after a good night's sleep, so he will head to bed at 8:00–8:30 p.m. on the night before a meet so as to offset the 5:30 a.m. wake-up. We know that Trystan does as well as he does in school because of his dedication to a regular sleep schedule that gives his brain time to rest and really learn all that he has taken in each day.

The point that hit home for my three sons (ages 17, 19, and 22) is that sleep can improve sports performance, test performance, and, really, performance in all aspects of their lives.

Summary and Action Plan for Exhausted Parents

Over the years, bedtimes have become later, resulting in less sleep, especially in light of early start times for school and sports activities. A later bedtime in itself is not necessarily a problem; after all, there is a normal shift among adolescents to later bedtimes and correspondingly later wake-up times. But when children are allowed to stay up too late or early school start times prevent sleeping later, sleep deficits accumulate. Depending on the cumulative sleep debt, catch-up sleep on weekends may or may not compensate for lost sleep on weekdays. One concrete step that parents can take to protect their child's sleep is to eliminate all electronic screen-based media in the bedroom after bedtime.

Bedtime resistance is more common than difficulty falling asleep. But difficulty falling asleep may be associated with anxiety and depression, and consultation with mental health professionals may be indicated. Many children who are short of sleep complain of aches and pains (headaches, stomachaches, chest pain, and limb pain), so if your child has any of these complaints, don't neglect to look beyond the immediate somatic symptoms and take sleep patterns into account.

CHAPTER 11

Solving Sleep Problems and Special Concerns

Sleep problems may occur at different ages, and you should read the earlier age-specific sections of this book to determine whether your child's sleep pattern is appropriate for his age. Some sleep problems, such as sleepwalking, sleep talking, or night terrors, appear to occur more frequently when children have abnormal sleep schedules, are otherwise sleep deprived, or have a fever. Sleepwalking, sleep talking, bruxism (teeth grinding), and night terrors tend to co-occur and run in families. Some of these common problems are bothersome to the family but are not necessarily harmful to the child. However, they might reflect an emotional problem; for example, Dr. Dieter Wolke found that "children who were bullied at age 8 or 10 years were more likely to have nightmares, night terrors, or sleepwalking at age 12 years."

One medical problem, severe and chronic snoring, may be especially hazardous to a child's health. Please read the section on poor-quality breathing even if your child has no specific sleep problems or if you think he does not snore. Snoring is sometimes not appreciated as a problem because the child has always snored, or because allergies developed when the child was older—an older child is usually in his own bedroom and the parents are unaware of how much snoring is occurring every night because they do not go into his bedroom after he has fallen asleep.

Sleepwalking

Between the ages of 6 and 16, about 5 percent of children sleepwalk between three and twelve times a year. An additional 5 to 10 percent of children walk in their sleep once or twice a year. Most commonly, episodes occur between the ages of 5 and 10 years. When it starts under age 10 and ends by age 15, sleepwalking is usually not associated with any emotional stress, personality types, or behavioral problems. Research has shown that there is a substantial genetic factor to sleepwalking, because it was found that the behavior is more common among identical twins than fraternal twins.

Sleepwalking episodes usually occur within the first two to three hours after falling asleep. The sleepwalk itself may last up to thirty minutes. Usually the sleepwalker appears to be little concerned about his environment and is unresponsive to verbal commands. His gait is not fluid and his movement is not purposeful. In addition to walking, other behaviors such as eating, dressing, and opening doors often occur.

Treatment consists only of safety measures to prevent sleepwalkers from falling down stairs or out of open windows. Try to remove toys or furniture from your child's path, but don't expect to be able to wake him. Contrary to popular belief, rousing a sleepwalker will not hurt the sleepwalker, but usually a sleepwalking child wakes spontaneously without any memory of the walk.

Sleep Talking

Sleep talkers do not make good conversationalists! They seem to talk to themselves and respond to questions with single-syllable answers. Adults appear annoyed or preoccupied. Children often repeat simple phrases like "get down" or "no more," as if they were remembering important stressful events that had occurred that day.

Between the ages of 3 and 10 years, about half of all children will talk in their sleep once a year. Older studies have suggested that sleepwalking and sleep talking tended to occur together and were more common in boys; however, newer studies do not support this association.

Confusional Arousals

In infants and toddlers, agitated behaviors with crying that may be intense and last five to fifteen minutes or longer may occur at night. Parents are unable to wake their child or to console them, and the child returns to sleep spontaneously.

Night Terrors

Your 3- to 10-year-old child utters a piercing scream, and you rush into his room. He appears wild-eyed, anxious, frightened. His pupils are dilated and sweat is covering his forehead, and as you pick him up to hug him you notice his heart is pounding and his chest heaving. He is inconsolable. Your heart is full of dread, and it almost seems as if some evil spirit has gripped your child. After five to fifteen minutes, the agitation and confused state finally subside. This is a night terror. Night terrors usually start between 4 and 12 years of age. When they start before puberty, they are not associated with any emotional or personality problems. Night terrors have nothing to do with seizures, convulsions, or epilepsy. Night terrors appear more often when a child has a fever or when sleep patterns are disrupted, such as on long trips, during school vacations, during holidays, or when relatives come to visit. Recurrent night terrors are also often associated with chronically abnormal sleep schedules.

Like sleepwalking, sleep talking, and confusional arousals, night terrors occur mainly during non-REM sleep and usually within the first few hours of going to sleep. They usually do not occur when we dream (during REM sleep); they are not bad dreams. In fact, children have no memory of them once they are awake.

Enabling our children to get more sleep is the treatment. I have observed that night terrors disappear when the parents moved the bedtime earlier by only thirty minutes.

Drug therapy is not warranted for most children with night terrors (nor, for that matter, for sleepwalking or sleep talking problems). Most children should be allowed to outgrow these problems without complex tests (such as CT scans), drug treatments, or psychotherapy.

Nightmares

In old English mythology, a nightmare was thought to be a female spirit or monster that beset people and animals at night, coming upon them when they are asleep and producing a feeling of dread or suffocation.

I have had nightmares of suffocation, strangulation, breathlessness, choking, being crushed or trapped, drowning, entrapment, and being buried alive—but only when I sleep on my back or have an alcoholic drink before going to bed. My wife says that at these times my breathing sounds like a diesel truck with a bad motor. When she pokes me to get me up, the nightmare ends, and I breathe normally again. You see, my nightmares occur when my upper airway is partially blocked, and this obstruction happens only when I sleep on my back or drink alcohol before bedtime. Occasionally I have less dramatic dreams of breathlessness while running, flying (without a plane, of course), or being chased. If my wife does not awaken me, I wake up to breathe, but I have no dream recall. Maybe some children have similar nightmares when they have bad colds or throat infections that partially obstruct their upper airway.

The child with a nightmare can be awakened and consoled, in contrast to the child with a night terror, which spontaneously subsides. About 30 percent of high school students have one nightmare a month. Adults who have more frequent nightmares (more than two per week) often have other sleep problems: frequent night awakenings, increased time required to fall asleep, and decreased sleep duration. They appear more anxious and distrustful, and experience fatigue in the morning.

But nightmares in most young children do not seem to be associated with any specific emotional or personality problems. However, two recent reports, one for children 5 to 8 years of age and the other for children 6 to 10 years of age, concluded that anxiety issues or other psychological problems are associated with nightmares. Analysis—guesswork, really—of dream content in disturbed children who have been referred to psychologists or psychiatrists should not be generalized to normal populations of children with the assumption that normal anxieties or fears represent a mental or emotional problem. We really do not know the exact value or limitations of dream interpretation. If you think your child is having a nightmare, shower him with hugs and kisses and try to awaken him.

What to do if the child begins coming into the parents' room, sometimes several times a night, complaining of nightmares? If you strongly suspect that your child is not feigning nightmares just to get extra attention at night, and the behavior does not subside in a reasonable amount of time, consider consulting with a child psychologist or psychiatrist.

Head Banging and Body Rocking

My third son banged his head against the crib every night after we moved into a new house. Actually, he struck his shoulder blades more than his head against the headboard of his crib. My solution was to use soft cushions to pad both ends and both sides completely. Now when he banged away there was no racket, no pain, and no parental attention. After a few days he stopped. Other parents are not so lucky.

About 5 to 10 percent of children will bang or roll their heads from side to side before falling asleep during their first few years. This usually starts at about 8 months of age. Boys behave this way more than girls. No behavioral or emotional problems are seen in these children as they develop, and they certainly have no neurological problems. Body rocking before falling asleep also occurs in normal children. All this rhythmic behavior usually stops before the fourth year if there are no underlying neurological diseases.

Bruxism

Teeth grinding, or bruxism, during sleep is common in children. At the Laboratory School at the University of Chicago, about 15 percent of the students were reported by their parents to have a history of bruxism. In the age range of 3 to 7 years, the percentage of bruxists was about 11 percent; between 8 and 12 years, it was 6 percent, and between 13 and 17 years, it dropped to about 2 percent. Teeth grinding does not occur during dreams or nightmares. There may be an association between anxiety and teeth grinding.

Poor-Quality Breathing: Allergies and Snoring

When you have a cold, you can't breathe easily during sleep, and you can't sleep easily, either. In turn, this makes you sleepy during the day, which can affect your mood and performance. When the cold finally disappears, you feel like your old self again, and your mood improves, as does your performance. Some children experience the same type of disrupted sleep *every night* because of allergies or snoring:

ALLERGIES

Allergies may cause difficulty breathing during sleep. Here's a partial list of symptoms among children with difficulty breathing during sleep.

Snoring
Stopping breathing during sleep
Restless sleep
Breathing through mouth when awake
Sweating when asleep
Excessive daytime sleepiness
Chronic runny nose
Frequent colds

Perhaps the chronic runny nose and the frequent colds are due to allergies—for example, to dust or the protein in cow's milk. Allergists have long associated food sensitivities or sensitivity to environmental allergens with behavioral problems, such as poor ability to concentrate, hyperactivity, tension, or irritability. Terms such as "tension-fatigue syndrome" or "allergic-irritability syndrome" are used by allergists to describe children who exhibit nasal or respiratory allergies, food allergies, and behavioral problems. Perhaps allergies cause behavioral problems in children by producing swollen respiratory membranes that partially obstruct breathing during sleep. The difficulty these children experience in breathing during sleep causes them to lose sleep and thus directly causes fatigue, irritability, and tension.

SNORING

Two of the world's leading sleep researchers, Dr. Christian Guilleminault and Dr. William C. Dement, published a landmark paper in 1976 that was the first careful study of how impaired breathing during sleep destroys good-quality sleep in children. They studied eight children ages 5 to 14 years, all of whom snored. All eight children snored loudly every night, and snoring had been present for several years. Snoring started in one child at 6 months, and while the snoring in most of the children was originally intermittent, it eventually became continuous. Here's how their symptoms were described:

> *Daytime drowsiness:* The report noted that "the children, particularly at school, tried desperately to fight it off, usually with success. To avoid falling asleep, the children tended to move about and gave the appearance of hyperactivity."
>
> *Bed-wetting:* All the children had been completely toilet trained, but seven started to wet their beds again.
>
> *Decreased school performance:* The teachers reported lack of attention, hyperactivity, and a general decrease in intellectual performance, particularly in the older children.
>
> *Morning headaches:* Headaches occurred only when they awoke in the morning; the headaches lessened or disappeared completely by late morning.
>
> *Mood and personality changes:* Half the children had received professional counseling or family psychotherapy for "emotional" problems. The report noted that "three children were particularly disturbed at bedtime; they consistently

avoided going to bed, fighting desperately against sleepiness. They refused to be left alone in their rooms while falling asleep and, if allowed, would go to sleep on the floor in the living room."

Weight problems: Five of the children were underweight, and two were overweight.

Not all children who snore have all of the problems described above, and these differences may be explained by differences in the severity and duration of the underlying problem. But overall we have a picture here of impaired mood and school performance, which deteriorated as the children grew older or as the snoring became more continuous or severe. Sleep is definitely not bliss for these children! After surgery to remove enlarged adenoids, tonsils, or both, these symptoms were quickly—and often dramatically—reduced or eliminated. For example, in one report, a 13-month-old boy was assessed as having the developmental level of an 11-month-old baby before surgery, but five months after surgery, his developmental level had jumped past his real age, to the level of a 20-month-old! So the good news is that these problems are reversible when the sleep deficits are corrected. One word of caution: If the problem has been long-standing, then once children are cured of their snoring or their allergies are under control, bad social or academic habits or chronic stresses in the family or school will still require the attention of professionals, such as psychologists, tutors, or family therapists. The treated child is now a more rested child, however, and is in a better position to respond to this extra effort.

But was this a new discovery? Not really. Medical texts written as early as 1914 acknowledged that snoring can disrupt sleep and cause behavior problems. As Dr. William Ballenger noted one hundred years ago:

> Restlessness during the night is a prominent symptom; the patient often throws the covers off during the unconscious rolling and tossing which is so characteristic. . . .

Daytime restlessness is also a characteristic sign. The child is fretful and peevish, or is inclined to turn from one amusement to another . . . the mental faculties are often much impaired . . . difficult attention is very often present. The child is listless and has difficulty in applying himself continuously to his play, studies, or other tasks, of which he soon tires. He has fits of abstraction.

A 1925 study identified enlarged adenoids and tonsils as a physical cause of poor sleep. Even a major pediatric professional journal cited "difficulty in breathing, such as seen with extreme enlargement of the adenoids," as a common cause of "infantile insomnia" as far back as 1951.

Why, then, has kids' snoring particularly been ignored? In part, this is another example of a medical concern that has taken a long time to be recognized by physicians and parents as a real problem (see Chapter 2). But also, could it be that there are more snorers around today? Perhaps yes, because although surgical removal of tonsils and adenoids is much less common today, it was for many years in the past a very popular procedure for recurrent throat infections; it also happened to "cure" snoring in children. And perhaps yes, because the air we breathe is increasingly polluted and our processed foods increasingly allergenic; this may cause reactive enlargement of adenoids or tonsils in more children.

Children with documented obstruction of breathing generally sleep less than normal children. At about age 4, the average duration of night sleep was only eight and a half hours in affected children, compared to ten and a quarter hours in healthy children.

In another study I performed, the total sleep duration for snorers was about half an hour less than that of children who did not snore. They also had night wakings that lasted longer, they went to bed later, and they took longer to fall asleep after going to bed. These affected children exhibited snoring, difficult or labored breathing, or mouth breathing when asleep. Parents described problems such as overactivity, hyperactivity, a short attention span, an inability to sit still, learning disabilities, or other academic difficulties in their snoring children.

Even in infants, snoring might be a problem. I studied a group of 141 normal infants between 4 and 8 months of age. In these infants, 12 percent exhibited snoring and 10 percent exhibited mouth breathing when asleep. These snoring infants slept one and a half hours less and awoke twice as often as infants who did not snore.

And as we have seen, a chronic sleep deficit of only *nineteen minutes* per night might cause impaired development (see Chapter 4).

Although snoring reflects difficulty breathing during sleep, it is not related to sudden infant death syndrome (SIDS).

The night waking in these snoring infants and the restless light sleep in older children probably represent protective arousals from sleep: that the child awakens or sleeps lightly in order to breathe better. When awake, the child breathes well, but the brain's control over breathing is blunted during deep sleep stages. So, to prevent asphyxiation, the child awakens frequently, cries out at night, and has trouble maintaining prolonged, consolidated deep sleep states. Here, the crying and waking at night and resistance to falling asleep are caused by a valid medical problem—not a behavioral problem, not nightmares, not a parenting problem.

All children snore a little, and frequent colds or a bad hay fever season might cause more snoring, which usually does no harm. Consider snoring a problem when it gets progressively worse, is chronic or continuous, disrupts your child's sleep, and affects daytime mood or performance. About 10 to 20 percent of children snore frequently.

The term "sleep-related breathing disorders," or SRBDs, was coined to describe those children who had snoring or heavy or loud breathing while sleeping, or who appeared to be struggling to breathe while sleeping, or who made a snorting sound and woke up. One research study conducted in 1997 directly connected SRBDs to attention deficit hyperactivity disorder (ADHD). They calculated that about 25 percent of children with ADHD would have their symptoms eliminated by correcting their habitual snoring or SRBD. In 1998, two studies showed that SRBD was associated with extremely poor academic performance in first grade (improvement occurred upon removal of tonsils and adenoids) and also that SRBD was associated with difficulties with behavioral sleep disorders such as fighting sleep at night or bedtime battles. By 2002, the terminology had changed to "sleep-disordered breathing," or SDB, but the message was the same. Inattention, hyperactivity, and behavioral and emotional difficulties are more common in children with SDB. However, the relationship between ADHD and SDB was controversial until a 2014 review by Dr. Karim Sedky, who concluded that "ADHD symptoms are related to SDB and improve after adenotonsillectomy."

If snoring appears to be disrupting your child's sleep, consult with your physician. Your child's doctor may have to do some tests to determine how serious the problem really is. Most children's hospitals have sleep centers to help diagnose and treat these problems.

Hyperactive Behavior

Attention deficit hyperactivity disorder (ADHD) is commonly called "hyperactivity." Hyperactivity in children is often not thought to be related to snoring or severe allergies, even though children suffering from ADHD have academic problems similar to those characteristic of children with snoring and poor sleep patterns. As discussed above, if the symptoms of ADHD are present, it is important to determine whether the child does or does not have difficulty in breathing during sleep.

Restless sleep, or increased amounts of movement during sleep, has been documented in hyperactive children. Could these turned-on school-age children be cranked up because of chronically poor sleep habits that started in infancy?

I studied a group of boys between 4 and 8 months old. Only boys were included, because most hyperactive school-age children are boys. Some infant boys had active sleep patterns—they moved throughout the night in a restless fashion, with many small movements of the hands, feet, or eyes. They also had difficult-to-manage temperaments: they were irregular and withdrawing, had high intensity, were slow to adapt, and were moody. This temperamental cluster is thought to be common among hyperactive children as well. The results showed that infant boys with more difficult temperaments and active sleep patterns also had briefer attention spans. Perhaps their motors were racing so fast, day and night, that they couldn't sleep quietly at night or concentrate for prolonged periods when awake during the day.

I conducted another study of 3-year-olds. It also showed that children who had increased motor activity when awake had a physically active sleep pattern. A child with active sleep patterns was more likely to be described as having symptoms of ADHD (restless or overactive, excitable, impulsive, disturbs other children, fails to finish things he starts, short attention span, constantly fidgeting, inattentive, easily distracted, demands must be met immediately, easily frustrated, cries often and easily, mood changes quickly and drastically, temper outbursts, explosive and unpredictable behavior).

Learning may suffer, then, in children who do not sleep well because they breathe poorly during sleep or sleep too little, and who in turn suffer from chronic fatigue that may cause hyperactivity. Of course, there may be other causes for school problems or hyperactivity, but disturbed sleep appears to be one that is both preventable and treatable.

Bed-wetting

Bed-wetting during sleep normally occurs in about 20 percent of children at age 4 and 10 percent at age 5. After age 5 or 6, bed-wetting during sleep might need to be treated. By the age of 10, it occurs in about 5 percent of children. The exact cause of bed-wetting is not known. It is not caused by emotional problems. It tends to occur more often in boys and has a tendency to be inherited. Pediatricians or pediatric urologists may offer bladder-training strategies or other treatments, but it is difficult to prove that one treatment works best, as most children outgrow the problem. Restricting fluids before bedtime does not work.

Moisture alarms are an effective treatment for bed-wetting. These alarms wake the child as he begins to urinate. This seems to disturb the sleeping brain, and so to prevent such an abrupt arousal from the alarm in the future, the brain controls the bladder better and prevents urination during sleep. Sometimes the alarm does not rouse the child, so the parent has to be able to hear the alarm in order to wake the child. The reason the child might sleep through the alarm is that bed-wetters appear to have very deep sleep. Even though older research suggests that bed-wetters are not more difficult to awaken than children who are not bed-wetters, this deep sleep may be a major part of the problem for some children.

In my experience, some children with too-late bedtimes or severe allergies causing difficulty breathing through the nose appear to be overtired during the day and wet at night. When they are helped to sleep better, they often appear to be better rested during the day and drier at night. The most dramatic "cures" of bed-wetting sometimes occur when enlarged adenoids or tonsils are removed. Now the child breathes easier during sleep, sleeps better, and becomes drier.

Special Events and Concerns

As if growing up were not hard enough, there are inevitable events that might significantly disrupt your child's healthy sleep habits. Other special concerns, such as frequent injuries, may well be the result of unhealthy sleep habits. Here are some examples.

CHANGES WITH DAYLIGHT SAVINGS TIME

When you move the clock an hour earlier or later, continue to put your child to sleep according to the new time. If her bedtime has been about 6:30 p.m. and you moved the clock ahead an hour, so her old 6:30 is now 7:30 p.m., still put her down to sleep at the new clock time of 6:30 p.m. You can ignore the time change because a lot of social cues in the family, such as active or quiet times, meals, bathing, and outdoor playtime, are adjusted along with the time change, and these social cues help regulate your child's sleep schedule.

NEW SIBLING

If you are expecting another child, it is best to maintain as much regularity as possible during the pregnancy and not move your young child to a bed until the new baby is about 4 months old, if then. Toward the end of the pregnancy, the mother is more tired and the older child becomes aware that his mother has less energy or patience. Receiving less attention or not as prompt a response is something that your older child will have to get used to. So don't kill yourself putting forth a heroic effort in a fruitless attempt to give your firstborn the same amount of attention that he received when he was an only child; it will only delay your older child's learning to adapt to the inevitable decrease in parental attention. When the newborn is about 4 months old, the developing biological rhythms in your baby permit a new and stable social rhythm in the household. Your older child now knows that there are approximate times when his mother is feeding the baby or putting it to sleep. The stability of these events makes the older child feel more secure. The transition from a crib to a bed is then easier. But consider leaving the crib up and empty for a while before the baby is shifted to the crib. The parents' understanding is that the older child is graduating to a big-kid bed, but the older child might not have the same opinion. Prepare yourself for the possibility that, either because of fearfulness in the big bed or because the older child now realizes he can easily get out of bed to explore the house, you might have to return him to the crib. Sometimes a crib tent is necessary (see Chapter 4) because your child is curious about the new baby at night but you do not have the energy to repeatedly do the silent return to sleep. Don't be inhibited because of a fear that you are causing a "regression" or sense of failure in your child by returning your baby from the bed to a crib. Under these circumstances, the new baby might have to go to a portable crib, another crib if the children are close together in age, or maybe some temporary larger substitute for the bassinet.

TWINS, TRIPLETS, AND MORE

Let's face it: having a baby is a blessing and a bother. With two or three babies at the same time, the blessings are two- or threefold, but the bother may be about ten or twenty times as great! The reason why the bother is so much greater is that you can't clone yourself. When one child is awake and wants to play but the other needs to be put to bed, or when one baby needs to be fed at the same time as the other needs to be changed, you've got a problem. Not everyone has family members or hired help to give them a break, and even if you are lucky in this regard, there are still times when both the mother and father are exhausted from not getting enough sleep (see Chapter 5). As discussed in my book *Healthy Sleep Habits, Happy Twins,* having twins is especially stressful for older mothers.

There is ample evidence that genetics contribute significantly to shaping our sleep patterns. Identical twins sleep more like each other than do fraternal twins, so there are limits on what we can do to modify the sleep schedules of fraternal twins if we attempt to synchronize them. The regularity of the mother's activity/rest cycles and her sleeping and eating patterns before the babies are born may substantially contribute to the regularity or irregularity of her babies' sleep patterns.

With twins, triplets, or more, the major principle is to start sleep training *early*. Early sleep training means starting around the time the babies are born, or around the time of their due date for children born early (many twins or triplets arrive before their due date). The first principle is to *avoid the overtired state*. Try to put your babies down for a nap, using method A (see Chapter 7), after a wakeful period of one or two hours. If they get overtired, it is harder for them to fall asleep. The more rested they are, the more adaptable they become later, and the more successful you will be in synchronizing their sleep schedules when they are older. Because their internal clock machinery is not really well developed during these first few weeks, you can't set their clocks to the same "time."

Counting from the due date, during the next 6 weeks you will notice more and more fussiness and wakefulness; by 6 weeks of age, it is mostly concentrated in the evening hours, about seven o'clock to ten o'clock. During these increasing spells of agitated or fussy wakefulness, do whatever you can to calm and comfort your babies. Remember, you can't spoil your babies, so during these spells do all the holding, hugging, nursing, or whatever works to keep your infants comfortable.

Around 6 weeks after the due date, when one baby awakes in the morning, you declare that the day is starting and night sleep has ended. This will usually occur between 6:00 and 8:00 a.m. At that time, awaken the other baby or babies. Remember, we are doing this at a few weeks of age to help synchronize their sleep schedules, but this maneuver of controlling the wake-up time may also be applied to older twins and triplets. If you are experienced parents, you might want to try to control the wake-up time when the children are much younger. If you are good at reading the babies' cues and you have identical twins, then you might be able to synchronize their schedules when they are even younger.

The next step is to keep the following interval of wakefulness ultra-short. We are going to try to put both children down for the first nap—together, in the same room or crib—after only *one hour* of wakefulness. Try as best you can to change, feed, and soothe them back to sleep within a total time of one hour. This means that you will probably have no time to play with them during this brief morning wakeful period. During this hour of wakefulness, if there is bright natural sunlight, open all your shades and expose them to this light, because exposure to bright morning light helps to set the sleep/wake clock. To sum up: start early, avoid the overtired state, use method A, and allow a very brief interval (only one hour) of wakefulness.

Now comes the hard part, especially if you are a first-time parent. Your hope is that your children will be able to learn some self-soothing skills even at this very young age. *Put your babies down to sleep after several minutes of soothing, whether or not they are in a deep sleep state.* Your children may be fully asleep, completely awake, or in a state between wakefulness and sleep at the time when you put them down. Your ultimate goal, however, is to put them down drowsy but awake.

If one or both babies cry as you walk away, leave them alone—but look at a clock so that you will know when they have been alone for five to ten minutes. Here are two common scenarios: Your babies cry very hard for a few minutes, then cry quietly for several minutes, and then fall asleep. Or possibly your babies cry hard for several minutes and do not appear to be able to fall asleep. Of course, one child may go one way and the other child another way. You are providing an opportunity for a midmorning nap for one or both children.

If one or both fall asleep, don't be surprised if the duration of the nap is brief; naps tend to lengthen only at 12 to 16 weeks of age, counting from the due date. Within any subsequent two-hour interval, try to put both children back down for a nap. This is because most young babies do not comfortably tolerate more than two hours of wakefulness.

If one or both do not fall asleep, rescue your baby or babies. You now have two choices. First, you may sense that after several minutes of hard crying your baby will now be able to fall asleep, so you repeat the process of soothing back to sleep. Or else the crying was so stressful for all of you that you will quickly go out for a walk, enjoy playing with and comforting your baby, and try this maneuver again another day. Remember, you want to give your babies the opportunity to learn how to soothe themselves to sleep. You are practicing *consistency* in how you soothe the baby to sleep and *timing* to avoid the overtired state.

If you had only one child, you might decide to always hold or nurse that child until he or she was in a deep sleep state and then either put the baby down alone or sleep with the baby in your bed or sofa (method B; see Chapter 7). The simple truth is that you cannot be consistent with method B if you have twins or triplets. So stick with method A. Because the process of falling asleep is learned behavior, your babies will learn faster if you are consistent in how you soothe them to sleep.

At night, an early bedtime is helpful because it regularizes and lengthens naps. Here, too, consistency in the style of soothing to sleep is helpful.

If you have older twins or triplets, between 4 and 15 months of age, control the wake-up time, expose them to bright light in the period after they wake up, and practice consistency in how you soothe your babies to sleep. Now your goal is to put them down for naps at about 9:00 a.m. and 1:00 p.m., and not to let them sleep at other times during the day. Expect your babies at 15 to 21 months of age to need a single nap between noon and 2:00 p.m.

The plan to have the babies asleep and awake at about the same time may initially fail, because there is a strong genetic component that influences how long babies sleep, how regular are the times when they need to sleep, and how self-soothing they are when put down to sleep. Therefore, you may be more successful in synchronizing sleep schedules with identical twins than with fraternal twins. But even identical twins can have their own personalities! Prepare yourself for the possibility that one twin may be a good sleeper (self-soothing, long sleep durations, regular sleep patterns) and the other twin the opposite.

As mentioned earlier, place your babies together in the same room, or even the same crib. Many of these babies seem to enjoy touching each other and sometimes appear to help the other one sleep by stroking, petting, or even putting a hand or finger in the mouth of the other. Later, if it becomes apparent that one twin or triplet is interfering with the sleep of another, then you have to try to separate the "bad sleeper" from the "good sleeper." Sometimes this is easier said than done because of the number of rooms in your house. Be creative. You might temporarily put one child in your bedroom for naps, or perhaps you have a large walk-in closet, or maybe there is some attic or basement space where you can create a nest for naps. This temporary separation might be needed until the "bad sleeper" settles down to a regular nap pattern, which usually evolves between 12 and 16 weeks after their due date. Also, please do not be surprised if the twins do a flip-flop and the one who had been a "good sleeper" becomes a "bad sleeper" and vice versa. The truth is that during the first few months, there is a lot of shifting around in daytime sleep patterns. All children sleep better during the day around 3 or 4 months of age, so be patient.

When I discussed this problem of synchronizing sleep schedules with mothers and fathers at a support group for parents of twins, some said they would wake up the good sleeper shortly after the sibling who slept less awoke, go out to have fun, and then put them both down together for the next sleep period. The risk is that the good sleeper might become overtired because the child's needs are not met. Other parents let the good sleeper finish the nap and later put them down together. Here the risk is that the bad sleeper becomes overtired from being up too long. One mother of twins really summed up the majority sentiment when she said, "You just have to compromise." Sometimes letting the good sleeper snooze a little longer before waking him up is all it takes to produce some regularity in the sleep routines.

Here's the conflict: you want to avoid the overtired state *and* you want to synchronize their sleeping patterns. Sleep logs, as described in Chapter 3, are very helpful to get a handle on how to strike a good compromise.

Each family with twins and triplets has its own strengths, resources, and stresses; please consider reviewing your situation with other parents of twins and triplets or your pediatrician before sleep problems develop.

My book *Healthy Sleep Habits, Happy Twins* provides more help and detailed information regarding helping twins sleep better.

MOVING

The only thing worse than moving is moving with children. You pack, they unpack. You clean up, they make a mess.

Your general goal should be to maintain as regular and consistent a pattern as possible when preparing for and following a move. Resist the temptation to drag the baby to the home improvement store or garden shop when he should be sleeping. If your child is young—say, less than 1 year old—quickly reestablish the bedtime rituals and sleep patterns that worked best before the move. Be firm, and after allowing a day or two for adjustment to the new surroundings, ignore any protest crying that may have evolved from the irregularity and inconsistency of the move. These young babies don't really care about the color of the walls or the new wallpaper in their bedroom; routines of the day and night provide security. If your child is older, say a few years, go slower. Fears of newness, excitement over novelty, and uncertainty regarding further changes may cause new problems of resistance to naps, difficulty falling asleep at night, or night waking. Be gentle, firm, and decisive. Reassurance, extra time at night, night-lights, and open doors have a calming or soothing effect. Be somewhat consistent in controlling this extra comfort so that the child does not learn that it is completely open-ended. For the older child, consider using a kitchen timer to control the amount of extra time for soothing. The timer helps the child to learn to expect that Mom or Dad will leave for the night after a predictable time period. Place the timer under a pillow or cushion to muffle the sound.

Anxiety or fear in your child regarding a move is natural, normal, and not something that should unduly alarm you. After several days, start a deliberate process of "social weaning" to encourage a return to your old, healthy sleep habits by gradually reducing the duration on the timer. This should usually take no more than several days in most instances.

VACATIONS AND CROSSING TIME ZONES

Think of a vacation with your child as sort of a semi-holiday. After all, you may spend a lot of time babysitting among the palms on sun-drenched beaches. I have spent many hours building simple sand castles with one son while trying to keep an eye on a non-swimmer son jumping over small waves. This intense concentration is not very relaxing!

Try to flow with your child: be flexible, forget schedules, try to have as much fun as possible, and don't worry much if your kids become tired. Irregularity and spontaneity are part of what make vacations fun.

When you cross two or more time zones, especially if you travel east, you might suffer the ill effects of jet lag. You are conditioned to sleep when it is dark, but activity/rest cycles and feeding habits also get messed up when you cross time zones. Children seem to be more sensitive to light, especially morning light, than adults are, so use this to help defeat jet lag. Sunlight helps regulate the internal timing mechanism. The day after you arrive (or the next day, if it is a very long trip) wake your child at the usual wake-up time. Do this both at your vacation destination, at the beginning of the trip, and when you return home after the vacation is over.

Scenario one: You leave your home very early in the morning because of holiday traffic and the extra time required because of airport security. You arrive at your destination, and it is now very late at night. By the time you claim your luggage, rent a car, drive to your hotel, and get settled, everyone is exhausted. It's been a long day crossing many time zones! So everyone sleeps in the next morning. If your child is napping, the late morning wake-up causes the nap(s) to be later. Therefore, maybe wake up your child after a one- to two-hour nap in order to protect a reasonably early bedtime. The *following morning,* either wake up your child at his customary wake-up time, to reestablish his regular sleeping schedule, or repeat the process of shortening the nap to more gradually get the bedtime to its regular early time. If your child is not napping, over the next day or days control the wake-up time by waking your child either a little or a lot earlier—and exposing him to bright sunlight, if available—until you get to your child's normal wake-up time.

Scenario two: The trip takes about half a day, and you arrive at your destination and get settled in by midafternoon or early evening. The *day after you arrive,* wake up your child at the usual time, try to give him a dose of bright sunlight, and immediately reestablish the customary sleep schedule.

Once you're home, it's boot camp again—back to the basics, with all the regular routines. Maybe you will do a reset (see Chapter 4). Repeat the strategies described above. Within a few days, if you are firm, consistent, and regular, your child will learn quickly that the vacation is over. If your child was well rested prior to this vacation, expect only one rough, crazy recovery day of protest crying. I tell families that one nasty reentry night may be the price you will pay for having a lovely family vacation. Trying to gradually soothe your child back to her previous good sleep routine over several days after a vacation often fails because your child fights sleep in order to enjoy your company, which she especially enjoyed during the vacation.

FREQUENT ILLNESSES

Night wakings routinely accompany frequent illnesses. First, let's have a clear understanding of what is happening. Video recordings of healthy young children in their homes at night show that many awakenings occur throughout the night, but the children usually return to sleep without any help. Fever can alter sleep patterns and can cause light sleep or more frequent awakenings. So it is not surprising that a painful illness with fever, such as an ear infection, causes an increased number of night wakings. These more frequent and prolonged arousals often require your intervention to soothe or calm your child back to sleep. Your child might now begin to associate your hugging, kissing, or holding at night with returning to sleep. This learning process might then produce an alteration in the child's behavior or expectations that continue long after the infection passes. Now we have a night-waking problem. Actually, awakening at night is *not* the problem. As we have seen, spontaneous awakenings are normal, as are increased awakenings with fever. Naturally, parents should go to their sick children at night. The real problem once the child is healthy again and not bothered by pain or fever is his learned difficulty in returning to sleep unassisted and attendant signaling behavior. How can you reteach your child to develop her own resources to return to sleep after awakening? Remember, parents are teachers and we teach health habits, even if the child might not initially cooperate or appreciate our efforts. Here are three options:

> *Option one:* Your child is sometimes healthy and signaling, but since he is also frequently ill—for example, because of

day care or older school-age siblings—you decide that you
will always respond and will simply wait for the child to
"outgrow" this habit. The problem with this option is that
the awakenings tend to become more frequent, because
your child learns to enjoy your company at night. After all,
who wants to be alone in a boring, dark, quiet room in the
middle of the night? Eventually, months or years later, the
child sleeps through the night and the parents can congrat-
ulate themselves for always having attended to their child's
crying at night. You have, however, paid a price. Parents
following this course of action often become sleep deprived
or chronically fatigued, and occasionally feel resentful
toward the child for not appreciating their dedicated efforts. In addition, the sleep fragmentation and sleep deprivation often produce a child who is more irritable, aroused,
agitated, and hyperexcitable, because the child is always
fighting chronic fatigue and drowsiness.

Option two: You might try to go to your child at night only
when you think she is really sick and leave her alone at
night when you think she is healthy. This is a strategy that
might fail, because you may often be uncertain whether an
illness is serious or just a minor concern. After all, at
7:00 p.m., you might decide that your child has only a minor
common cold and that you are going to ignore her crying,
but by 2:00 a.m. you begin to worry about the possibility of
an ear infection. Is it still reasonable to ignore the crying?
What usually occurs is intermittent reinforcement: you
sometimes go to your child and sometimes do not go. This
behavior generally teaches your child to cry longer and
louder when she awakens at night, because she learns that
only loud and persistent crying will bring her parents, while
quiet or brief crying usually fails to get their attention.

Option three: Work closely with your pediatrician to devise a
reasonable strategy whereby frequent visits or phone calls

permit a clearer distinction between colds that aren't serious and more distressing or disturbing illnesses. Generally speaking, your child's playfulness, sociability, activity, and appetite during the day are good clues, because common colds do not cause much change in your child's behavior when awake. Then, in a planned and deliberate fashion, your child is left alone more and more at night, so that she learns to return to sleep without your help even when there is a mild cough or sniffle. When an acute illness develops that is associated with high fever or severe pain, of course, do whatever comforts your child best, both night and day.

Common colds typically last seven to ten days, and one infection may be winding down when another one starts up. Overlapping or closely spaced colds give the illusion that a single infection lasts for several weeks or even months! However, the acute phase of each individual common cold is associated with more pain and fever and typically lasts twenty-four to seventy-two hours. During this time, your child needs more attention and perhaps medication. Typically, by the fifth day, the worst is over, though some symptoms may continue for another few days. When the acute phase of the illness has passed, start again to give your child less and less attention at night even though mild symptoms are continuing. This pattern of giving your child more attention at night with each new common cold for one to three nights and less or no attention for the next two days, or more, may occur more than once a month during the cold season. This is especially true if there is a school-age older sibling or your young child is in day care. But remember, most children sleep through mild colds. If your child with a cold suddenly becomes sicker with new symptoms or apparent worsening of symptoms, attend to him immediately and call his physician, because the cold may have caused a painful ear infection.

Research has shown that sleep loss itself can cause impairments in our immune system, which is the body's defense mechanism to prevent infections. So it's a vicious circle: illnesses might disturb sleep, and not sleeping well makes us more vulnerable to becoming sick.

MOTHER RETURNS TO WORK

The quality of the caregiver is what is important, not whether the person delivering the care is or is not the biological parent. Some adults develop sensitivity to children's needs and appreciate the benefits of regularity, consistency, and structure in their child care activities. Some do not.

> **Write down specific instructions for sleep routines so that the grandmother, the babysitter, the nanny, or the day care provider knows what soothes your child best.**

Do not assume that when the mother returns to work outside the home, your child's sleep habits will suffer. Keep data: track the schedule of naps when she is cared for by someone else, ask the nanny to keep a sleep log so you know exactly what is going on, watch for signs of tiredness in the early evening that might suggest nap deprivation.

Sometimes a nanny is a very nurturing person who wants to hold your baby all the time. But at some point you'll want to be able to use method A (see Chapter 7), which means putting your child down for naps after soothing whether or not she is asleep. If the nanny refuses to do this, then your child will not be able to learn to soothe herself to sleep. If the caregiver does not protect naps, or if the mother upon returning from work keeps her child up too late, the child is likely to show new signs of being overtired and have difficulty falling asleep. Sometimes this new behavior is misinterpreted as anxiety in the baby caused by the absence of the mother during the day! Not only does this produce unnecessary guilt in the mother, but it obscures the real cause: insufficient sleep for the child.

To help your child sleep better in different places, such as when she is in day care, when the family is on vacation, after a move, or when you bring her to your workplace, try to build an environment of familiarity by using certain cues only for sleeping:

The same music box

The same stuffed animal or blanket

A spray of perfume that is used only at sleep times

Your child will then learn to associate these sensations with falling asleep, and this will help reduce the disruptive effect of the novelty of any new surroundings. None of these items, however, will work in the absence of regularity and consistency of parent care.

Please don't let your guilt about being away so much during the day cause you to keep your child up too late. Please take care not to reinforce night wakings by giving in to your natural desire for sweet nocturnal private time with your baby. Please do not induce nap deprivation on weekends by cramming in too many activities in an effort to make up for "lost time" during the week. And don't let household errands, chores, or nonessential social events rob you and your child of unstructured, low-intensity playtime. The most common mistake is to keep your child up past the time of tiredness; your child needs sleep just like she needs food. Don't withhold sleep any more than you would withhold food.

HOME OFFICE

Parents who work at home are closer to their children throughout the day, and some parents have a similar situation when they are able to bring their baby to their workplace. The general problem is that some parents try to schedule their child's sleep around their work. In the beginning, with a newborn baby who naturally sleeps a lot, parents sometimes have the illusion that it will always be smooth going. This is especially true if you have an easy-temperament baby. Unfortunately, the ebb and flow of the baby's developing sleep rhythms cannot be molded to fit a work schedule. An exception might be made if both parents are working together and there is always one available to attend to the baby.

Let's say that you have a home office and have hired someone to assist you with the care of your baby. Please do not expect to work, care for your baby, and breast-feed on any regular schedule. Your baby can smell you; she will know you are there! When she is hungry and wants to be fed, even though she might not see you, she senses your presence and expects you to feed her—now, not later. If you decided to feed formula instead of breast milk, then others will be able to help out more with the feedings. Expect to make lots of compromises between your needs, the baby's needs, and the expectations of the person helping you care for your child.

One thing you can do to make it easier is to start early to respect your child's need to sleep, and be very careful to avoid the overtired state. Starting as soon as you come home from the hospital is best. The reason for starting early is that a well-rested baby is more adaptable to schedule changes that might occur when you try to coordinate baby care and working in your home office. Also, if you are breast-feeding, introduce a single bottle per day of expressed breast milk or formula at about two weeks of age. It does not have to be at the same time each day. If you do this, your baby will be able to take a bottle. If you wait a longer time to introduce a bottle, your baby may decide that he will take only the breast, and you lose some flexibility. The single bottle will not confuse your baby or cause weaning to occur.

It's not easy being a parent; it's harder when you have to work outside the home. The home office option is not available to everyone, but with planning and an attitude of flexibility and willingness to compromise, many mothers and fathers find the rewards are more than worth the effort. Even when children outgrow naps, the home office is a possibility.

Some parents try to set up a mini-nursery or nest in their office or store for their babies to sleep. The truth is that it is difficult to answer phones or do business with clients when your baby needs your attention. Perhaps for a few months, your child might seem to fit in, but it will become increasingly more difficult as he becomes more social, more alert, and more demanding of your attention. Again, an exception might be when both parents are working together, so that one is always available for the baby.

DUAL-CAREER FAMILIES

When both parents are working outside the home, the major problem is that the child tends to be put to sleep too late. Sometimes this occurs because by the time the child is picked up from day care and brought home, it is already past the child's biological time for night sleep to start. Occasionally this is further complicated by having to awaken your child in the morning to get to day care on time or by the day care facility not being able to maintain a routine and environment conducive to good-quality day sleep. At other times, both parents return home late from work, and they naturally want to play with their child before feeding, bathing, and bedtime.

If your child goes to sleep past the time of biological sleep onset, then she gradually becomes overtired. If she is young, naps might be extra long to partially compensate for going to bed too late. Later, when your older child begins to outgrow naps, the problems associated with the too-late bedtime begin to develop. Research has clearly shown that even with a fixed amount of sleep deficit, the child's irritability, fussiness, and short temper do not stay fixed; rather, they increase (see "Cumulative Sleepiness" in Chapter 1). Everything gets worse, but this process may develop very slowly. Eventually bedtime battles and night waking emerge, perhaps for the first time. Many parents assume that there is some other problem, such as teething pain, separation anxiety, insecurity because of the mother returning to work, the "terrible twos," nightmares, or the stress of a move or new sibling. Parents often do not see that their child has very slowly become overtired because, several months before, the bedtime was allowed to become slightly too late.

MAJOR POINT

Constant sleep deficits cause increasing amounts of impaired functioning during wakefulness.

Q: *When should my child go to sleep at night?*
A: Before she becomes overtired.

If you think your child might be overtired in the late afternoon or early in the evening, try putting her to sleep twenty minutes earlier than you currently do. If she falls asleep at this earlier time, then you will know that you have been putting her to bed too late. After several days, consider moving her bedtime another twenty minutes earlier if she still looks overtired. Remember, the way your child behaves or appears to you is more important than any recommended sleep duration or bedtime for "average" children (see "Sleep Recommendations" in Chapter 1). Common inhibiting fears about putting your child to bed early are that he will start the day too early and will love you less because you are spending less time with him. Not true! Because sleep begets sleep, if your child becomes better rested, he will be better able to fall asleep and stay asleep. He will not get up earlier and earlier because of an earlier bedtime. You will prevent or eliminate bedtime battles and night waking for attention. Naps will tend to become longer and more regular if your child goes to bed earlier. One common scenario is that because of a too-late bedtime, the child takes a single too-long midmorning nap, which causes him to be extremely tired by 4:00 or 5:00 p.m. A temporarily very early bedtime will often shorten the midmorning nap so that the child is able to take a restorative midday nap between noon and 2:00 p.m. and subsequently be able to stay up a little later.

REMEMBER

Sleep begets sleep. It's not logical that earlier bedtimes allow children to sleep later in the morning: it's biological.

Q: *I miss my baby so much during the day—why can't I spend more time with her at night? The only time I have to love my baby is late at night. Won't she miss me?*

A: If she becomes overtired, her company will not be much fun. She will not enjoy or benefit as much from your social interaction because both of you will become increasingly fatigued. Her evolving bedtime battles and night waking will eventually produce an overtired family. At the price of seeing her less at night, she will stay better rested, sweeter, and more charming, and you will mutually enjoy each other's company more in the morning and on the weekends.

Sometimes dual-career parents have to allow the sitter or the parent who comes home early to bathe, feed, and dress their child for bed; immediately after the arrival of the parent who comes home late, the child is quietly soothed to sleep. With our busy lifestyles, it may be difficult to coordinate a work schedule with a child's biological needs. If this is the case for you, your baby's needs must come first. You would not withhold food when the body needs it simply because it is inconvenient to feed your child, and you try to anticipate when your child will become hungry in order to feed her before she becomes overly hungry. Similarly, try not to withhold sleep when the brain needs it, and try to anticipate when your child will become tired before she becomes overtired.

Occasionally it happens that a sitter or day care center is protecting and maintaining good-quality naps on weekdays, but on weekends everything falls apart. Dual-career families might try to do too much playing with their children on weekends to compensate for being with them less during the week, or they may simply not respect the child's need to nap because there are so many errands that have to be done. Either way, these children are often so overtired that they appear to be in pain. Every pediatrician gets some of these calls Sunday night or Monday morning because the parents often believe there is a painful ear infection. Severe *sleep inertia* can cause a child to awaken from an extra-long nap and scream as if in severe pain. Also, *night terrors* are often more common when children become severely overtired. On busy weekends, you should not feed your baby on the run; you need to find a quiet time to feed. Same thing for naps; don't nap on the run.

INJURIES

Injuries occur to children of all ages. Some can be prevented, but some cannot. Examples of preventable injuries include leaving a 4-month-old infant alone on a changing table from which she falls, poisonings occurring when safety seals are not used or medicines are left lying around, or electrical shocks from uncovered wall sockets. A non-preventable injury is truly an accident—for example, those resulting from an earthquake or a lightning bolt.

The truth is, though—and I realize this sounds harsh to many parents' ears—that most so-called childhood accidents are really preventable injuries that occur because of parental neglect or the lack of parental forethought. These injuries can be one consequence of home routines that create tired children—and tired *families*.

But is there such a thing as an accident-prone child? To determine if traits within a child can cause him to suffer frequent injuries, various studies have examined babies before injuries start to occur. (After a child has had several injuries, a "halo" effect develops, and adults are more likely to perceive traits in the child—clumsiness, lack of self-control, and so on—that "explain" why he has had so many injuries.)

One study included two hundred babies between 4 and 8 months of age. Some of the infants were difficult to manage. As we saw earlier, these infants were called "difficult" because they were irregular, not very adaptable, initially withdrawing, and negative in mood. During the next two years, difficult babies were much more likely to have cuts requiring sutures than were babies with easy-to-manage temperaments. This study showed that during the first 2 years of life, about one-third of the difficult children had cuts deep or severe enough to require stitches, while only 5 percent of easy babies had similar cuts.

Remember also my data: at 4 to 8 months of age, difficult babies slept about three hours less than easy babies, and at age 3 years, the difference was about one and a half hours. By age 3, the briefer the sleep, the more active, excitable, impulsive, inattentive, and easily distracted the child appeared—the perfect description of an accident-prone child. Little wonder, then, that these tired children fell more often, sustaining deep cuts.

Obviously, for both the "difficult" kids and all other children, chronic fatigue can lead to more injuries, such as cuts and falls. More sleep is the remedy.

Another study that supports this connection between fatigue and injury included more than seven thousand children who were 1 to 2 years old. Researchers compared children who frequently woke up at night with those who slept through the night. Among the night wakers, 40 percent had injuries requiring medical attention, compared to only 17 percent of the good sleepers. The parents of the children who were night wakers reported that they immediately went to their child when they heard a cry in order to prevent further crying. There was a tendency for the mothers of night wakers to feel more irritable in general and "out of control." One sign of family tension was that these mothers felt unable to confide in their husbands; the association of marital difficulties with disturbed sleep has been mentioned in many studies (see Chapter 3).

Maybe the parents who don't supervise sleep patterns so that their child can have his sleep needs met are the same ones who don't supervise children at play in order to protect their physical safety.

The message is clear: if your child is often injured, it's not necessarily because he is careless or clumsy—he may be exhausted instead.

I have seen many children who were so overtired that they fell down only a stair or two or fell from a very low height. But because they hit their head and were later noted to be sleepy or wobbly, the parents worried about a head injury or concussion. In fact, it was the overtired state that produced both the fall and the wobbliness. What these children needed was more sleep, not a head CT scan!

OVERWEIGHT, EXERCISE, AND DIET

Overweight (See Chapter 2)

Difficult-to-manage children fuss and cry a lot. One way to quiet them is to put food in their mouths. One theory is that fussiness might have some evolutionary value, ensuring survival in times when food is scarce. This was shown to be the case among the Masai of East Africa during drought conditions in 1974, when babies who cried more, and were perceived to be stronger, were fed more. But in a 1985 study by Dr. William Carey, conducted in a white, middle-class Pennsylvania pediatric practice, the babies with a more difficult temperament (who tend to have short sleep durations) tended to be fatter. Perhaps this connection between fussiness and being fed sets the stage for obesity in later years.

In my own pediatric practice, fat babies are almost always overtired babies. That's because their mothers have incorrectly attributed their babies' crying to hunger instead of fatigue. These mothers are always feeding their babies, then telling me that their babies can't sleep because they're always hungry! The major point here? Overfeeding the crying child to keep him quiet could cause unhealthy weight gain or obesity.

This overfeeding habit may actually begin innocently enough in some children at 3 to 4 months of age, when nutritional feedings in the middle of the night give way to recreational feedings. Later, the bottle or breast is used as a pacifier and the frequent sipping and snacking causes excessive weight gain. Please try to become sensitive to the difference between nutritive and non-nutritive feeding. Overdoing milk or juice bottles is a common way babies learn to not "like" eating solids. After all, they are getting calories, so they have no appetite to motivate them to eat solid foods when they are older. For children between 5 and 7 years, we now have direct evidence that the more tired the child is, the more likely it is that he will be overweight or obese.

Q: *If I give my child a bottle at naps or at bedtime, will I make him fat? When should I not include a bottle in the bedtime ritual?*

A: Sucking or sipping a bottle before falling asleep comforts most babies and even older children. There is no harm in doing this, and there is no particular age when you should stop as long as (1) you prop the baby, not the bottle, so he drinks in your arms, (2) the rate of weight gain is not too fast, and (3) frequent or prolonged feedings are not part of a sleep problem.

A 2012 paper by Dr. E. de Jong showed that a late bedtime causing short sleep duration was associated with being overweight among 4- to 8-year-old boys and among 9- to 13-year-old boys and girls. For all children, short sleep duration was strongly associated with more television viewing and computer use.

Exercise

Recent research has shown that adolescents with high levels of physical activity have longer total sleep time, fewer wakings at night, fewer symptoms of insomnia, and higher sleep quality. Additionally, it is possible that exercise reduces anxiety. On the other hand, strenuous exercise, especially common among teenagers, might mask an underlying problem of chronically insufficient sleep. The chronically or severely overtired adolescent is sometimes described as living in a "twilight zone": frequent episodes of drowsiness, "micro-sleeps," lethargy, depression, apathy, cognitive impairment, and proneness to accidents. Counteracting measures that fight the fatigued state are internal stimulation (heightened emotionality, such as anger or elation) or external stimulation such as exercise. So, exercise may be helpful, but it will not solve an underlying sleep problem.

Diet

Diet should influence sleep, because food provides the chemical building blocks for the brain's neurotransmitters. But studies in infants and adults do not show support for any strong link between sleep and diet.

CHILD ABUSE

Let's get one ugly fact out in the open: when we are very, very tired of hearing our baby cry to fight sleep at night, we might like to shut him up. We don't act on our feelings; we don't harm our baby. But at nighttime, the thought might have occurred to us: "What if I weren't in so much control? Might I . . . ?"

The tired, difficult-to-manage infant whose howling at night will not stop can become a target for abuse or infanticide. Crying is the behavior that seems to trigger child abuse in some parents, and crying at night instead of sleeping is the historical context for infanticide.

So when your baby gets all cranked up late at night with desperate, angry, or relentless screaming when she should be asleep, and you feel like a tightly wound spring, don't be surprised if you feel you want to "get even" or "shut her up for good." If you and your child don't get the sleep you need, you may have experienced these intense feelings of anger, resentment, or ill will toward your child. That doesn't make you a bad person. The important thing is to be aware of what you are feeling and why. If you feel the need for help, contact your pediatrician, social workers at local hospitals, or the following organizations.

National Committee to Prevent Child Abuse
1-800-244-5373

Parents Without Partners
1-800-637-7974

When we ourselves are extremely sleep deprived, it can be difficult for us to see that the sleep problems in our family are solvable. There is no shame or failure in calling for help.

ATOPIC DERMATITIS AND ECZEMA

Atopic dermatitis is a chronic skin condition that causes severe itching. Itching of the skin can cause restlessness during sleep because a lot of the scratching goes on during light and REM sleep. As a result, children wake frequently throughout the night. Some studies have shown that these children have difficulty waking up for school, difficulty staying awake in the afternoon, and major discipline problems. However, one study that used sleep lab recordings and video recordings during sleep of atopic children showed that the sleep abnormalities of frequent arousals actually did not occur with the act of scratching. This study was performed when the skin condition was in remission, so it is possible that during flare-up there might be more intense itching that interfered with sleep consolidation. If your child is often scratching his skin, talk to your pediatrician or ask for a referral to a dermatologist.

References

Abe, K., Oda, N., and Amatomi, M. (1984). Natural history and predictive significance of head-banging, head-rolling and breath-holding spells. *Developmental Medicine and Child Neurology, 26,* 644–648.

Abe, K., Sasaki, H., Takebayashi, K., Seki, F., and Nambu, H. (1978). The development of circadian rhythm of human body temperature. *Journal of Interdisciplinary Cycle Research, 9,* 211–216.

Acebo, C., and Carskadon, M. A. (2002). Influence of irregular sleep patterns on waking behavior. In M. A. Carskadon (ed.), *Adolescent Sleep Patterns: Biological, Social, and Psychological Influences* (220–235). Cambridge: Cambridge University Press.

Aldrich, C. A., Sung, C., and Knop, C. (1945). The crying of newly born babies. I. The community phase. *Journal of Pediatrics, 26,* 313–335.

Aldrich, C. A., Sung, C., Knop, C., Stevens, G., and Burchell, M. (1945). The crying of newly born babies. II. The individual phase. *Journal of Pediatrics, 27,* 89–96.

Aldrich, C. A., Sung, C., and Knop, C. (1945). The crying of newly born babies. III. The early period at home. *Journal of Pediatrics, 27,* 428–435.

Anders, T. F., Carskadon, M. A., Dement, W. C., and Harvey, K. (1978). Sleep habits of children and the identification of pathologically sleepy children. *Child Psychiatry and Human Development, 9,* 56–63.

Anders, T. F., Carskadon, M. A., and Dement, W. C. (1980). Sleep and sleepiness in children and adolescents. *Pediatric Clinics of North America, 27,* 29–43.

Anders, T. F., and Keener, M. A. (1985). Developmental course of nighttime sleep-wake patterns in full-term and premature infants during the first year of life: Part I. *Sleep, 8,* 173–192.

Anders, T. F., Keener, M. A., and Kramer, H. (1985). Sleep-wake state organization, neonatal assessment and development in premature infants during the first year of life: Part II. *Sleep, 8,* 193–206.

Anderson, D. R. (1979). Treatment of insomnia in a 13-year-old boy by relaxation training and reduction of parental attention. *Journal of Behavior Therapy and Experimental Psychiatry, 10,* 263–265.

Anderson, O. W. (1951). The management of "infantile insomnia." *Journal of Pediatrics, 38,* 394–401.

Archbold, K. H., Pituch, K. J., Panahi, P., and Chervin, R. D. (2002). Symptoms of sleep disturbances among children at two general pediatric clinics. *Journal of Pediatrics, 140,* 97–102.

Armstrong, K. L., Van Haeringen, A. R., Dadds, M. R., and Cash, R. (1998). Sleep deprivation or postnatal depression in later infancy: Separating the chicken from the egg. *Journal of Paediatrics and Child Health, 34,* 260–262.

Arvola, T., Tahvanainen, A., and Isolauri, E. (2000). Concerns and expectations of parents with atopic infants. *Pediatric Allergy and Immunology, 11,* 183–188.

Asnes, R. S., Santulli, R., and Bemporad, J. R. (1981). Psychogenic chest pain in children. *Clinical Pediatrics, 20,* 788–791.

Atkinson, E., Vetere, A., and Grayson, K. (1995). Sleep disruption in young children. The influence of temperament on the sleep patterns of pre-school children. *Child: Care, Health and Development, 21,* 233–246.

Bader, G., Nevéus, T., Kruse, S., and Sillén, U. (2002). Sleep of primary enuretic children and controls. *Sleep, 25,* 579–583.

Baekeland, F., and Lasky, R. (1966). Exercise and sleep patterns in college athletes. *Perceptual and Motor Skills, 23,* 1203–1207.

Ballenger, W. L. (1914). *Diseases of the Nose, Throat and Ear, Medical and Surgical,* 4th ed. Philadelphia: Lea and Febiger.

Barr, R. G., Kramer, M. S., and Pless, I. B. (1989). Feeding and temperament as determinants of early infant crying/fussing behavior. *Pediatrics, 84,* 514–521.

Bates, J. E., Viken, R. J., Alexander, D. B., Beyers, J., and Stockton, L. (2002). Sleep and adjustment in preschool children: Sleep diary reports by mothers relate to behavior reports by teachers. *Child Development, 73,* 62–75.

Baum, K. T., Desai, A., Field, J., Miller, L. E., Rausch, J., and Beebe, D. W. (2014). Sleep restriction worsens mood and emotion regulation in adolescents. *Journal of Child Psychology and Psychiatry, 55,* 180–190.

Bayer, J. K., Hiscock, H., Hampton, A., and Wake, M. (2007). Sleep problems in young infants and maternal mental and physical health. *Journal of Paediatrics and Child Health, 43,* 66–73.

Beal, V. A. (1969). Termination of night feeding in infancy. *Journal of Pediatrics, 75,* 690–692.

Belechri, M., Petridou, E., and Trichopoulos, D. (2002). Bunk versus conventional beds: A comparative assessment of fall injury risk. *Journal of Epidemiology and Community Health, 56,* 413–417.

Bell, J. F., and Zimmerman, F. J. (2010). Shortened nighttime sleep duration in early life and subsequent childhood obesity. *Archives of Pediatrics and Adolescent Medicine, 164,* 840–845.

Beltramini, A. U., and Hertzig, M. E. (1983). Sleep and bedtime behavior in preschool-aged children. *Pediatrics, 71,* 153–158.

Berger, R. H., Miller, A. L., Seifer, R., Cares, S. R., and Lebourgeois, M. K. (2012). Acute sleep restriction effects on emotion responses in 30- to 36-month-old children. *Journal of Sleep Research, 21,* 235–246.

Bernstein, P., Emde, R., and Campos, J. (1973). REM sleep in four-month infants under home and laboratory conditions. *Psychosomatic Medicine, 35,* 322–329.

Blader, J. C., Koplewicz, H. S., Abikoff, H., and Foley, C. (1997). Sleep problems of elementary school children. A community survey. *Archives of Pediatrics and Adolescent Medicine, 151,* 473–480.

Blum, N. J., Taubman, B., Tretina, L., and Heyward, R. Y. (2002). Maternal ratings of infant intensity and distractibility: Relationship with crying duration in the second month of life. *Archives of Pediatrics and Adolescent Medicine, 156,* 286–290.

Boergers, J., Gable, C. J., and Owens, J. A. (2014). Later school start time is associated with improved sleep and daytime functioning in adolescents. *Journal of Developmental and Behavioral Pediatrics, 35,* 11–17.

Bonnet, M. H. (1985). Effect of sleep disruption on sleep, performance, and mood. *Sleep, 8,* 11–19.

Boon, W. H. (1982). The crying baby. *Journal of the Singapore Paediatric Society, 24,* 145–147.

Bootzin, R. R. (1973). Stimulus control treatment for insomnia. *Proceedings of the American Psychological Association, 7,* 395–396.

Bootzin, R. R., and Perlis, M. L. (1992). Nonpharmacologic treatments of insomnia. *Journal of Clinical Psychiatry, 53* (Suppl.), 37–41.

Brazelton, T. B. (1962). Crying in infancy. *Pediatrics, 29,* 579–588.

Breslow, L. (1957). A clinical approach to infantile colic: A review of 90 cases. *Journal of Pediatrics, 50,* 196–206.

Brown, S. L., and Stool, S. E. (1982). Behavior manifestations of sleep apnea in children. *Sleep, 5,* 200–201.

Busby, K., Firestone, P., and Pivik, R. T. (1981). Sleep patterns in hyperkinetic and normal children. *Sleep, 4,* 366–383.

Busby, K., and Pivik, R. T. (1983). Sleep patterns in children of superior intelligence. *Journal of Child Psychology and Psychiatry, 24, 587–600.*

Butte, N. F., Jensen, C. L., Moon, J. K., Glaze, D. G., and Frost, J. D. (1992). Sleep organization and energy expenditure of breast-fed and formula-fed infants. *Pediatric Research, 32, 514–519.*

Butte, W., Robertson, C., and Phelan, P. (1985). Snoring in children: Is it pathological? *Medical Journal of Australia, 143, 335–336.*

Byars, K. C., Yolton, K., Rausch, J., Lanphear, B., and Beebe, D. W. (2012). Prevalence, patterns, and persistence of sleep problems in the first 3 years of life. *Pediatrics, 129, e276–e284.*

Cai, D. J., Mednick, S. A., Harrison, E. M., Kanady, J. C., and Mednick, S. C. (2009). REM, not incubation, improves creativity by priming associative networks. *Proceedings of the National Academy of Sciences, 106, 10130–10134.*

Camfield, C. S., Chaplin, S., Doyle, A.-B., Shapiro, S. H., Cummings, C., and Camfield, P. R. (1979). Side effects of phenobarbital in toddlers: Behavioral and cognitive aspects. *Journal of Pediatrics, 95, 361–365.*

Canivet, C., Jakobsson, I., and Hagander, B. (2000). Infantile colic. Follow-up at four years of age: Still more "emotional." *Acta Paediatrica, 89, 13–17.*

Carey, W. B. (1972). Clinical applications of infant temperament measurements. *Journal of Pediatrics, 81, 823–828.*

Carey, W. B. (1968). Maternal anxiety and infantile colic: Is there a relationship? *Clinical Pediatrics, 7, 590–595.*

Carey, W. B. (1985). Temperament and increased weight gain in infants. *Journal of Developmental and Behavioral Pediatrics, 6, 128–131.*

Carey, W. B., and McDevitt, S. C. (1978). Revision of the infant temperament questionnaire. *Pediatrics, 61, 735–739.*

Carskadon, M. A. (ed.) (2002). *Adolescent Sleep Patterns: Biological, Social, and Psychological Influences.* Cambridge: Cambridge University Press.

Carskadon, M. A., Vieiera, C., and Acebo, C. (1993). Association between puberty and delayed phase preference. *Sleep, 16,* 258–262.

Cason, H. (1935). The nightmare dream. *Psychological Monographs, 46,* i–51.

Cellucci, A. J., and Lawrence, P. S. (1978). Individual differences in self-reported sleep variable correlations among nightmare sufferers. *Journal of Clinical Psychology, 34,* 721–725.

Chervin, R. D., Archbold, K. H., Dillon, J. E., Panahi, P., Pituch, K. J., Dahl, R. E., and Guilleminault, C. (2002). Inattention, hyperactivity, and symptoms of sleep-disordered breathing. *Pediatrics, 109,* 449–456.

Chervin, R. D., Dillon, J. E., Bassetti, C., Ganoczy, D. A., and Pituch, K. J. (1997). Symptoms of sleep disorders, inattention, and hyperactivity in children. *Sleep, 20,* 1185–1192.

Christophersen, E. R. (1998). *Beyond Discipline: Parenting That Lasts a Lifetime,* 2nd ed. (127–128). Shawnee Mission, Kansas: Overland Press.

Christophersen, E. R. (2002). Diagnosis and management of sleep problems. In E. R. Christophersen and S. M. VanScoyoc, *Treatments That Work with Children.* Washington, DC: American Psychological Association.

Clarkson, S., Williams, S., and Silva, P. A. (1986). Sleep in middle childhood—a longitudinal study of sleep problems in a large sample of Dunedin children aged 5–9 years. *Journal of Paediatrics and Child Health, 22,* 31–35.

Clifford, T. J., Campbell, M. K., Speechley, K. N., and Gorodzinsky, F. (2002). Infant colic: Empirical evidence of the absence of an association with source of early infant nutrition. *Archives of Pediatrics and Adolescent Medicine, 156,* 1123–1128.

Clifford, T. J., Campbell, M. K., Speechley, K. N., and Gorodzinsky, F. (2002). Sequelae of infant colic: Evidence of transient infant distress and absence of lasting effects on maternal mental health. *Archives of Pediatrics and Adolescent Medicine, 156,* 1183–1188.

Cobb, K. (2002). Missed ZZZ's, more disease?: Skimping on sleep may be bad for your health. *Science News, 162,* 152–154.

Collins, D. D., Scoggin, C. H., Zwillich, C. W., and Weil, J. V. (1978). Hereditary aspects of decreased hypoxic response. *Journal of Clinical Investigation, 62,* 105–110.

Conners, C. K. (1973). Rating scale for use in drug studies with children. *Psychopharmacology Bulletin, 10* (Special Issue), 24–84.

Coons, S., and Guilleminault, C. (1982). Development of sleep-wake patterns and non–rapid eye movement sleep stages during the first six months of life in normal infants. *Pediatrics, 69,* 793–798.

Coons, S., and Guilleminault, C. (1984). Development of consolidated sleep and wakeful periods in relation to the day/night cycle in infancy. *Developmental Medicine and Child Neurology, 26,* 169–176.

Coons, S., and Guilleminault, C. (1985). Motility and arousal in near miss sudden infant death syndrome. *Journal of Pediatrics, 107,* 728–732.

Coren, S., and Searleman, A. (1985). Birth stress and self-reported sleep difficulty. *Sleep, 8,* 222–226.

Coulter, D. L., and Allen, R. J. (1982). Benign neonatal sleep myoclonus. *Archives of Neurology, 39,* 191–192.

Crockenberg, S. B., and Smith, P. (1982). Antecedents of mother-infant interaction and infant irritability in the first three months of life. *Infant Behavior and Development, 5,* 105–119.

Cullen, K. J. (1976). A six-year controlled trial of prevention of children's behavior disorders. *Journal of Pediatrics, 88,* 662–666.

Czeisler, C. A., Richardson, G. S., Coleman, R. M., Zimmerman, J. C., Moore-Ede, M. C., Dement, W. C., and Weitzman, E. D. (1981). Chronotherapy: Resetting the circadian clocks of patients with delayed sleep phase insomnia. *Sleep, 4,* 1–21.

Czeisler, C. A., Weitzman, E., Moore-Ede, M. C., Zimmerman, J. C., and Knauer, R. S. (1980). Human sleep: Its duration and organization depend on its circadian phase. *Science, 210,* 1264–1267.

Dahl, R. E., Pelham, W. E., and Wierson, M. (1991). The role of sleep disturbances in attention deficit disorder symptoms: A case study. *Journal of Pediatric Psychology, 16,* 229–239.

Daiss, S. R., Bertelson, A. D., and Benjamin, L. T. (1986). Napping versus resting: Effects on performance and mood. *Psychophysiology, 23,* 82–88.

Deisher, R. W., and Goers, S. S. (1954). A study of early and later introduction of solids into the infant diet. *Journal of Pediatrics, 45,* 191–199.

De Jong, E., Stocks, T., Visscher, T. L., HiraSing, R. A., Seidell, J. C., and Renders, C. M. (2012). Association between sleep duration and overweight: The importance of parenting. *International Journal of Obesity, 36,* 1278–1284.

Dement, W. C., and Carskadon, M. A. (1982). Current perspectives on daytime sleepiness: The issues. *Sleep, 5* (Suppl. 2), S56–S66.

Deneberg, V. H., and Thoman, E. B. (1981). Evidence for a functional role for active (REM) sleep in infancy. *Sleep, 4,* 185–191.

DeVries, M. W. (1984). Temperament and infant mortality among the Masai of East Africa. *American Journal of Psychiatry, 141,* 1189–1194.

De Zambotti, M., Covassin, N., De Min Tona, G., Sarlo, M., and Stegagno, L. (2011). Sleep onset and cardiovascular activity in primary insomnia. *Journal of Sleep Research, 20,* 318–325.

DiMario, F. J., Jr., and Emery, E. S. (1987). The natural history of night terrors. *Clinical Pediatrics, 26,* 505–511.

Dinges, D. F., and Broughton, R. J. (eds.) (1989). *Sleep and Alertness: Chronobiological, Behavioral, and Medical Aspects of Napping.* New York: Raven Press.

Dinges, D. F., Pack, F., Williams, K., Gillen, K. A., Powell, J. W., Ott, G. E., Aptowicz, C., and Pack, A. I. (1997). Cumulative sleepiness, mood disturbance, and psychomotor vigilance performance decrements during a week of sleep restricted to 4–5 hours per night. *Sleep, 20,* 267–277.

Dixon, K. N., Monroe, L. J., and Jakim, S. (1981). Insomniac children. *Sleep, 4,* 313–318.

Dobson, D., Lucassen, P. L., Miller, J. J., Vlieger, A. M., Prescott, P., and Lewith, G. (2012). Manipulative therapies for infantile colic. *Cochrane Database of Systematic Reviews,* 12:CD004796.

Dollinger, S. J. (1985). Effects of a paradoxical intervention on a child's anxiety about sleep- and sports-related performance. *Perceptual and Motor Skills, 61,* 83–86.

Douglas, J., and Richman, N. (1984). *My Child Won't Sleep.* Hammondsworth, Middlesex, England: Penguin Books.

Douglas, P. S., and Hill, P. S. (2011). The crying baby; what approach? *Current Opinion in Pediatrics, 23,* 523–529.

Dreyfus-Brisac, C., and Monod, N. (1965). Sleep of premature and full-term neonates—A polygraphic study. *Proceedings of the Royal Society of Medicine, 58,* 6–7.

Dunst, C. J., and Lingerfelt, B. (1985). Maternal ratings of temperament and operant learning in two- to three-month-old infants. *Child Development, 56,* 555–563.

Earls, F. (1980). Prevalence of behavior problems in 3-year-old children. *Archives of General Psychiatry, 37,* 1153–1157.

Ednick, M., Cohen, A. P., McPhail, G. L., Beebe, D., Simakajornboon, N., and Amin, R. S. (2009). A review of the effects of sleep during the first year of life on cognitive, psychomotor, and temperament development. *Sleep, 32,* 1449–1458.

Elias, M. F., Nicolson, N. A., Bora, C., and Johnston, J. (1986). Sleep/wake patterns of breast-fed infants in the first 2 years of life. *Pediatrics, 77,* 322–329.

Emde, R. N., Gaensbauer, T. J., and Harmon, R. J. (1976). Emotional expression in infancy; a biobehavioral study. *Psychological Issues, 10,* 1–200.

Emde, R. N., and Metcalf, D. R. (1970). An electroencephalographic study of behavioral rapid eye movement states in the human newborn. *Journal of Nervous and Mental Disease, 150,* 376–386.

Emde, R. N., Swedberg, J., and Suzuki, B. (1975). Human wakefulness and biological rhythms after birth. *Archives of General Psychiatry, 32,* 780–783.

Emde, R. N., and Walker, S. (1976). Longitudinal study of infant sleep: Results of 14 subjects studied at monthly intervals. *Psychophysiology, 13,* 456–461.

Epstein, R., Chillag, N., and Lavie, P. (1998). Starting times of school: Effects on daytime functioning of fifth-grade children in Israel. *Sleep, 21,* 250–256.

Espie, C. A., and Lindsay, W. R. (1985). Paradoxical intention in the treatment of chronic insomnia: Six case studies illustrating variability in therapeutic response. *Behaviour Research and Therapy, 23,* 703–709.

Etzel, B. C., and Gewirtz, J. L. (1967). Experimental modification of caretaker-maintained high-rate operant crying in a 6- and a 20-week-old infant (*Infans tyrannotearus*): Extinction of crying with reinforcement of eye contact and smiling. *Journal of Experimental Child Psychology, 5,* 303–317.

Fagen, J. W., Ohr, P. S., Fleckenstein, L. K., and Ribner, D. R. (1985). The effect of crying on long-term memory in infancy. *Child Development, 56,* 1584–1592.

Falbe, J., Davison, K. K., Franckle, R. L., Ganter, C., Gortmaker, S. L., Smith, L., Land, T., and Taveras, E. M. (2015). Sleep duration, restfulness, and screens in the sleep environment. *Pediatrics, 135,* e367–e375.

Fallone, G. P., Seifer, R., Acebo, C., and Carskadon, M. A. (2000). Prolonged sleep restriction in 11- and 12-year-old children: Effects on behavior, sleepiness, and mood. *Sleep, 23* (Suppl. 2), A28.

Fernandez-Mendoza, J., Vgontzas, A. N., Calhoun, S. L., Vgontzas, A., Tsaoussoglou, M., Gaines, J., Liao, D., Chrousos, G. P., and Bixler, E. O. (2014). Insomnia symptoms, objective sleep duration and hypothalamic-pituitary-adrenal activity in children. *European Journal of Clinical Investigation, 44,* 493–500.

Fibiger, W., Singer, G., Miller, A. J., Armstrong, S., and Datar, M. (1984). Cortisol and catecholamine changes as functions of time-of-day and self-reported mood. *Neuroscience and Biobehavioral Reviews, 8*, 523–530.

Fischetti, M. (2014). Sleeping through high school. *Scientific American, 311*, 27.

Fish, B. (1963). The maturation of arousal and attention in the first months of life: A study of variations in ego development. *Journal of the American Academy of Child and Adolescent Psychiatry, 2*, 253–270.

Flemming, B. M. (1925). A study of sleep of young children. *Journal of the American Association of University Women, 19*, 25–28.

Folkard, S., Hume, K. I., Minors, D. S., Waterhouse, J. M., and Watson, F. L. (1985). Independence of the circadian rhythm in alertness from the sleep/wake cycle. *Nature, 313*, 678–679.

Foster, J. C., Goodenough, F. L., and Anderson, J. E. (1928). The sleep of young children. *Journal of Genetic Psychology, 35*, 201–218.

France, K. G. (1992). Behavior characteristics and security in sleep-disturbed infants treated with extinction. *Journal of Pediatric Psychology, 17*, 467–475.

France, K. G., Blampied, N. M., and Wilkinson, P. (1991). Treatment of infant sleep disturbance by trimeprazine in combination with extinction. *Journal of Developmental and Behavioral Pediatrics, 12*, 308–314.

Freedman, D. G. (1979). Ethnic differences in babies. *Human Nature, 2*, 36–43.

Fukuda, K., and Ishihara, K. (2002). Routine evening naps and night-time sleep patterns in junior high and high school students. *Psychiatry and Clinical Neurosciences, 56*, 229–230.

Fukuda, K., and Sakashita, Y. (2002). Sleeping pattern of kindergartners and nursery school children: Function of daytime nap. *Perceptual and Motor Skills, 94*, 219–228.

Fukumoto, M., Mochizuki, N., Takeishi, M., Nomura, Y., and

Segawa, M. (1981). Studies of body movements during night sleep in infancy. *Brain and Development, 3,* 37–43.

Gaillard, J. M. (1985). Neurochemical regulation of the states of alertness. *Annals of Clinical Research, 17,* 175–184.

Garrison, M. M., and Christakis, D. A. (2000). A systematic review of treatments for infant colic. *Pediatrics, 106,* 184–190.

Gau, S. S.-F., and Soong, W.-T. (1995). Sleep problems of junior high school students in Taipei. *Sleep, 18,* 667–673.

Giganti, F., Fagioli, I., Ficca, G., and Salzarulo, P. (2001). Polygraphic investigation of 24-h waking distribution in infants. *Physiology and Behavior, 73,* 621–624.

Glod, C. A., Teicher, M. H., Polcari, A., McGreenery, C. E., and Ito, Y. (1997). Circadian rest-activity disturbances in children with seasonal affective disorder. *Journal of the American Academy of Child and Adolescent Psychiatry, 36,* 188–195.

Golley, R. K., Maher, C. A., Matricciani, L., and Olds, T. S. (2013). Sleep duration or bedtime? Exploring the association between sleep timing behaviour, diet and BMI in children and adolescents. *International Journal of Obesity, 37,* 546–551.

Gómez, R. L., Bootzin, R. R., and Nadel, L. (2006). Naps promote abstraction in language-learning infants. *Psychological Science, 17,* 670–674.

Greenhill, L., Puig-Antich, J., Goetz, R., Hanlon, C., and Davies, M. (1983). Sleep architecture and REM sleep measures in prepubertal children with attention deficit disorder with hyperactivity. *Sleep, 6,* 91–101.

Gregory, A. M., Caspi, A., Moffitt, T. E., and Poulton, R. (2006). Family conflict in childhood: A predictor of later insomnia. *Sleep, 29,* 1063–1067.

Gregory, A. M., and O'Connor, T. G. (2002). Sleep problems in childhood: A longitudinal study of developmental change and association with behavioral problems. *Journal of the American Academy of Child and Adolescent Psychiatry, 41,* 964–971.

Gregory, A. M., Rijsdijk, F. V., Lau, J. Y., Dahl, R. E., and Eley, T. C.

(2009). The direction of longitudinal associations between sleep problems and depression symptoms: A study of twins aged 8 and 10 years. *Sleep, 32,* 189–199.

Gregory, A. M., Willis, T. A., Wiggs, L., Harvey, A. G., and the STEPS team. (2008). Presleep arousal and sleep disturbances in children. *Sleep, 31,* 1745–1747.

Groeger, J. A., Viola, A. U., Lo, J. C., von Schantz, M., Archer, S. N., and Dijk, D. J. (2008). Early morning executive functioning during sleep deprivation is compromised by a *PERIOD3* polymorphism. *Sleep, 31,* 1159–1167.

Gruber, R., Cassoff, J., Frenette, S., Wiebe, S., and Carrier, J. (2012). Impact of sleep extension and restriction on children's emotional lability and impulsivity. *Pediatrics, 130,* e1155–e1161.

Gruber, R., Laviolette, R., Deluca, P., Monson, E., Cornish, K., and Carrier, J. (2010). Short sleep is associated with poor performance on IQ measures in healthy school-age children. *Sleep Medicine, 11,* 289–294.

Grunwaldt, E., Bates, T., and Guthrie, D. (1960). The onset of sleeping through the night in infancy: Relation to introduction of solid food in the diet, birth weight, and position in the family. *Pediatrics, 26,* 667–668.

Guilleminault, C., and Dement, W. C. (1977). 235 cases of excessive daytime sleepiness. Diagnosis and tentative classification. *Journal of Neurological Sciences, 31,* 13–27.

Guilleminault, C., Eldridge, F. L., Simmons, F. B., and Dement, W. C. (1976). Sleep apnea in eight children. *Pediatrics, 58,* 23–30.

Gunnar, M. R., Malone, S., Vance, G., and Fisch, R. O. (1985). Coping with aversive stimulation in the neonatal period: Quiet sleep and plasma cortisol levels during recovery from circumcision. *Child Development, 56,* 824–834.

Guteilus, M. F., Kirsch, A. D., MacDonald, S., Brooks, M. R., and McErlean, T. (1977). Controlled study of child health supervision: Behavioral results. *Pediatrics, 60,* 294–304.

Hagenauer, M. H., and Lee, T. M. (2013). Adolescent sleep patterns in humans and laboratory animals. *Hormones and Behavior,* *64,* 270–279.

Hall, B., Chesters, J., and Robinson, A. (2012). Infantile colic: A systematic review of medical and conventional therapies. *Journal of Paediatrics and Child Health, 48,* 128–137.

Harper, R. M., Leake, B., Miyahara, L., Mason, J., Hoppenbrouwers, T., Sterman, M. B., and Hodgman, J. (1981). Temporal sequencing in sleep and waking states during the first 6 months of life. *Experimental Neurology, 72,* 294–307.

Harrison, G. A. (1985). Stress, catecholamines, and sleep. *Aviation, Space, and Environmental Medicine, 56,* 651–653.

Hauri, P., and Fisher, J. (1986). Persistent psychophysiologic (learned) insomnia. *Sleep, 9,* 38–53.

Hauri, P., and Olmstead, E. (1980). Childhood-onset insomnia. *Sleep, 3,* 59–65.

Hayasaki, Y. (1927). On the sleeping hours at school, children of 6 to 20 years. *Psychological Abstracts, 1,* 439.

Hayes, M. J., Parker, K. G., Sallinen, B., and Davare, A. A. (2001). Bedsharing, temperament, and sleep disturbance in early childhood. *Sleep, 24,* 657–662.

Heine, R. G., Cameron, D. J. S., Chung, W. C., Hill, D. J., and Catto-Smith, A. G. (2002). Cause and effect of unhappy coexistence. GERD does not cause crying. *Journal of Pediatrics, 140,* 14–19.

Henderson, J. M. T., France, K. G., Owens, J. L., and Blampied, N. M. (2010). Sleeping through the night: The consolidation of self-regulated sleep across the first year of life. *Pediatrics, 126,* e1081–e1087.

Hicks, R. A., and Pellegrini, R. J. (1977). Anxiety levels of short and long sleepers. *Psychological Reports, 41,* 569–570.

Hicks, R. A., and Pellegrini, R. J. (1991). The changing sleep habits of college students. *Perceptual and Motor Skills, 72,* 1106.

Hill, D. J., and Hosking, C. S. (2000). Infantile colic and food hypersensitivity. *Journal of Pediatric Gastroenterology and Nutrition, 30* (Suppl.), S67–S76.

Hiscock, H., Cook, F., Bayer, J., Le, H. N. D., Mensah, F., Cann, W., Symon, B., and St. James-Roberts, I. (2014). Preventing early infant sleep and crying problems and postnatal depression: A randomized trial. *Pediatrics, 133,* e346–e354.

Hiscock, H., and Wake, M. (2001). Infant sleep problems and postnatal depression: A community-based study. *Pediatrics, 107,* 1317–1322.

Hiscock, H., and Wake, M. (2002). Randomised controlled trial of behavioural infant sleep intervention to improve infant sleep and maternal mood. *British Medical Journal, 324,* 1062–1065.

Hoddes, E., Zarcone, V., Smythe, H., Phillips, R., and Dement, W. C. (1973). Quantification of sleepiness: A new approach. *Psychophysiology, 10,* 431–436.

Howarth, E., and Hoffman, M. S. (1984). A multidimensional approach to the relationship between mood and weather. *British Journal of Psychology, 75,* 15–23.

Huber, R., Mäki, H., Rosanova, M., Casarotto, S., Canali, P., Casali, A. G., Tononi, G., and Massimini, M. (2013). Human cortical excitability increases with time awake. *Cerebral Cortex, 23,* 332–338.

Hugh, S. C., Wolter, N. E., Propst, E. J., Gordon, K. A., Cushing, S. L., and Papsin, B. C. (2014). Infant sleep machines and hazardous sound pressure levels. *Pediatrics, 133,* 1–5.

Hunsley, M., and Thoman, E. B. (2002). The sleep of co-sleeping infants when they are not co-sleeping: Evidence that co-sleeping is stressful. *Developmental Psychobiology, 40,* 14–22.

Hunziker, U. A., and Barr, R. G. (1986). Increased carrying reduces infant crying: A randomized controlled trial. *Pediatrics, 77,* 641–648.

Hysing, M., Harvey, A. G., Torgersen, L., Ystrom, E., Reichborn-Kjennerud, T., and Sivertsen, B. (2014). Trajectories and predictors of nocturnal awakenings and sleep duration in infants. *Journal of Developmental and Behavioral Pediatrics, 35,* 309–316.

Iglowstein, I., Jenni, O. G., Molinari, L., and Largo, R. H. (2003). Sleep duration from infancy to adolescence: Reference values and generational trends. *Pediatrics, 111,* 302–307.

Illingworth, R. S. (1954). "Three months' colic." *Archives of Disease in Childhood, 29,* 167–174.

Illingworth, R. S. (1955). Crying in infants and children. *British Medical Journal, 1,* 75–78.

Jacklin, C. N., Snow, M. E., Cozahapt, M., and Maccoby, E. E. (1980). Sleep pattern development from 6 through 33 months. *Journal of Pediatric Psychology, 5,* 295–302.

Johs, M. W., Gay, T. J. A., Masterton, J. P., and Bruce, D. W. (1971). Relationship between sleep habits, adrenocortical activity and personality. *Psychosomatic Medicine, 33,* 499–508.

Jones, D. P. H., and Verduyn, C. M. (1983). Behavioral management of sleep problems. *Archives of Disease in Childhood, 58,* 442–444.

Kahn, A., Mozin, M. J., Casimir, G., Montauk, L., and Blum, D. (1985). Insomnia and cow's milk allergy in infants. *Pediatrics, 76,* 880–884.

Kahn, A., Van de Merckt, C., Rebuffat, E., Mozin, M. J., Sottiaux, M., Blum, D., and Hennart, P. (1989). Sleep problems in healthy preadolescents. *Pediatrics, 84,* 542–546.

Kahyama, J., Shiike, T., and Hasegawa, T. (2000). Young children who are late sleepers sleep less than early sleepers. *Sleep, 23* (Abstract Suppl. 2), A198–A199.

Kales, A., Bixler, E. O., Vela-Bueno, A., Cadieux, R. J., Soldatos, C. R., and Kales, J. D. (1984). Biopsychobehavioral correlates of insomnia: Part III. Polygraphic findings of sleep difficulty and their relationship to psychopathology. *International Journal of Neuroscience, 23,* 43–56.

Kales, A., Soldatos, C. R., Caldwell, A. B., Kales, J. D., Humphrey, F. J., Charney, D. S., and Schweitzer, P. K. (1980). Somnambulism: Clinical characteristics and personality patterns. *Archives of General Psychiatry, 37,* 1406–1410.

Kaley, F., Reid, V., and Flynn, E. (2012). Investigating the biographic, social and temperamental correlates of young infants' sleeping, crying and feeding routines. *Infant Behavior and Development, 35,* 596–605.

Karacan, I., Wolff, S. M., Williams, R. L., Hursch, C. J., and Webb, W. B. (1968). The effects of fever on sleep and dream patterns. *Psychosomatics, 9,* 331–339.

Karelitz, S., Fisichelli, V. R., Costa, J., Karelitz, R., and Rosenfeld, L. (1964). Relation of crying activity in early infancy to speech and intellectual development at age three years. *Child Development, 35,* 769–777.

Keefe, M. R., Kotzer, A. M., Froese-Fretz, A., and Curtin, M. (1996). A longitudinal comparison of irritable and nonirritable infants. *Nursing Research, 45,* 4–9.

Keener, M. A., Zeanah, C. H., and Anders, T. F. (1988). Infant temperament, sleep organization, and nighttime parental interventions. *Pediatrics, 81,* 762–771.

Kelly, Y., Kelly, J., and Sacker, S. (2013). Changes in bedtime schedules and behavioral difficulties in 7 year old children. *Pediatrics, 132,* e1184–e1193.

Keyes, K. M., Maslowsky, J., Hamilton, A., and Schulenberg, J. (2015). The great sleep recession: Changes in sleep duration among US adolescents, 1991–2012. *Pediatrics, 135,* 460–468.

Kilgore, W. D., Kahn-Greene, E. T., Lipizzi, E. L., Newman, R. A., Kamimori, G. H., and Balkin, T. J. (2008). Sleep deprivation reduces perceived emotional intelligence and constructive thinking skills. *Sleep Medicine, 9,* 517–526.

Kim, S. J., Lee, Y. J., Cho, S. J., Cho, I. H., Lim, W., and Lim, W. (2011). Relationship between weekend catch-up sleep and poor performance on attention tasks in Korean adolescents. *Archives of Pediatrics and Adolescent Medicine, 165,* 806–812.

Kirjavainen, J., Kirjavainen, T., Huhtala, V., Lehtonen, L., Korvenranta, H., and Kero, P. (2001). Infants with colic have a normal sleep structure at 2 and 7 months of age. *Journal of Pediatrics, 138,* 218–223.

Kirmil-Gray, K., Eagleston, J. R., Gibson, E., and Thoresen, C. E. (1985). Sleep disturbance in adolescents: Sleep quality, sleep habits, beliefs about sleep, and daytime functioning. *Journal of Youth and Adolescence, 13,* 375–384.

Klackenberg, G. (1982). Sleep behaviour studied longitudinally. *Acta Paediatrica Scandinavica, 71,* 501–506.

Klackenberg, G. (1982). Somnambulism in childhood—prevalence, course, and behavioral correlations: A prospective longitudinal study (6–16 years). *Acta Paediatrica Scandinavica, 71,* 495–499.

Klatskin, E. H., Jackson, E. B., and Wilkin, L. C. (1956). The influence of degree of flexibility in maternal child care practices on early child behavior. *American Journal of Orthopsychiatry, 26,* 79–93.

Klein, G. L., Ziering, R. W., Girsh, L. S., and Miller, M. F. (1985). The allergic irritability syndrome: Four case reports and a position statement from the Neuroallergy Committee of the American College of Allergy. *Annals of Allergy, 55,* 22–24.

Klein, K. E., Herrmann, R., Kuklinski, P., and Hans, M. W. (1977). Circadian performance rhythms: Experimental studies in air operations. In R. R. Mackie (ed.), *Vigilance: Theory, Operational Performance, and Physiological Correlates* (NATO Conference Series III, Human Factors, Vol. 3, 111–132). New York: Plenum Press.

Kohyama, J., Shiike, T., Ohinata-Sugimoto, J., and Hasegawa, T. (2002). Potentially harmful sleep habits of 3-year-old children in Japan. *Journal of Developmental and Behavioral Pediatrics, 23,* 67–70.

Kolata, G. (1982). Food affects human behavior. *Science, 218,* 1209–1210.

Kotagal, S. (2008). Parasomnias of childhood. *Current Opinion in Pediatrics, 20,* 659–65.

Kravath, R. E., Pollak, C. P., and Borowiecki, B. (1977). Hypoventilation during sleep in children who have lymphoid airway obstruction treated by nasopharyngeal tube and T and A. *Pediatrics, 59,* 865–871.

Kurth, S., Achermann, P., Rusterholz, T., and LeBourgeois, M. K. (2013). Development of brain EEG connectivity across early childhood: Does sleep play a role? *Brain Sciences, 3,* 1445–1460.

Kurtoglu, S., Uzüm, K., Hallac, I. K., and Coskum, A. (1997). 5-hydroxy-3-indole acetic acid levels in infantile colic: Is serotoninergic tonus responsible for this problem? *Acta Paediatrica, 86,* 764–765.

Lam, J. C., Mahone, E. M., Mason, T. B. A., and Scharf, S. M. (2011). The effects of napping on cognitive function in preschoolers. *Journal of Developmental and Behavioral Pediatrics, 32,* 90–97.

Lang, C., Brand, S., Feldmeth, A. K., Holsboer-Trachsler, E., Pühse, U., and Gerber, M. (2013). Increased self-reported and objectively assessed physical activity predict sleep quality among adolescents. *Physiology and Behavior, 120,* 46–53.

Largo, R. H., and Hunziker, U. A. (1984). A developmental approach to the management of children with sleep disturbances in the first three years of life. *European Journal of Pediatrics, 142,* 170–173.

Larson, M. C., Gunnar, M. R., and Hertsgaard, L. (1991). The effects of morning naps, car trips, and maternal separation on adrenocortical activity in human infants. *Child Development, 62,* 362–372.

Latz, S., Wolf, A. W., and Lozoff, B. (1999). Cosleeping in context: Sleep practices and problems in young children in Japan and the United States. *Archives of Pediatrics and Adolescent Medicine, 153,* 339–346.

Lavigne, J. V., Arend, R., Rosenbaum, D., Smith, A., Weissbluth, M., Binns, H. J., and Christoffel, K. K. (1999). Sleep and behavior problems among preschoolers. *Journal of Developmental and Behavioral Pediatrics, 20,* 164–169.

Lehtonen, L., Korhonen, T., and Korvenranta, H. (1994). Temperament and sleeping patterns in colicky infants during the first year of life. *Journal of Developmental and Behavioral Pediatrics, 15,* 416–420.

Lester, B. M., and Boukydis, C. F. Z. (eds.) (1985). *Infant Crying: Theoretical and Research Perspectives.* New York: Plenum Press.

Leung, A. K., and Robson, W. L. (1990). Head banging. *Journal of the Singapore Paediatric Society, 32,* 12–17.

Lewis, M. (1997). *Altering Fate: Why the Past Does Not Predict the Future.* New York: Guilford Press.

Lind, M. G., and Lundell, B. P. W. (1982). Tonsillar hyperplasia in children: A cause of obstructive sleep apneas, CO_2 retention, and retarded growth. *Archives of Otolaryngology, 108,* 650–654.

Liu, X., Sun, Z., Uchiyama, M., Shibui, K., Kim, K., and Okawa, M. (2000). Prevalence and correlates of sleep problems in Chinese schoolchildren. *Sleep, 23,* 1053–1062.

Liu, X., Uchiyama, M., Okawa, M., and Kurita, H. (2000). Prevalence and correlates of self-reported sleep problems among Chinese adolescents. *Sleep, 23,* 27–34.

Lodemore, M., Petersen, S. A., and Wailoo, M. P. (1991). Development of night time temperature rhythms over the first six months of life. *Archives of Disease in Childhood, 66,* 521–524.

Lonstein, J. S. Regulation of anxiety during the postpartum period. (2007). *Frontiers in Neuroendocrinology, 28,* 115–141.

Louis, J., Cannard, C., Bastuji, H., and Challamel, M.-J. (1997). Sleep ontogenesis revisited: A longitudinal 24-hour home polygraphic study on 15 normal infants during the first two years of life. *Sleep, 20,* 323–333.

Lounsbury, M. L., and Bates, J. E. (1982). The cries of infants of differing levels of perceived temperamental difficultness:

Acoustic properties and effects on listeners. *Child Development, 53,* 677–686.

Lozoff, B., Smith, J. B., Kaciroti, N., Clark, K. M., Guevara, S., and Jimenez, E. (2013). Functional significance of early-life iron deficiency: Outcomes at 25 years. *Journal of Pediatrics, 163,* 1260–1266.

Lozoff, B., Wolf, A. W., and Davis, N. S. (1984). Cosleeping in urban families with young children in the United States. *Pediatrics, 74,* 171–182.

Lozoff, B., Wolf, A. W., and Davis, N. S. (1985). Sleep problems seen in pediatric practice. *Pediatrics, 75,* 477–483.

Lucey, D. R., Hauri, P., and Snyder, M. L. (1981). The wakeful "type A" student. *International Journal of Psychiatry in Medicine, 10,* 333–337.

Lyons, T. J., and Oates, R. K. (1993). Falling out of bed: A relatively benign occurrence. *Pediatrics, 92,* 125–127.

Macknin, M. L., Piedmonte, M., Jacobs, J., and Skibinski, C. (2000). Symptoms associated with infant teething: A prospective study. *Pediatrics, 105,* 747–752.

Mah, C. D., Mah, K. D., Kerzirian, E. J., and Dement, W. C. (2011). The effects of sleep extension on the athletic performance of collegiate basketball players. *Sleep, 34,* 943–950.

Mahowald, M. W., and Schenck, C. H. (1992). Dissociated states of wakefulness and sleep. *Neurology, 42* (Suppl. 6), 44–51.

Manber, R., Bootzin, R. R., Acebo, C., and Carskadon, M. A. (1996). The effects of regularizing sleep-wake schedules on daytime sleepiness. *Sleep, 19,* 432–441.

Mangat, D., Orr, W. C., and Smith, R. O. (1977). Sleep apnea, hypersomnolence, and upper airway obstruction secondary to adenotonsillar enlargement. *Archives of Otolaryngology, 103,* 383–386.

Manni, R., Ratti, M. T., Marchioni, E., Castelnovo, G., Murelli, R., Sartori, I., Galimberti, C. A., and Tartara, A. (1997). Poor sleep in adolescents: A study of 869 17-year-old Italian secondary school students. *Journal of Sleep Research, 6,* 44–49.

Mantz, J., Muzet, A., and Neiss, R. (1995). Sleep in 6-year-old children: Survey in school environment. *Archives of Pediatrics, 2,* 215–220.

Marks, G. A., Shaffery, J. P., Oksenberg, A., Speciale, S. G., and Roffwarg, H. P. (1995). A functional role for REM sleep in brain maturation. *Behavioural Brain Research, 69,* 1–11.

Martin, J., Hiscock, H., Hardy, P., Davey, B., and Wake, M. (2007). Adverse associations of infant and child sleep problems and parent health: An Australian population study. *Pediatrics, 119,* 947–955.

Martin, S. E., Engleman, H. M., Deary, I. J., and Douglas, N. J. (1996). The effect of sleep fragmentation on daytime function. *American Journal of Respiratory and Critical Care Medicine, 153,* 1328–1332.

Matheny, A. D., and Dolan, A. B. (1974). Childhood sleep characteristics and reading achievement. *JSAS Catalog of Selected Documents in Psychology, 4,* 76.

Matheny, A. P., Jr., Wilson, R. S., Dolan, A. B., and Krantz, J. Z. (1981). Behavioral contrasts in twinships: Stability and patterns of differences in childhood. *Child Development, 52,* 579–588.

Matricciani, L., Blunden, S., Rigney, G., Williams, M. T., and Olds, T. S. (2013). Children's sleep needs: Is there sufficient evidence to recommend optimal sleep for children? *Sleep, 36,* 527–534.

Matricciani, L., Olds, T., and Petkov, J. (2012). In search of lost sleep: Secular trends in the sleep time of school-aged children and adolescents. *Sleep Medicine Reviews, 16,* 203–211.

Mauer, K. W., Staats, B. A., and Olsen, K. D. (1983). Upper airway obstruction and disordered nocturnal breathing in children. *Mayo Clinic Proceedings, 58,* 349–353.

Maziade, M., Boudreault, M., Côté, R., and Thivierge, J. (1986). Influence of gentle birth delivery procedures and other perinatal circumstances on infant temperament: Developmental and social implications. *Journal of Pediatrics, 108,* 134–136.

McGraw, K., Hoffmann, R., Harker, C., and Herman, J. H. (1999).

The development of circadian rhythms in a human infant. *Sleep, 22*, 303–310.

Meyer, J. E., and Thaler, M. M. (1971). Colic in low birthweight infants. *American Journal of Diseases of Children, 122*, 25–27.

Middlemiss, W., Granger, D. A., Goldberg, W. A., and Nathans, L. (2012). Asynchrony of mother-infant hypothalamic-pituitary-adrenal axis activity following extinction of infant crying responses induced during the transition to sleep. *Early Human Development, 88*, 227–232.

Miller, A. L., Lumeng, J. C., and LeBourgeois, M. K. (2015). Sleep patterns and obesity in childhood. *Current Opinion in Endocrinology, Diabetes and Obesity, 22*, 41–47.

Minde, K., Faucon, A., and Falkner, S. (1994). Sleep problems in toddlers: Effects of treatment on their daytime behavior. *Journal of the American Academy of Child and Adolescent Psychiatry, 33*, 1114–1121.

Minde, K., Popiel, K., Leos, N., Falkner, S., Parker, K., and Handley-Derry, M. (1993). The evaluation and treatment of sleep disturbances in young children. *Journal of Child Psychology and Psychiatry, 34*, 521–533.

Mindell, J. A., and Barrett, K. M. (2002). Nightmares and anxiety in elementary-aged children: Is there a relationship? *Child: Care, Health and Development, 28*, 317–322.

Mindell, J. A., Bartle, A., Ahn, Y., Ramamurthy, M. B., Huong, H. T., Kohyama, J., Li, A. M., Ruangdaraganon, N., Sekartini, R., Teng, A., and Goh, D. Y. (2013). Sleep education in pediatric residency programs: A cross-cultural look. *BMC Research Notes, 6*, 130.

Mindell, J. A., Kuhn, B., Lewin, D. S., Meltzer, L. J., and Sadeh, A. (2006). Behavioral treatment of bedtime problems and night wakings in infants and young children. *Sleep, 29*, 1263–1276.

Mindell, J. A., Sadeh, A., Wiegand, B., How, T. H., and Goh, D. Y. (2010). Cross-cultural differences in infant and toddler sleep and maternal mood. *Sleep Medicine, 11*, 274–280.

Mindell, J. A., Telofski, L. S., Wiegand, B., and Kurtz, E. S. (2009). A nightly bedtime routine: Impact on sleep in young children. *Sleep, 32,* 599–606.

Minors, D. S., and Waterhouse, J. M. (1984). The sleep-wakefulness rhythm, exogenous and endogenous factors (in man). *Experientia, 40,* 410–416.

Monnier, M., and Gaillard, J. M. (1980). Biochemical regulation of sleep. *Experientia, 36,* 21–24.

Montgomery-Downs, H. E., and Gozal, D. (2006). Toddler behavior following polysomnography: Effects of unintended sleep disturbance. *Sleep, 29,* 1282–1287.

Moon, R. Y. (2011). SIDS and other sleep-related infant deaths: Expansion of recommendations for a safe infant sleeping environment. *Pediatrics, 128,* 1030–1039.

Moore, B. A., Friman, P. C., Fruzzetti, A. E., and MacAleese, K. (2007). Brief report: Evaluating the Bedtime Pass Program for child resistance to bedtime—a randomized, clinical trial. *Journal of Pediatric Psychology, 32,* 283–287.

Morgenthaler, T. I., Owens, J., Alessi, C., Boehlecke, B., Brown, T. M., Coleman, J., Jr., Friedman, L., Kapur, V. K., Lee-Chiong, T., Pancer, J., and Swick, T. J. (2006). Practice parameters for behavioral treatment of bedtime problems and night wakings in infants and young children. *Sleep, 29,* 1277–1281.

Morrison, D. N., McGee, R., and Stanton, W. R. (1992). Sleep problems in adolescence. *Journal of American Academy of Child and Adolescent Psychiatry, 31,* 94–99.

Neelon, S. E. B., Duffey, K., and Slining, M. M. (2014). Regulations to promote healthy sleep practices in child care. *Pediatrics, 134,* 1167–1174.

Neumann, M., and Jacobs, K. W. (1992). Relationship between dietary components and aspects of sleep. *Perceptual and Motor Skills, 75,* 873–874.

Nevéus, T., Cnattingius, S., Olsson, U., and Hetta, J. (2001). Sleep habits and sleep problems among a community sample of schoolchildren. *Acta Paediatrica, 90,* 1450–1455.

Nicassio, P. M., and Buchanan, D. C. (1981). Clinical application of behavior therapy for insomnia. *Comprehensive Psychiatry, 22,* 512–521.

Nikolopoulou, M., and St. James-Roberts, I. (2003). Preventing sleeping problems in infants who are at risk of developing them. *Archives of Disease in Childhood, 88,* 108–111.

Nixon, G. M., Thompson, J. M. D., Han, D. Y., Becroft, D. M., Clark, P. M., Robinson, E., Waldie, K. E., Wild, C. J., Black, P. N., and Mitchell, E. A. (2008). Short sleep duration in middle childhood: Risk factors and consequences. *Sleep, 31,* 71–78.

Norvenius, G., Widerlöv, E., and Lönnerholm, G. (1979). Phenylpropanolamine and mental disturbances. *Lancet, 2,* 1367–1368.

Novosad, C., Freudigman, K., and Thoman, E. B. (1999). Sleep patterns in newborns and temperament at eight months: A preliminary study. *Journal of Developmental and Behavioral Pediatrics, 20,* 99–105.

O'Connor, L. H., and Feder, H. H. (1984). Estradiol and progesterone influence a serotonin mediated behavioral syndrome (myoclonus) in female guinea pigs: Comparison with steroid effects on reproductive behavior. *Brain Research, 293,* 119–125.

Ogden, T. H. (1985). The mother, the infant and the matrix: Interpretations of aspects of the work of Donald Winnicott. *Contemporary Psychoanalysis, 21,* 346–371.

Okami, P., Weisner, T., and Olmstead, R. (2002). Outcome correlates of parent-child bedsharing: An eighteen-year longitudinal study. *Journal of Developmental and Behavioral Pediatrics, 23,* 244–253.

Olafsdottir, E., Forshei, G., Fluge, G., and Markestad, T. (2001). Randomised controlled trial of infantile colic treated with chiropractic spinal manipulation. *Archives of Disease in Childhood, 84,* 138–141.

Olds, T. S., Maher, C. A., and Matricciani, L. (2011). Sleep duration or bedtime? Exploring the relationship between sleep habits and weight status and activity patterns. *Sleep, 34,* 1299–1307.

Onishi, S., Miyazawa, G., Nishimura, Y., Sugiyama, S., Yamakawa, T., Inagaki, H., Katoh, T., Itoh, S., and Isobe, K. (1983). Postnatal development of circadian rhythm in serum cortisol levels in children. *Pediatrics, 72,* 399–404.

Øster, J., and Nielsen, A. (1972). Growing pains: A clinical investigation of a school population. *Acta Paediatrica Scandinavica, 61,* 329–334.

Owens, J., Maxim, R., McGuinn, M., Nobile, C., Msall, M., and Alario, A. (1999). Television-viewing habits and sleep disturbance in school children. *Pediatrics, 104,* e27.

Owens, J., Opipari, L., Nobile, C., and Spirito, A. (1998). Sleep and daytime behavior in children with obstructive sleep apnea and behavioral sleep disorders. *Pediatrics, 102,* 1178–1184.

Owens, J. A. (2009). Pharmacotherapy of pediatric insomnia. *Journal of the American Academy of Child and Adolescent Psychiatry, 48,* 99–107.

Owens, J. A. (2014). School start times for adolescents. *Pediatrics, 134,* 642–649.

Owens, J. A., Belon, K., and Moss, P. (2010). Impact of delaying school start time on adolescent sleep, mood, and behavior. *Archives of Pediatrics and Adolescent Medicine, 164,* 608–614.

Owens-Stively, J., Frank, N., Smith, A., Hagino, O., Spirito, A., Arrigan, M., and Alario, A. J. (1997). Child temperament, parenting discipline style, and daytime behavior in childhood sleep disorders. *Journal of Developmental and Behavioral Pediatrics, 18,* 314–321.

Papousek, M., and von Hofacker, N. (1998). Persistent crying in early infancy: A non-trivial condition of risk for the developing mother-infant relationship. *Child: Care, Health and Development, 24,* 395–424.

Parmelee, A. H. (1977). Remarks on receiving the C. Anderson Aldrich Award. *Pediatrics, 59,* 389–395.

Parmelee, A. H., Schulz, H. R., and Disbrow, M. A. (1961). Sleep patterns of the newborn. *Journal of Pediatrics, 58,* 241–250.

Parmelee, A. H., Wenner, W. H., and Schulz, H. R. (1964). Infant sleep patterns: From birth to 16 weeks of age. *Journal of Pediatrics, 65,* 576–582.

Paulozzi, L., and Sells, M. (2002). Variation in homicide risk during infancy—United States, 1989–1998. *Morbidity and Mortality Weekly Report, 51,* 187–189.

Petzoldt, J., Wittchen, H.-U., Wittch, J., Einsle, F., Hofler, M., and Martini, J. (2014). Maternal anxiety disorders predict excessive crying: A prospective longitudinal study. *Archives of Disease in Childhood, 99,* 800–806.

Pierce, P. P. (1948). Delayed onset of "three months'" colic in premature infants. *American Journal of Diseases of Children, 75,* 190–192.

Ponsonby, A.-L., Dwyer, T., Gibbons, L. E., Cochrane, J. A., and Wang, Y.-G. (1993). Factors potentiating the risk of sudden infant death syndrome associated with the prone position. *New England Journal of Medicine, 329,* 377–382.

Porrino, L. J., Rapoport, J. L., Behar, D., Sceery, W., Ismond, D. R., and Bunney, W. E. (1983). A naturalistic assessment of the motor activity of hyperactive boys. I. Comparison with normal controls. *Archives of General Psychiatry, 40,* 681–687.

Posadzki, P., Lee, M. S., and Ernst, E. (2013). Osteopathic manipulative treatment for pediatric conditions: A systematic review. *Pediatrics, 132,* 140–152.

Price, A. M. H., Brown, J. E., Bittman, M., Wake, M., Quach, J., and Hiscock, H. (2014). Children's sleep patterns from 0 to 9 years: Australian population longitudinal study. *Archives of Disease in Childhood, 99,* 119–125.

Price, V. A., Coates, T. J., Thoresen, C. E., and Grinstead, O. A. (1978). Prevalence and correlates of poor sleep among adolescents. *American Journal of Diseases of Children, 132,* 583–586.

Radbill, S. X. (1965). Teething in fact and fancy. *Bulletin of the History of Medicine, 39,* 339–345.

Radesky, J. S., Silverstein, M., Zuckerman, B., and Christakis, D. A.

(2014). Infant self-regulation and early childhood media exposure. *Pediatrics, 133,* e1172–e1178.

Radesky, J. S., Zuckerman, B., Silverstein, M., Rivara, F. P., Barr, M., Taylor, J. A., Lengua, L. J., and Barr, R. G. (2013). Inconsolable intent crying and maternal postpartum depressive symptoms. *Pediatrics, 131,* e1857–e1864.

Räihä, H., Lehtonen, L., Korhonen, T., and Korvenranta, H. (1996). Family life 1 year after infantile colic. *Archives of Pediatrics and Adolescent Medicine, 150,* 1032–1036.

Randazzo, A. C., Muehlbach, M. J., Schweitzer, P. K., and Walsh, J. K. (1998). Cognitive function following acute sleep restriction in children ages 10–14. *Sleep, 21,* 861–868.

Randazzo, A. C., Schweitzer, P. K., and Walsh, J. K. (1998). Cognitive function following 3 nights of sleep restriction in children 10–14. *Sleep, 21* (Suppl.), A249.

Rautava, P., Lehtonen, L., Helenius, H., and Sillanpää, M. (1995). Infantile colic: Child and family three years later. *Pediatrics, 96,* 43–47.

Rebelsky, F., and Black, R. (1972). Crying in infancy. *Journal of Genetic Psychology, 121,* 49–57.

Reding, G. R., Zepelin, H., Robinson, J. E., Smith, V. H., and Zimmerman, S. O. (1968). Sleep pattern of bruxism: A revision. *Psychophysiology, 4,* 396.

Reid, A., Maldonado, C. C., and Baker, F. C. (2002). Sleep behavior of South African adolescents. *Sleep, 25,* 423–427.

Reid, G. J., Hong, R. Y., and Wade, T. J. (2009). The relationship between common sleep problems and emotional and behavioral problems among 2- and 3-year-olds in the context of known risk factors for psychopathology. *Journal of Sleep Research, 18,* 49–59.

Reid, M. J., Walter, A. L., and O'Leary, S. G. (1999). Treatment of young children's bedtime refusal and nighttime wakings: A comparison of "standard" and graduated ignoring procedures. *Journal of Abnormal Child Psychology, 27,* 5–16.

Reijneveld, S. A., Brugman, E., and Hirasing, R. A. (2001). Excessive infant crying: The impact of varying definitions. *Pediatrics, 108,* 893–897.

Reimão, R., and Lefévre, A. B. (1980). Prevalence of sleep-talking in childhood. *Brain and Development, 2,* 353–357.

Reppert, S. M. (1985). Maternal entrainment of the developing circadian system. *Annals of the New York Academy of Sciences, 453,* 162–169.

Reuveni, H., Chapnick, G., Tal, A., and Tarasiuk, A. (1999). Sleep fragmentation in children with atopic dermatitis. *Archives of Pediatrics and Adolescent Medicine, 153,* 249–253.

Reyner, L. A., and Horne, J. A. (2013). Sleep restriction and serving accuracy in performance tennis players, and effects of caffeine. *Physiology and Behavior, 120,* 93–96.

Rhoades, K. A., Leve, L. D., Harold, G. T., Mannering, A. M., Neiderhiser, J. M., Shaw, D. S., Natsuaki, M. N., and Reiss, D. (2012). Marital hostility and child sleep problems: Direct and indirect associations via hostile parenting. *Journal of Family Psychology, 26,* 488–498.

Richman, N. (1981). A community survey of one- to two-year-olds with sleep disruptions. *Journal of the American Academy of Child Psychiatry, 20,* 281–291.

Richman, N., Douglas, J., Hunt, H., Lansdown, R., and Levere, R. (1985). Behavioural methods in the treatment of sleep disorders—a pilot study. *Journal of Child Psychology and Psychiatry, 26,* 581–590.

Roane, B. M., and Taylor, D. J. (2008). Adolescent insomnia as a risk factor of early adult depression and substance abuse. *Sleep, 31,* 1351–1356.

Roberts, R. E., Roberts, C. R., and Chen, I. G. (2002). Impact of insomnia on future functioning of adolescents. *Journal of Psychosomatic Research, 53,* 561–569.

Robertson, R. M. (1974). Solids and "sleeping through." *British Medical Journal, 1,* 200.

Roehrs, T. A., Tietz, E. I., Zorick, F. J., and Roth, T. (1984). Daytime sleepiness and antihistamines. *Sleep, 7,* 137–141.

Roenneberg, T., Allebrandt, K. V., Merrow, M., and Vetter, C. (2012). Social jetlag and obesity. *Current Biology, 22,* 939–943.

Rosenfeld, A. A., Wenegrant, A. O., Haavik, D. K., Wenegrant, B. C., and Smith, C. R. (1982). Sleeping patterns in upper-middle-class families when the child awakens ill or frightened. *Archives of General Psychiatry, 39,* 943–947.

Russo, R. M., Gururaj, V. J., and Allen, J. E. (1976). The effectiveness of diphenhydramine HCl in pediatric sleep disorders. *Journal of Clinical Pharmacology, 16,* 284–288.

Ryu, J. E. (1985). Effect of maternal caffeine consumption on heart rate and sleep time in breast-fed infants. *Developmental Pharmacology and Therapeutics, 8,* 355–363.

Sadeh, A. (1997). Sleep and melatonin in infants: A preliminary study. *Sleep, 20,* 185–191.

Sadeh, A., Gruber, R., and Raviv, A. (2002). Sleep, neurobehavioral functioning, and behavior problems in school-age children. *Child Development, 73,* 405–417.

Sadeh, A., Mindell, J. A., Luedtke, K., and Wiegand, B. (2009). Sleep and sleep ecology in the first 3 years: A web-based study. *Journal of Sleep Research, 18,* 60–73.

Salzarulo, P., and Chevalier, A. (1983). Sleep problems in children and their relationship with early disturbances of the waking-sleeping rhythms. *Sleep, 6,* 47–51.

Salzarulo, P., Fagioli, I., Salomon, F., Duhamel, J. F., and Ricour, C. (1979). Alimentation continué et rythme veille-sommeil chez l'enfant. [Continuous feeding and the waking-sleeping rhythm in children.] *Archives Françaises de Pédiatrie, 36* (Suppl.), 26–32.

Sandyk, R. (1992). Melatonin and maturation of REM sleep. *International Journal of Neuroscience, 63,* 105–114.

Scharf, R. J., Demmer, R. T., Silver, E. J., and Stein, R. E. K. (2013). Nighttime sleep duration and externalizing behaviors of preschool children. *Journal of Developmental and Behavioral Pediatrics, 34,* 384–391.

Scher, A. (2008). Maternal separation anxiety as a regulator of infants' sleep. *Journal of Child Psychology and Psychiatry and Allied Disciplines, 49,* 618–625.

Scher, A., Epstein, R., Sadeh, A., Tirosh, E., and Lavie, P. (1992). Toddlers' sleep and temperament: Reporting bias or a valid link: A research note. *Journal of Child Psychology and Psychiatry and Allied Disciplines, 33,* 1249–1254.

Scher, A., Hall, W. A., Zaidman-Zait, A., and Weinberg, J. (2010). Sleep quality, cortisol levels, and behavioral regulation in toddlers. *Developmental Psychobiology, 52,* 44–53.

Scher, A., Tirosh, E., and Lavie, P. (1998). The relationship between sleep and temperament revisited: Evidence for 12-month-olds: A research note. *Journal of Child Psychology and Psychiatry and Allied Disciplines, 39,* 785–788.

Schmitt, J., Chen, C.-M., Apfelbacher, C., Romanos, M., Lehmann, I., Herbarth, O., Schaaf, B., Kraemer, U., von Berg, A., Wichmann, H.-E., Heinrich, J., and the LISA-plus Study Group. (2011). Infant eczema, infant sleeping problems, and mental health at 10 years of age: The prospective birth cohort study LISAplus. *Allergy, 66,* 404–411.

Schneider-Helmert, D., and Spinweber, C. L. (1986). Evaluation of L-tryptophan for treatment of insomnia: A review. *Psychopharmacology, 89,* 1–7.

Schulz, H., Massetani, R., Fagioli, I., and Salzarulo, P. (1985). Spontaneous awakening from sleep in infants. *Electroencephalography and Clinical Neurophysiology, 61,* 267–271.

Schulz, H., Salzarulo, P., Fagioli, I., and Massetani, R. (1983). REM latency: Development in the first year of life. *Electroencephalography and Clinical Neurophysiology, 56,* 316–322.

Sears, W. (1995). *Nighttime Parenting: How to Get Your Baby and Child to Sleep.* New York: New American Library.

Sedky, K., Bennett, D. S., and Carvalho, K. S. (2014). Attention deficit hyperactivity disorder and sleep disordered breathing in pediatric populations: A meta-analysis. *Sleep Medicine Reviews, 18,* 349–356.

Seehagen, S., Konrad, C., Herbert, J. S., and Schneider, S. (2015). Timely sleep facilitates declarative memory consolidation in infants. *Proceedings of the National Academy of Sciences of the United States of America, 112,* 1625–1629.

Sekine, M., Yamagami, T., Handa, K., Saito, T., Nanre, S., Kawaminami, K., Tokui, N., Yoshida, K., and Kagamimori, S. (2002). A dose-response relationship between short sleeping hours and childhood obesity: Results of the Toyama Birth Cohort Study. *Child: Care, Health and Development, 28,* 163–170.

Shamir, R., St. James-Roberts, I., Di Lorenzo, C., Burns, A. J., Thapar, N., Indrio, F., Riezzo, G., Raimondi, F., Di Mauro, A., Francavilla, R., Leuchter, R. H., Darque, A., Hüppi, P. S., Heine, R. G., Bellaïche, M., Levy, M., Jung, C., Alvarez, M., and Hovish, K. (2013). Infant crying, colic, and gastrointestinal discomfort in early childhood: A review of the evidence and most plausible mechanisms. *Journal of Pediatric Gastroenterology and Nutrition, 57* (Suppl. 1), S1–45.

Shaver, B. A. (1973). Maternal personality and early adaptation as related to infantile colic. In P. M. Schereshefsky and L. J. Yarrow (eds.), *Psychological Aspects of a First Pregnancy and Early Postnatal Adaptation* (209–215). New York: Raven Press.

Shimada, M., Takahashi, K., Segawa, M., Higurashi, M., Samejim, M., and Horiuchi, K. (1999). Emerging and entraining patterns of the sleep-wake rhythm in preterm and term infants. *Brain and Development, 21,* 468–473.

Short, M. A., Gradisar, M., Wright, H., Lack, L. C., Dohnt, H., and Carskadon, M. A. (2011). Time for bed: Parent-set bedtimes associated with improved sleep and daytime functioning in adolescents. *Sleep, 34,* 797–800.

Simola, P., Liukkonen, K., Pitkäranta, A., Pirinen, T., and Aronen, E. T. (2014). Psychosocial and somatic outcomes of sleep problems in children: A 4-year follow-up study. *Child: Care, Health and Development, 40,* 60–67.

Simonds, J. F., and Parraga, H. (1982). Prevalence of sleep disorders and sleep behaviors in children and adolescents. *Journal of the American Academy of Child and Adolescent Psychiatry, 21,* 383–388.

Simonds, J. F., and Parraga, H. (1984). Sleep behaviors and disorders in children and adolescents evaluated at psychiatric clinics. *Journal of Developmental and Behavioral Pediatrics, 5,* 6–10.

Sivertsen, B., Harvey, A. G., Reichborn-Kjennerud, T., Torgersen, L., Ystrom, E., and Hysing, M. (2015). Later emotional and behavioral problems associated with sleep problems in toddlers. *Journal of the American Medical Association Pediatrics, 169,* 575–582. Published online April 13, 2015. doi:10.10001/jamapediatrics.2015.0187.

Skjeie, H., Skonnord, T., Fetveit, A., and Brekke, M. (2013). Acupuncture for infantile colic: A blinding-validated, randomized controlled multicenter trial in general practice. *Scandinavian Journal of Primary Health Care, 31,* 190–196.

Smedje, H., Broman, J. E., and Hetta, J. (2001). Short-term prospective study of sleep disturbances in 5- to 8-year-old children. *Acta Paediatrica, 90,* 1456–1463.

Snow, M. E., Jacklin, C. N., and Maccoby, E. E. (1980). Crying episodes and sleep-wakefulness transitions in the first 26 months of life. *Infant Behavior and Development, 3,* 387–394.

Soffer-Dudek, N., Sadeh, A., Dahl, R. E., and Rosenblat-Stein, S. (2011). Poor sleep quality predicts deficient emotion information processing over time in early adolescence. *Sleep, 34,* 1499–1508.

Spock, Benjamin. (1983). *Baby and Child Care.* New York: Pocket Books.

Spring, B., Maller, O., Wurtman, J., Digman, L., and Cozolino, L. (1982–1983). Effects of protein and carbohydrate meals on mood and performance: Interactions with sex and age. *Journal of Psychiatric Research, 17,* 155–167.

Spruyt, K., Aitken, R. J., So, K., Charlton, M., Adamson, T. M., and Horne, R. S. C. (2008). Relationship between sleep/wake patterns, temperament and overall development in term infants over the first year of life. *Early Human Development, 84,* 289–296.

Spruyt, K., Molfese, D. L., and Gozal, D. (2011). Sleep duration, sleep regularity, body weight, and metabolic homeostasis in school-aged children. *Pediatrics, 127,* e345–e352.

St. James-Roberts, I., Alvarez, M., Csipke, E., Abramsky, T., Goodwin, J., and Sorgenfrei, E. (2006). Infant crying and sleeping in London, Copenhagen and when parents adopt a "proximal" form of care. *Pediatrics, 117,* e1146–e1155.

St. James-Roberts, I., Alvarez, M., and Hovish, K. (2013). Emergence of a developmental explanation for prolonged crying in 1- to 4-month-old infants: Review of the evidence. *Journal of Pediatric Gastroenterology and Nutrition, 57* (Suppl. 1), S30–S36.

St. James-Roberts, I., Conroy, S., and Hurry, J. (1997). Links between infant crying and sleep-waking at six weeks of age. *Early Human Development, 48,* 143–152.

St. James-Roberts, I., and Peachey, E. (2011). Distinguishing infant prolonged crying from sleep-waking problems. *Archives of Disease in Childhood, 96,* 340–344.

St. James-Roberts, I., and Plewis, I. (1996). Individual differences, daily fluctuations, and developmental changes in amounts of infant waking, fussing, crying, feeding, and sleeping. *Child Development, 67,* 2527–2540.

St. James-Roberts, I., Roberts, M., Hovish, K., and Owen, C. (2015). Video evidence that London infants can resettle themselves back to sleep after waking in the night, as well as sleep for long periods, by 3 months of age. *Journal of Developmental and Behavioral Pediatrics, 36,* 324–329.

Ståhlberg, M.-R. (1984). Infantile colic: Occurrence and risk factors. *European Journal of Pediatrics, 143,* 108–111.

Steinsbekk, S., and Wichstrøm, L. (2015). Stability of sleep disorders from preschool to first grade and their bidirectional relationship with psychiatric symptoms. *Journal of Developmental and Behavioral Pediatrics, 36,* 243–251.

Stenger, K. (1956). Therapy of spastic bronchitis. *Medizinische Klinik, 51,* 1451–1455.

Stepanski, E., Lamphere, J., Badia, P., Zorick, F., and Roth, T. (1984). Sleep fragmentation and daytime sleepiness. *Sleep, 7,* 18–26.

Stéphan-Blanchard, E., Telliez, F., Léké, A., Djeddi, D., Bach, V., Libert, J.-P., and Chardon, K. (2008). The influence of *in utero* exposure to smoking on sleep patterns in preterm neonates. *Sleep, 31,* 1683–1689.

Stifter, C. A., and Braungart, J. (1992). Infant colic: A transient condition with no apparent effects. *Journal of Applied Developmental Psychology, 13,* 447–462.

Still, G. F. (1931). *The History of Pediatrics.* London: Oxford University Press.

Stone, M. R., Stevenson, D., and Faulkner, G. E. J. (2013). Maintaining recommended sleep throughout the week is associated with increased physical activity in children. *Preventive Medicine, 56,* 112–117.

Sullivan, C. E., Murphy, E., Kozar, L. F., and Phillipson, E. A. (1979). Ventilatory responses to CO_2 and lung inflation in tonic versus phasic REM sleep. *Journal of Applied Physiology: Respiratory, Environmental and Exercise Physiology, 47,* 1305–1310.

Sundell, C. E. (1922). Sleeplessness in infants. *Practitioner, 109,* 89–92.

Sung, V., Collett, S., de Gooyer, T., Hiscock, H., Tang, M., and Wake, M. (2013). Probiotics to prevent or treat excessive infant crying: Systematic review and meta-analysis. *Journal of the American Medical Association Pediatrics, 167,* 1150–1157.

Sung, V., Hiscock, H., Tang, M. L. K., Mensah, F. K., Nation, M. L., Satzke, C., Heine, R. G., Stock, A., Barr, R. G., and Wake, M. (2014). Treating infant colic with the probiotic *Lactobacillus reuteri:* Double blind, placebo controlled randomised trial. *British Medical Journal, 348,* g2107.

Takasu, N. N., Takenaka, Y., Fujiwara, M., and Toichi, M. (2012). Effects of regularizing sleep-wake schedules on daytime autonomic functions and psychological states in healthy university students with irregular sleep-wake habits. *Sleep and Biological Rhythms 10*, 84–93.

Tan, T. L., Kales, J. D., Kales, A., Soldatos, C. R., and Bixler, E. O. (1984). Biopsychobehavioral correlates of insomnia. IV: Diagnosis based on DSM-III. *American Journal of Psychiatry, 141*, 357–362.

Tandon, P., Gupta, M. L., Barthwal, J. P., Gupta, T. K., Parmar, S. S., and Bhargava, K. P. (1983). Role of monoamine oxidase-B in medroxyprogesterone acetate (17-acetoxy-6 alpha-methyl-4-pregnene-3, 20-dione) induced changes in brain dopamine levels of rats. *Steroids, 42*, 231–239.

Tasanen, A. (1968). General and local effects of the eruption of deciduous teeth. *Annales Paediatriae Fenniae, 14* (Suppl. 29).

Taveras, E. M., Gillman, M. W., Peña, M.-M., Redline, S., and Rifas-Shiman, S. L. (2014). Chronic sleep curtailment and adiposity. *Pediatrics, 133*, 1013–1022.

Terman, L. M. (1925). *Genetic studies of genius:* Vol. 1. *Mental and physical traits of a thousand gifted children.* Palo Alto: Stanford University Press.

Terman, L. M., and Hocking, A. (1913). The sleep of school children: Its distribution according to age, and its relation to physical and mental efficiency. Part 1: The distribution of sleep according to age. *Journal of Educational Psychology, 4*, 138–147.

Teti, D. M., and Crosby, B. (2012). Maternal depressive symptoms, dysfunctional cognitions, and infant night waking: The role of maternal nighttime behavior. *Child Development, 83*, 939–953.

Teti, D. M., Kim, B.-R., Mayer, G., and Countermine, M. (2010). Maternal emotional availability at bedtime predicts infant sleep quality. *Journal of Family Psychology, 24*, 307–315.

Thomas, A., and Chess, S. (1984). Genesis and evolution of behavioral disorders: From infancy to early adult life. *American Journal of Psychiatry, 141*, 1–9.

Thomas, A., Chess, S., and Birch, H. G. (1968). *Temperament and Behavior Disorders in Childhood*. New York: New York University Press.

Tikotzky, L., Sadeh, A., and Glickman-Gavrieli, T. (2011). Infant sleep and paternal involvement in infant caregiving during the first 6 months of life. *Journal of Pediatric Psychology, 36,* 36–46.

Tononi, G., and Cirelli, C. (2013). Perchance to Prune. *Scientific American, 309,* 34–39.

Troxel, W. M., Trentacosta, C. J., Forbes, E. E., and Campbell, S. B. (2013). Negative emotionality moderates associations among attachment, toddler sleep, and later problem behaviors. *Journal of Family Psychology, 27,* 127–136.

Twenge, J. M. (2015). Time period and birth cohort differences in depressive symptoms in the U.S., 1982–2013. *Social Indicators Research, 12,* 437–454.

van der Helm, E., Gujar, N., and Walker, M. P. (2010). Sleep deprivation impairs the accurate recognition of human emotions. *Sleep, 33,* 335–342.

Van Tassel, E. B. (1985). The relative influence of child and environmental characteristics on sleep disturbances in the first and second years of life. *Journal of Developmental and Behavioral Pediatrics, 6,* 81–86.

Vendrame, M., and Kothare, S. V. (2011). Epileptic and nonepileptic paroxysmal events out of sleep in children. *Journal of Clinical Neurophysiology, 28,* 111–119.

von Kries, R., Toschke, A. M., Wurmser, H., Sauerwald, T., and Koletzko, B. (2002). Reduced risk for overweight and obesity in 5- and 6-y-old children by duration of sleep—a cross-sectional study. *International Journal of Obesity and Related Metabolic Disorders, 26,* 710–716.

Vriend, J. L., Davidson, F. D., Corkum, P. V., Rusak, B., Chambers, C. T., and McLaughlin, E. N. (2013). Manipulating sleep duration alters emotional functioning and cognitive performance in children. *Journal of Pediatric Psychology, 38,* 1058–1069.

Wake, M., Hesketh, K., and Lucas, J. (2000). Teething and tooth eruption in infants: A cohort study. *Pediatrics, 106,* 1374–1379.

Watamura, S. E., Sebanc, A. M., and Gunnar, M. R. (2002). Rising cortisol at childcare: Relations with nap, rest, and temperament. *Developmental Psychobiology, 40,* 33–42.

Watanabe, K., Inokuma, K., and Negoro, T. (1983). REM sleep prevents sudden infant death syndrome. *European Journal of Pediatrics, 140,* 289–292.

Webb, W. B., and Agnew, H. W. (1974). Regularity in the control of the free-running sleep-wakefulness rhythm. *Aerospace Medicine, 45,* 701–704.

Webb, W. B., and Campbell, S. S. (1983). Relationships in sleep characteristics of identical and fraternal twins. *Archives of General Psychiatry, 40,* 1093–1095.

Weideman, C. L., Bush, D. L., Yan-Go, F. L., Clark, G. T., and Gornbein, J. A. (1996). The incidence of parasomnias in child bruxers versus nonbruxers. *Pediatric Dentistry, 18,* 456–460.

Weiler, N. (2014). A bedtime story. *Stanford Magazine,* September/October, 65.

Weinraub, M., Bender, R. H., Friedman, S. L., Susman, E. J., Knoke, B., Bradley, R. H., Houts, R., and Williams, J. (2012). Patterns of developmental change in infants' nighttime sleep awakenings from 6 through 36 months of age. *Developmental Psychology, 48,* 1511–1528.

Weissbluth, L., and Weissbluth, M. (1992). Infant colic: The effect of serotonin and melatonin on circadian rhythms on the intestinal smooth muscle. *Medical Hypotheses, 39,* 164–167.

Weissbluth, M. (1981). Infantile colic and near-miss sudden infant death syndrome. *Medical Hypotheses, 7,* 1193–1199.

Weissbluth, M. (1981). Sleep duration and infant temperament. *Journal of Pediatrics, 99,* 817–819.

Weissbluth, M. (1982). Modification of sleep schedule with reduction of night waking: A case report. *Sleep, 5,* 262–266.

Weissbluth, M. (1984). *Crybabies.* New York: Arbor House.

Weissbluth, M. (1984). Is drug treatment of night terrors warranted? *American Journal of Diseases of Children, 138,* 1086.

Weissbluth, M. (1984). Sleep duration, temperament, and Conners' ratings of three-year-old children. *Journal of Developmental and Behavioral Pediatrics, 5,* 120–123.

Weissbluth, M. (1985). How sleep affects school performance. *Gifted Children Monthly, 6,* 14–15.

Weissbluth, M. (1986–2006). Infant colic. In S. S. Gellis and B. M. Kagan (eds.), *Current Pediatric Therapy,* 12th–18th eds. Philadelphia: W. B. Saunders.

Weissbluth, M. (1987). Sleep and the colicky infant. In C. Guilleminault (ed.), *Sleep and Its Disorders in Children* (129–140). New York: Raven Press.

Weissbluth, M. (1995). Colic. In R. Ferber and M. Kryger (eds.), *Principles and Practice of Sleep Medicine in the Child* (75–78). Philadelphia: W. B. Saunders.

Weissbluth, M. (1995). Naps in children: 6 months–7 years. *Sleep, 18,* 82–87.

Weissbluth, M., Brouillette, R. T., Liu, K., and Hunt, C. E. (1982). Sleep apnea, sleep duration, and infant temperament. *Journal of Pediatrics, 101,* 307–310.

Weissbluth, M., Christoffel, K. K., and Davis, A. T. (1984). Treatment of infantile colic with dicyclomine hydrochloride. *Journal of Pediatrics, 104,* 951–955.

Weissbluth, M., Davis, A. T., and Poncher, J. (1984). Night waking in 4- to 8-month-old infants. *Journal of Pediatrics, 104,* 477–480.

Weissbluth, M., Davis, A. T., Poncher, J., and Reiff, J. (1983). Signs of airway obstruction during sleep and behavioral, developmental, and academic problems. *Journal of Developmental and Behavioral Pediatrics, 4,* 119–121.

Weissbluth, M., Hunt, C. E., Brouillette, R. T., Hanson, D., David, R. J., and Stein, I. M. (1985). Respiratory patterns during sleep and temperament ratings in normal infants. *Journal of Pediatrics, 106,* 688–690.

Weissbluth, M., and Liu, K. (1983). Sleep patterns, attention span, and infant temperament. *Journal of Developmental and Behavioral Pediatrics, 4,* 34–36.

Weissbluth, M., Poncher, J., Given, G., Schwab, J., Mervis, R., and Rosenberg, M. (1981). Sleep duration and television viewing. *Journal of Pediatrics, 99,* 486–488.

Weissbluth, M., and Weissbluth, L. (1992). Colic, sleep inertia, melatonin and circannual rhythms. *Medical Hypotheses, 38,* 224–228.

Weitzman, E. D., Czeisler, C. A., Coleman, R. M., Spielman, A. J., Zimmerman, J. C., Dement, W. C., Richardson, G., and Pollak, C. P. (1981). Delayed sleep phase syndrome. A chronobiological disorder with sleep-onset insomnia. *Archives of General Psychiatry, 38,* 737–746.

Wessel, M. A., Cobb, J. C., Jackson, E. B., Harris, G. S., and Detwiler, A. C. (1954). Paroxysmal fussing in infants, sometimes called "colic." *Pediatrics, 14,* 421–435.

White, B. P., Gunnar, M. R., Larson, M. C., Donzella, B., and Barr, R. G. (2000). Behavioral and physiological responsivity, sleep, and patterns of daily cortisol production in infants with and without colic. *Child Development, 71,* 862–877.

Williams, C. D. (1959). The elimination of tantrum behavior by extinction procedures. *Journal of Abnormal and Social Psychology, 59,* 269.

Winnicott, D. W. (1965). The capacity to be alone. In D. W. Winnicott, *The Maturational Processes and Facilitating Environment* (29–36). New York: International Universities Press.

Witting, W., Mirmiran, M., Bos, N. P. A., and Swaab, D. F. (1993). Effect of light intensity on diurnal sleep-wake distribution in young and old rats. *Brain Research Bulletin, 30,* 157–162.

Wladimirova, G. (1993). Study of cyclic structure of daytime sleep in normal infants aged 2 to 12 months. *Acta physiologica et pharmacoligica Bulgarica, 9,* 62–69.

Wolke, D., Gray, P., and Meyer, R. (1994). Excessive infant crying: A controlled study of mothers helping mothers. *Pediatrics, 94,* 322–332.

Wolke, D., and Lereya, S. T. (2014). Bullying and parasomnias: A longitudinal cohort study. *Pediatrics, 134,* e1040–e1048.

Wolke, D., Meyer, R., Ohet, B., and Riegel, K. (1995). Co-morbidity of crying and feeding problems with sleeping problems in infancy: Concurrent and predictive associations. *Early Development and Parenting, 4,* 191–207.

Wolke, D., Rizzo, P., and Woods, S. (2002). Persistent infant crying and hyperactivity problems in middle childhood. *Pediatrics, 109,* 1054–1060.

Wolverton, M. (2013). Chasing slumber. *Psychology Today,* 73–77.

Wright, L., Woodcock, J., and Scott, R. (1970). Treatment of sleep disturbance in a young child by conditioning. *Southern Medical Journal, 63,* 174–176.

Wright, P., MacLeod, H. A., and Cooper, M. J. (1983). Waking at night: The effect of early feeding experience. *Child: Care, Health and Development, 9,* 309–319.

Yogman, M. W., and Zeisel, S. H. (1985). Nutrients, neurotransmitters and infant behavior. *American Journal of Clinical Nutrition, 42,* 352–360.

Youngstedt, S. D., O'Connor, P. J., and Dishman, R. K. (1997). The effects of acute exercise on sleep: A quantitative synthesis. *Sleep, 20,* 203–214.

Zeskind, P. S., and Huntington, L. (1984). The effects of within-group and between-group methodologies in the study of perceptions of infant crying. *Child Development, 55,* 1658–1665.

Index

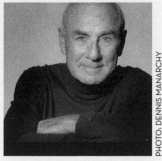

Marc Weissbluth, M.D., has been a pediatrician since 1973. A leading researcher on sleep and children, he founded the original Sleep Disorders Center at Children's Memorial Hospital (now the Ann and Robert H. Lurie Children's Hospital of Chicago) and is a Professor of Clinical Pediatrics, Emeritus, at the Northwestern University Feinberg School of Medicine. Dr. Weissbluth discovered that sleep is linked to temperament and that sleep problems are related to infant colic, and he coined the now-familiar phrase "sleep training" to describe his method for helping children learn how to fall asleep. His finding that changing the time a child is put to bed dramatically decreases the number of night awakenings was published in the prestigious journal *Sleep* in 1982. His landmark seven-year study on the development and disappearance of naps, also published in *Sleep* in 1995, highlighted the importance of daytime sleep. Since its original publication in 1987, *Healthy Sleep Habits, Happy Child* has sold more than a million copies and, in 12 foreign editions, helped millions of families the world over. Dr. Weissbluth was acknowledged by the American Academy of Pediatrics for his extensive contributions to the chapter "Your Child's Sleep" in their popular book for parents, *Caring for Your Baby and Young Child: Birth to Age 5*. Dr. Weissbluth is also the author of *Your Fussy Baby* and *Healthy Sleep Habits, Happy Twins,* and the producer of a CD, *Sweet Baby: Lullabies to Soothe Your Newborn*. Married to his wife, Linda, since 1965, he is the father of four sons and eight grandchildren—and they are all good sleepers. Dr. and Mrs. Weissbluth live in Chicago.

drweissbluth.com

About the Type

This book was set in Sabon, a typeface designed by the well-known German typographer Jan Tschichold (1902–74). Sabon's design is based upon the original letter forms of sixteenth-century French type designer Claude Garamond and was created specifically to be used for three sources: foundry type for hand composition, Linotype, and Monotype. Tschichold named his typeface for the famous Frankfurt typefounder Jacques Sabon (c. 1520–80).